MEDIC ADMINISTRATION FOR FRONT-LINE DOCTORS

SECOND EDITION

by C ANDREW PEARSON
OBE, MB, ChB, DTM, FMCGP (Nig), FWACP

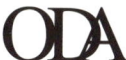

The publishers are grateful to the UK Overseas Development Administration for a grant towards the cost of producing this book.

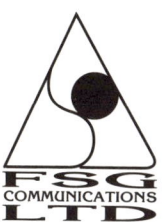

To all who are, or would like to be, front-line doctors.

© C A Pearson 1995

All rights reserved. No part of this publication may be reproduced, stored in a retrieval system, or transmitted, in any form or by any means electronic, mechanical, photocopying, or otherwise, without the prior permission of the publisher.

Published by:
FSG Communications Ltd, publishers of *Africa Health* journal,
Vine House, Fair Green, Reach,
Cambridge CB5 0JD, UK.

Price: £5.00 plus £2.50 postage and packing — developing countries
 £10.00 plus £2.00 postage and packing — elsewhere.

First published 1990
Second edition 1995

ISBN 1 8871188 03 2

Printed in Great Britain by Warwick Printing Co Ltd, Theatre Street, Warwick CV34 4DR

CONTENTS

	Page
Foreward By Professor Olikoye Ransome-Kuti	**vi**
Preface	vii

Chapter 1
The place of the Doctor in Hospital Administration   1
    Definition of administration
    The doctor's role in the basic leadership team
    Sharing time for clinical work and administration

Chapter 2
Management Structures   9
    Questions to ask on being given responsibility
    Government, private sector and voluntary agency structures
    Democratic control through boards, committees and hospital officers
        with defined powers

Chapter 3
Handling Money   23
    Attitudes to public money
    Basic requirements of a good accounting system
    Computerisation – yes or no?
    Audit and budgeting
    Accounting in branch centres

Chapter 4
A Therapeutic Community   51
    Personnel management
    Staff appointments and housing
    The hospital environment; staff health
    Staff consultation and discipline
    Personal factors

Chapter 5
Medical Records   67
    Yardsticks for evaluation of good records; making changes
    Out-patient records, general and special
    In-patient charts, admission register, hospital statistics and annual
        report

Chapter 6
Infrastructure and Maintenance 93
Water, power and emergency supplies
Maintenance staff: Care of instruments, equipment and buildings

Chapter 7
Supporting Services 117
Transport, vehicles and drivers, and methods of communication
Laundry and kitchen services
The mortuary, waste-disposal and sanitation with, and without, adequate water

Chapter 8
Improving and Extending Hospital Buildings 143
Protection from the elements – sun, rain, wind, lightning and fire
Planning for growth, proper use of the site
Out-patients, theatre, maternity and children's ward extensions

Chapter 9
Hospital Supplies and Technical Services 173
Drugs and surgical sundries; local manufacture
Central stores for laboratory and blood bank, theatre, CSSD, wards and X-ray department

Chapter 10
Training 197
Staff advancement as a policy; personal initiatives and hospital-based training programmes
Opportunities for labour staff, artisans, technical staff
Nursing and midwifery – hospital aspects
Involvement in physician training; the general practice programme; chaplains

Chapter 11
Primary Health Care Outreach 213
Concern for the community, new attitudes needed
Primary care facility networks; VHW training
The hospital as base for preventive health care, growth charts, family planning, immunisation
Manpower and money for community health
Illustrative programmes

Chapter 12
Wider Responsibilities 231
District planning and national health administration
Working within the realities, yet maintaining a vision for the future
The doctor's responsibility in society, keeping up-to-date, sharing in clinical research and the professional associations; ethical, and family considerations

Appendices 249
    1. Constitution of the community hospital
    2. Policy for cleaning and decontamination of equipment or environment
    3. Model list of essential drugs
    4. Essential reagents for rural medical laboratories
    5. Notes for elective medical students from overseas
    6. Guidelines for general practice training hospitals
    7. Ethics and religion
    8. Guidelines for 'front-line parents'
    9. Specimen short essay type questions on medical administration

References 278

Index 280

FOREWORD

by Professor Olikoye Ransome-Kuti
Formerly Federal Minister of Health, Nigeria

Since the World Health Organisation's Declaration of Alma Ata in 1978, countries throughout the world and particularly in developing countries have proclaimed health policies aimed at making relevant and affordable primary health care services available to all its citizens. Hitherto, efforts were put into the provision of tertiary health services strongly supported by the academic medical and specialist leadership and available only to those in urban areas, and particularly for the elite.

To facilitate putting the primary health care services in place, the World Health Organisation advocates its implementation, starting at the village level until a district or local government area is totally covered. The highest referral points for problems which cannot be solved in the community or health centres at the district level are general or district hospitals which constitute the nation's secondary health care system. These facilities have, sadly, been neglected over the years; moreover scant attention has been given to define the skills required of the health personnel, particularly the doctors, who provide these services. They, therefore, form a very weak link in the health service chain from primary to tertiary.

The doctors in these hospitals are in the frontline. They often work single-handedly or with one or two other colleagues assisted by nurses and other health personnel. Apart from leading the provision of the services, much of the medical administration devolves on them. Such a doctor needs to be a good, broadly-based clinician and a competent administrator. This book goes a long way to meet his need. Andrew Pearson writes from long experience, mainly of the voluntary agency hospital, but also in the public service. He also has an appreciation of the private sector. From his time in Nigeria he speaks with some authority on the crucial link between the hospital, and the primary care services of the community in which it is set. While in Nigeria, he championed the cause of the front-line doctor and initiated a training programme designed to give such a person the skills to function effectively in a district or general hospital. That training is incorporated into the programme of the Nigeria National Postgraduate Medical College, through its Faculty of General Medical Practice, and has guided the writing of this book. His concern has always been for the patient whose problems are beyond the skills of health personnel at the village or health centre level, and the doctor to whom the patient is referred at the general hospital.

The book is refreshingly free from jargon. We may not agree with all its recommendations, but we can all learn from them.

I am glad to commend this book for close and honest study – and for necessary action.

O O R-K 1989

PREFACE

If the reader has already been involved with hospitals in the developing world then much of this book will be covering familiar ground. You have travelled this way before. For those coming to it afresh it will serve as an introduction to some aspects of what can be one of the most satisfying jobs in the world, that of the 'front-line doctor'. The book has been written from personal experience, first in China for five years, then in Nigeria. This preface gives the background to the three main fields of medical care which have filled the 30 years in Nigeria.

Wesley Guild Hospital (WGH)

Within three months of being appointed to WGH Ilesha, 75 miles east of Ibadan in southwest Nigeria in 1952, my senior colleague returned to UK and left me as the medical superintendent in full charge. There was one other missionary doctor as fresh as I was, but fortunately an experienced matron who had been there 25 years, three sisters and a small core of nurses, clerical assistants and labour staff. The hospital had already been established 40 years, and then had 70 beds, but with no other professional staff – no pharmacist, no accountant, no administrator, and no qualified technical staff in the laboratory or X-ray room. There was electricity from a generator, the first in the town, but no mains water, only rain water from roof tanks and a well, and bucket latrines. For maintenance purposes there was no mechanic or engineer, and it was rumoured that the previous doctor in charge was as likely to be found under the hospital lorry repairing a shock absorber, as in the theatre repairing a hernia. That is how it was in those days. The doctor had no option but to be the leader of his team, doing the best he could for his patients, and his staff, and in the maintenance of the facilities with which he was provided.

During the next 20 years the hospital was rebuilt on a new and larger site and grew to 200 beds, with increasing specialisation within the hospital, and outreach in primary care facilities all around. By 1975 the combined staff totalled over 400, and apart from specialist medical staff included a fine team of nursing sisters and staff nurses, qualified nurse tutors, pharmacist, laboratory superintendent, radiographer, clerical and maintenance staff. Administration became more complex, but was still physician-led. There was close cooperation between the voluntary agency and the state government. The hospital management committee had representatives from the community, local government, state and university, as well as the church proprietors. The system evolved worked efficiently enough. The hospital had an enviable reputation throughout the country, and in some respects, internationally as well.

Ibarapa Community Health Programme, College of Medicine, Ibadan

After the takeover of WGH Ilesha in 1975 to be part of the Ife University Teaching Hospital Complex, I transferred to Igbo-Ora, 60 miles west of Ibadan, to be the Chief Medical Officer of the Ibarapa Programme. Though now a university doctor, with teaching responsibilities for the visiting medical students on their community health posting, clinical service was given entirely within the government system as 'acting PMO' of Eruwa District Hospital and senior doctor for Igbo-Ora Rural Health Centre, and the Ibarapa Local Government health facilities. The insight given into the nature of medical administration under government and university proved invaluable.

Director of Training, Faculty of General Medical Practice, National Postgraduate Medical College, Nigeria

For my final two years in Nigeria, 1983–85, I was based in Lagos, but travelled the entire country in the process of setting up the training programme in general practice. This involved sharing with other fellows of the faculty in the inspection of hospitals applying to be approved for taking trainees. These included those areas of university teaching hospitals to be used for GP training, state general and specialist hospitals, army hospitals, mission hospitals and private hospitals. The opportunity to see such a wide variety of institutions was illuminating. Rather to my own surprise I came to appreciate for the first time the many excellent hospitals and dedicated doctors in the private sector, both in cities and rural areas all over the country.

Some of the lessons learned over these 30 years are, I believe, worth passing on. As experience is my sole qualification for going in to print, Nigerian examples predominate. However, I am sure that the ideas put forward are of wider applicability. Every situation is different, but the underlying principles remain the same.

The need to write the book has been made particularly urgent by the development of postgraduate training for general medical practice in Nigeria. Trainees are preparing themselves for work in secondary care, and the district level of primary care, and at this level medical administration is inescapable. Some will arrive in situations where patterns have been set to which they have to adapt, but they may feel the need for change. Others may find themselves setting up a new district hospital or comprehensive health centre, and wonder how to begin. Or they may still be undergoing the postgraduate training, an essential part of which is knowledge of medical administration and hospital maintenance. They may find the specimen exam questions at the end of the book a useful stimulus.

Doctors making a long-term career at this level have been few. For most it has been a temporary step along the way before moving back to the teaching hospital to prepare for a specialty, or out into an urban-based private practice. Governments in many developing countries have been hard put to fill the vacancies in provincial and district hospitals, and have often had to recruit from other countries which produce doctors in excess of their needs, but not always well motivated or well prepared for service in a tropical environment. Church based hospitals, particularly those in rural areas, have had difficulty in attracting national doctors to long-term service in their mission set-up, despite good personal motivation.

However, now that such hospitals of adequate quality in Nigeria have been approved for postgraduate training for a Fellowship in General Medical Practice, they no longer have any shortage of doctors applying for registrar posts. This is a new and exciting situation. These doctors are being specifically prepared for a career in secondary care hospitals, or the district level of primary care, and they are there by choice, and not compulsion.

There are some who consider that physicians have little or no place in the primary care services of developing countries. This is to ignore the desperate need for them at the district level where the distinction between comprehensive health centre and small hospital becomes blurred. The World Health Organisation, in its technical report on *Health manpower requirements for the achievement of health for all by the year 2000* (No. 717, 1985), recognises the present deficiencies in physician manpower in many countries, particularly at the district level, yet notes how vital it is to attract doctors into such work if the whole health service structure is to work as it should. As the report says:

> 'Effective planning and administration at district level is especially important, since this may be the lowest level of the health system in communication with central government, as well as being the highest level in direct contact with communities.'

A doctor in such work needs to be a first rate clinician, with a wide range of medical and surgical expertise, able to maintain good service far from specialist assistance, and to provide wise consultative opinion to the rest of the primary care team with whom he is working. In addition he needs to be familiar with good management techniques, passing on responsibilities to others according to their ability. Both his clinical and administrative skills will increase with time, and his ability to inspire community support, and effective self-reliant action, will grow. To fill such posts with junior or short-term staff, or poorly motivated foreign doctors, is generally unsatisfactory and self-defeating. The Nigerian programme gives some grounds for hope that the 'front-line doctors' it produces will be able to enjoy such careers, with real job satisfaction. Other countries could usefully develop the same type of programme.

This is not a complete textbook on management of health services, but it does aim to highlight those areas where a doctor in primary/secondary care should accept responsibility for medical administration, and see it not just as a burden, but as an opportunity to solve problems, promote change and provide better health care for his patients, and for the community as a whole.

The book should be of particular help to the following groups:
1. Doctors in training for the Fellowship in General Medical Practice in Nigeria, and any similar programme which may be developed in West Africa or other developing countries.

2. Government medical officers appointed as physician in charge of a provincial or district general hospital, or a comprehensive health centre at the district-level of primary health care.

3. Doctors placed in charge of a church-based hospital, possibly taking over from an expatriate missionary doctor returning home.

4. Doctors running, or planning to set up, their own private medical centre, especially if in a rural area far from other colleagues.

5. Administrators in ministries of health, and those in teaching hospitals who may have responsibilities for outlying hospitals and health centres to which students go for part of their training, and where 'front-line doctors' are employed.

6. Those in training to become hospital administrators, who need to appreciate

the role a doctor, who is adequately prepared, can play in the administrative team.

7. Senior health workers in the primary health care team who have to take their share of medical administration in situations where there is no doctor present full time.

In the writing of this book, the established convention of using 'he' as the third person singular pronoun has been adopted throughout, in preference to the ungainly 'he/she'. It is of course recognised that women too are represented amongst hospital staff and play an increasingly important role in the delivery of health services.

The scene in all developing countries is rapidly changing, and not always for the better when faced by economic recession, and mounting population pressures. Some of the ideas expressed here may appear dated. Time has moved on. Other ideas may seem frankly idealistic, given the frustrations of the day. However, nothing has been included which has not been found to work well at the time and place indicated. Any opinions expressed are, of course, my own.

If the book helps to bring fresh heart to those who continue to give such valuable service in the small hospitals of developing countries, and encourages those preparing to join them, it will have served a worthwhile purpose.

Preface to the Second Edition

The First Edition found its way to many developing countries around the world, and has been well-received. It was experience in Nigeria which first convinced me of the need to write the book, so naturally the majority of the examples quoted were drawn from that country. However, since first publication in 1990. I have had the opportunity to see something of the work of front-line doctors in other places, such as Zambia, Nepal, Philippines, China and Western Samoa. Useful suggestions as to what might be added have been given during these travels, and also through journal reviews. Problems in medical administration are largely the same the world over, but the attempt has been made to make the Second Edition a little less Nigerian, and more truly international, without losing the emphasis on what has been found to work well in practice.

Some of the changes reflect the new technology which is beginning to reach the district hospital, even in poorer countries. Imaging by ultrasound is no longer a rarity. Computerisation of accounts is spreading. Testing for HIV, though a dilemma because of cost, has necessarily been included, and also the counselling of AIDs patients in terminal care. The growing realisation of the need for community-based rehabilitation has been reflected, with emphasis on the support which a district centre can give in terms of physiotherapy, limb-fitting and the provision of other aids. More has been added on water-purification, and the local manufacture of health care equipment. The WHO's Essential Drug List is now taken as the start for the making of a hospital formulary, and a note given on alternative methods of dispensing from the pharmacy to the wards. There has been an update on books and learning resources, and methods for running a small hospital library.

An important development in the last five years has been the growing influence of the World Health Organisation's *Division for Strengthening Health Services*. This has been emphasising the role of the first referral hospital within the district health system, and defining secondary care and the vital work of the 'front-line doctor'. WHO has also been pressing many countries to give a greater degree of decentralisation of management from the state capital to the district hospital and related health services. These points are in line with the original theme of this book, and it has been good to be able to include reference to such developments.

The need to provide relevant postgraduate education to prepare doctors to make a career at district level is also becoming more widely recognised. Several countries, for example, Nepal, Zambia, Malaysia and India, have now joined Nigeria in embarking on this, and *Action in International Medicine (AIM)* has begun networking information between them. Training district doctors for medical administration remains an essential part of the exercise. Hopefully, this book will continue to be of value to all in the front-line of district health care, whether in governmental or non-governmental institutions, in all countries where the resources are stretched and the needs so great.

C A Pearson
2 Springfield Road,
Bury St Edmunds,
Suffolk IP33 3AN, UK.

ACKNOWLEDGEMENTS

This book has been a long time in gestation. Twelve years ago Professor Ralph Hendrickse of Liverpool urged me to put my mind to the task. He knew the hospital in Ilesha well and felt that the lessons learned there through practical experience should be made more widely available.

In finally producing the book, many have helped. These include former colleagues at Ilesha, Joan Stephenson, Steve Athey and Lawrence Beyer, in relation to the pharmacy and the laboratory; and John Mellanby who gave us such valuable service as consultant and engineer. Assistance has also been received from Bill Brieger, John Hodson, Yombo and Tinu Awojobi, Ros Everett, Ken Hamilton, Paul Johnson, Gary Parkes and Jean Pearson.

We are indebted to the following individuals, organisations and publishers for the use of certain illustrations, tables and technical detail:

Chapman and Hall, London, publishers of *Control of Hospital Infection*, EJL Lowbury, 1981, for source of the policy for cleaning and decontamination of equipment or environment; modified for Appendix 2.

World Health Organisation, Geneva, for the part of *A model list of essential drugs* (seventh revision), found in the Technical Report Series, 1992 used in Appendix 3.

Editor of *Tropical Doctor,* Royal Society of Medicine, London, for the essential reagents tables in the issue of 1986, 16: 58-60, used in Appendix 4.

Oxford University Press, publishers of *Medical care in developing countries*, by M King, 1966, for the diagram on solar water heating used in Figure 6.8.

Macmillan, UK publishers of *District health care* by Amonoo-Lartson *et al,* 1984, for the diagram on matching needs to resources used in Figure 12.1.

World Bank, Washington, publishers of *Ventilated improved pit latrines: recent developments in Zimbabwe* by P R Morgan and D D Mara, 1982; for diagram of a VIP latrine, used in Figure 7.11.

Road Research Laboratory, Crowthorne, Berkshire, UK, publishers of booklet by Jacobs and Sayer containing road-accident fatality rates in various developing countries 1978, used in Figure 7.3.

Conference of Missionary Societies, Edinburgh House, London SW1W 9BL, publishers and authors of *A model health centre,* for diagrams on orientation of buildings, ventilation of the roof space, and site plans, used in Figures 8.1, 8.3 and 15.17.

Christian Medical Fellowship, 157 Waterloo Road, London SE1 8XN, for statement on Christian ethics in medical practice, used in Appendix 7.

Coordinator of Studies, Ibarapa Programme, Department of P S M, College of Medicine, Ibadan, Nigeria; for his Notes for elective medical students, used in Appendix 5.

Faculty of General Medical Practice, National Postgraduate Medical College, Nigeria, Lagos; producers of *Guidelines for General Practice Training Hospitals,* Parts I and II, used in Appendix 6.

TALC, St Albans, Hertfordshire, for picture of direct recording scale, used in Figure 11.3.

The picture on p.57 is by Janne Andrew. Other drawings are by the author.

CHAPTER 1

The Place of the Doctor in Hospital Administration

Administration is a skill, like driving a car. It has to be learned. It is not an end in itself, but a means to an end. A person who purchases a car for the first time, may ask the salesman to show him where the controls are, fill up with petrol, and then drive off, hopefully depending on common-sense and learning as he goes. Such a person may be lucky and survive, and not cause too much havoc to other drivers and pedestrians on the road; or he may not. He would be wiser to have driving lessons first, taking the wheel under trained supervision, and learning the finer points of safe and courteous driving – for his own and everyone else's benefit.

Many professionals find that, in the course of their job, they sooner or later have to 'take the wheel', provide leadership, and exercise administrative skills. The senior architect finds himself heading a firm designing buildings; the engineer is placed in charge of a construction company putting up bridges; the teacher is promoted headmaster; the university professor is made vice-chancellor. In the same way a doctor may be appointed medical superintendent or principal medical officer in charge of a hospital.

Some professionals have no choice but to learn administration the hard way – 'on the job'. They may have a natural aptitude and cope well; or they may be a disaster, and, among professionals, doctors are no exception to this generalisation. Hence this book. Doctors are well advised to seek some instruction in administrative skills.

Defining our terms

Administration or management?

Some prefer one term, some another, but in reality, *good administration is good management.* The terms are, according to Chambers' dictionary, interchangeable. Administration has been defined by Wilmott (1) in one short sentence in which every word carries significance:

> 'It is the skill shown in managing people, money, materials and time in such a way as to produce the desired goals.'

It is worth reading that definition through again.

The place of the doctor

The amount of administration for which a doctor may be responsible will obviously vary according to his seniority, and the size of the team with which he works, and whether he is in a large or small hospital, in a comprehensive health centre with few other professionals around, or virtually on his own in a private practice.

The doctor in a clinic

At the simplest level, consider the doctor who sets up a private clinic. The service which he can give strictly on his own will be very limited. Inevitably he will soon require assistance – a records clerk, a cleaner, a nursing aid. As work increases, and he employs qualified nursing staff, or technical staff for a laboratory or small X-ray unit, and trained clerical staff for the office, so the complexity grows. A full time administrative assistant will soon be needed. The success of the practice will depend much on good administration, so that limited resources are used wisely, the staff all feel members of a team, and the patients find a happy atmosphere, which engenders confidence, so enabling the doctor to do his primary work of healing. The doctor remains in charge. He has to lead, and he leads from his position beside the patient.

The early stage of the venture may be depicted with the doctor and patient central, and the nurse aide, clerk, and cleaner in a single ring around them (figure 1.1).

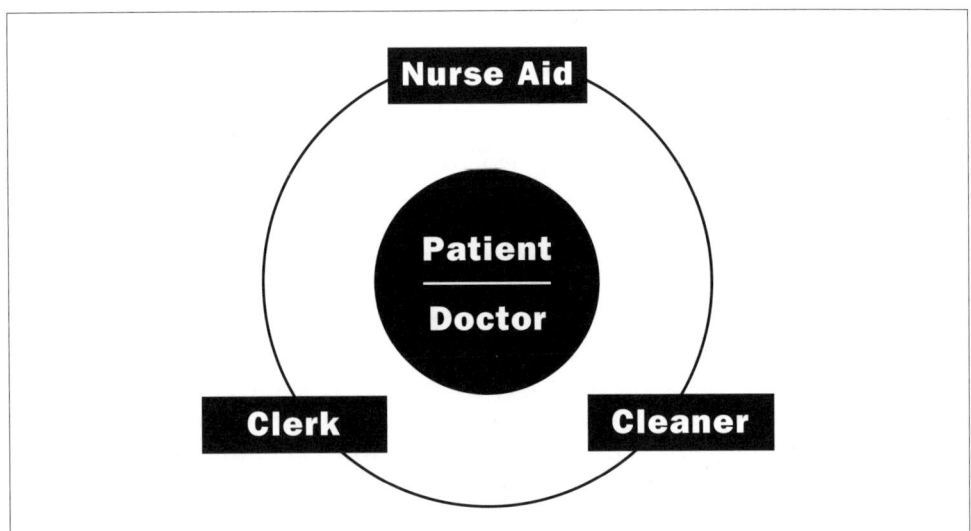

Figure 1.1 *The doctor and patient in the clinic situation*

The doctor in a hospital
The initial clinic may expand to become a health centre, or a small hospital. The size of the staff grows, but the same pattern still applies. The doctor and his patients remain central, with the staff around them in concentric rings of diminishing responsibility (figure 1.2).

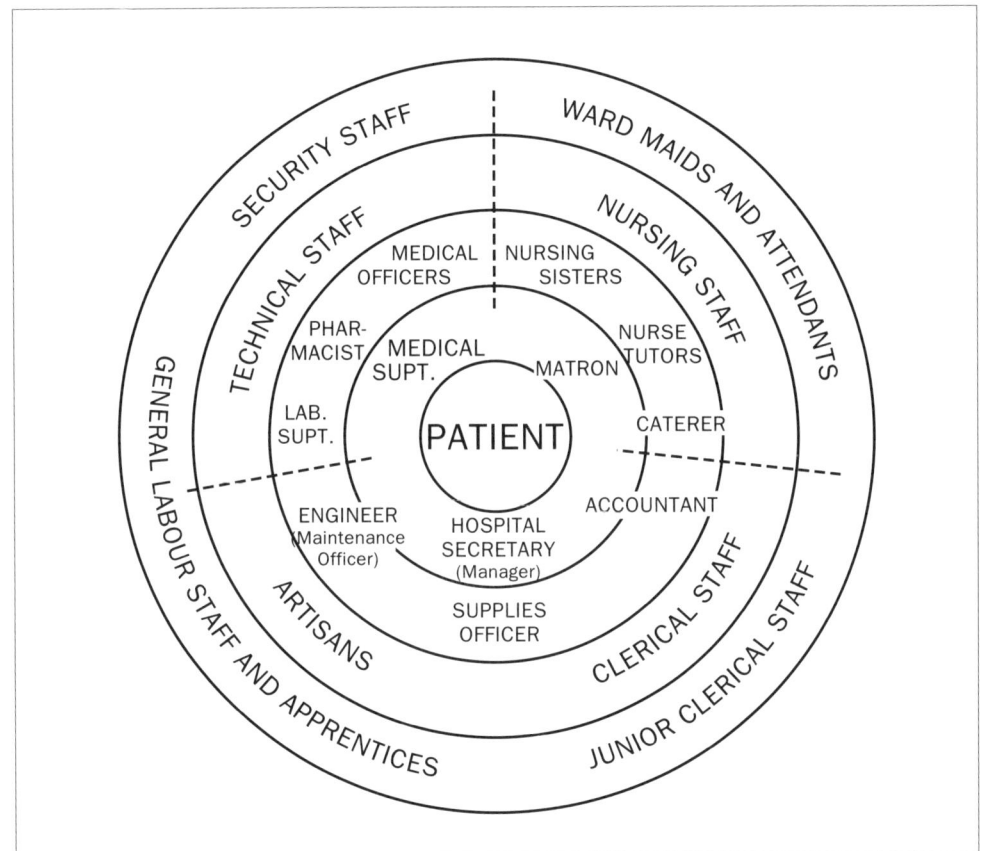

Figure 1.2 *The doctor in a small hospital*

The picture is equally true of the doctor in a voluntary agency or public service hospital. The doctor is still best thought of as leading from the centre, not from above with everybody else below, as in the traditional 'responsibility pyramid'. He is there, not primarily to command, but to unify the efforts of the whole health team, and see that all pull in one direction.

The basic leadership team

It is a matter of experience that the three people who carry the greatest responsibility in a hospital are the most senior doctor, the most senior nurse and the most senior administrator. Their titles may vary, but let us call them:

the medical superintendent,
the matron,
the hospital administrator.

It is these three who form the *basic leadership team.*

The medical superintendent, and his medical colleagues, are in final charge of the care of patients. They decide the diagnosis, prescribe the treatment, and all 'life and death decisions' have to be made by them. They carry the final legal responsibility.

The matron is in charge of the nursing service, and in general charge of nurse training, together with the nurse tutors. The nursing staff and students make up the largest segment of the hospital staff, and much of the success and effectiveness of the hospital depends upon them.

The hospital administrator is in immediate charge of all the clerical and accounting staff, and often indirectly in charge of all the maintenance and labouring staff as well. The smooth functioning of the hospital system depends upon him. His overall responsibilities may indeed be much greater.

Good teamwork between all three is essential, but, in the last resort, one of them has to be the executive head. On this there is more than one school of thought, and we need to look at the debate more closely.

Who should be in charge?
It is the patient who is central, and, as we have seen, in the early stages of a health institution, it is the person in final charge of patient care who takes the lead in administration. In health facilities which include doctors on the staff, it will generally be the most senior doctor who takes charge. In smaller centres with no doctor, such as primary health centre or maternity home, the most senior person in clinical contact with patients may be a midwife, nurse or community health officer. He or she will be the on-the-spot person in charge. Administration will be in their hands, and they will do it well. Medical responsibility will be further up the line of referral.

Some maternity centres run by a nursing sister have achieved excellent standards. However problems have tended to arise when the centre has expanded to become a hospital, and one or more doctors are employed on contract. How should the administrative responsibilities be shared between them? Should the nursing sister hand over to the doctor the task of leadership? Most commonly this dilemma has occurred in Catholic hospitals run by an order of nuns with nursing qualifications, under the authority of the mother superior of their convent. The senior contract doctor may not share the same ethos and ideals, so the senior nursing sister retains administrative control. This may work reasonably well for a while, but the situation can give rise to strained relationships. Happy is the order which can produce its own 'sister doctor' to be medical superintendent. Some orders, such as the Medical Missionaries of Mary, accept the need for the most senior contract doctor to be medical superintendent anyway, and trust that with one of their sisters as matron, or hospital administrator, the purposes for which the hospital was started will be upheld by the administrative team as a whole.

The argument for having a non-medical hospital administrator as executive head

It is claimed that because doctors put in charge prefer to give the best of their time to clinical work, they inevitably skimp on administration. Only a full-time administrator can do justice to the work. Furthermore, as the doctors are not the only professionals in the health team the administrators say it is better for a non-physician to hold the balance between the doctors and the nurses, pharmacists, laboratory scientists, accountants and the rest. Srinivasan, and his team of health administration educators, have written cogently from their Indian experience (2). Of the non-physician administrator taking charge they say:

> 'It is not the status or power that is of primary concern. His competence in ably steering the many groups towards the provision of inexpensive timely and accessible service to the community, with particular attention to needy groups in the community, is the single most overriding attribute we should look for. It is surely a full-time job.'

The vital place of the hospital administrator within the basic leadership team is fully acknowledged, and there is no doubt about the load of responsibility requiring a full-time person. The debate has been as to whether he should be executive head. In some situations it has been the doctors themselves who have been unwilling to shoulder the burdens of administration and leadership – the endless committees, the mountains of paper, and the perpetual crises! The administrators have then argued, 'You concentrate on the clinical work which only you can do, and for which you were trained. Leave us to manage the administration. We will come to you for advice when we need it. We will take charge'.

So, the doctors have handed over the leadership role. In many developed countries this is the present position. However the doctors do find they have lost the power to influence many vital decisions which affect the welfare of their patients. The situation may feel like being on an ocean-going ship with no captain. Control has been handed over to the engineers who know how to make the ship work well, but with no captain on the bridge to assure the passengers that the ship will go to the destination promised.

Physician administration
In developing countries, particularly in secondary care hospitals, doctors should have no doubt about the importance of their leadership role. In other professional activities there has never been any question. As already noted, it is the experienced teacher who is called on to head a school, not the bursar, because it is the teachers who are immediately responsible for the children. So too, the doctor, who is primarily responsible for the patients, should expect to be called on to head the hospital. In Nigeria, even the authorities who used to run teaching hospitals with a director of administration as executive head have now accepted the need for a chief medical director to be in overall charge. The need for skilled physician administration is the basis of this book.

What makes a good medical administrator?

The doctor called upon to lead may begin with some trepidation. He may wonder how his additional responsibilities will affect his clinical work. He may begin to realise how little he knows about the health needs of the community all around and the way in which the hospital relates to them. He may feel woefully inadequate, and anxious to tap the experience of others, or receive additional training.

The place of clinical work
The advantage of being involved in patient care
It is an advantage for a medical administrator to retain some regular clinical responsibilities, and to take his share, with other doctors, in emergency and weekend call duties. Far from diminishing his ability to administer it will enhance it because he will be there with the patients whose needs are at the heart of the whole thing.

He will be more aware of the problems that directly affect patient care – shortage of junior staff, broken equipment, absence of essential drugs etc. His priorities for urgent action will be those measures which promote better medical care, subject to available finance. His leadership will be the more credible, and the more effective, as he stands beside the patient, rather than in some remote office. A 1987 publication of the Nuffield Provincial Hospitals Trust by Hoffenberg *et al* (3) states:

> 'Doctors are best placed to shift the emphasis . . . to health outcome and patient satisfaction. For this reason alone medical participation in management is imperative. By ensuring that resources are devoted optimally to serve the interests of the patients, doctors will find that their own clinical freedom is maximised'.

A balanced timetable

Administrative responsibilities also demand that the doctor in charge should make himself available in the office at certain hours, such as at the beginning of each working day, and in the afternoon. People should know where and when he can be found for administrative consultation. If routine or emergency clinical duties persistently prevent this, then he is too busy.

It must be recognised that some doctors find it very difficult to keep the balance. Providing the best clinical service, and keeping up to date with new developments, can be an all-consuming passion. Simply to emerge occasionally from the theatre or wards to deal peremptorily with the latest crisis is a highly unsatisfactory style of medical administration. Such a doctor should, if possible, take on additional medical staff, and reduce his clinical work load. Or alternatively more administrative reponsibility should be passed over to a medical colleague, or to one of the other members of the basic management team. If the doctor succeeds in this, and retains the leadership, the devolution of duties should be within the limits which will allow him still to be accountable, and in touch with all major developments.

Practical examples

1. The medical superintendent of a 640-bed specialist hospital in Hong Kong, employing 70 doctors and 300 nurses, still made time to continue his special interest in the treatment of children with hare-lip. All such cases were referred to him for operation and care, but with such a big institution, the rest of his time had to be spent on administration.

2. The author's own practice at Wesley Guild Hospital, Ilesha, where the number of doctors in the 1970s varied from two to eight, was, when there was a full complement, to limit himself to medical out-patient clinics, and the care of the 10-bed isolation ward. His special interests included tuberculosis and leprosy. He took an equal share with the other doctors on the emergency duty roster. When any of the specialist doctors were away on leave, he generally had to step into their shoes and act as surgeon, obstetrician or paediatrician until their return. In addition he joined with all the doctors in taking a share in the monthly visits to a branch maternity hospital 100km away, and the rural health centres and clinics providing primary health care, which were given administrative supervision from Ilesha. It was good all round general practice experience, and administrative duties were interwoven at many levels.

Appreciation of the health needs of the community

The doctor will be wise if he develops an attitude which looks beyond the hospital walls. District hospitals and primary health care services should be related. The broad issues involved are touched on in Chapter 11, but dealt with more fully in books with this specific field in mind. For example,

Amonoo-Lartson (4), in *District Health Care*, writes for the doctor given the task officially of evaluating the health needs of the district, and preparing a Health Plan for implementation by all the health workers in the area, in cooperation with the community. Such an opportunity to promote radical change may seem far from the situation which the reader of this book is facing; but some should be prepared for it. Amonoo-Lartson's book shows that there are differences between the management problems in a hospital and those met in primary care (pp 20–21).

Even if the doctor's official responsibilities are confined to the hospital, he should retain a community orientation, and support self-reliant action in the community wherever he can.

Administrative training

We all have to learn administration, and we do it from senior colleagues in other institutions, from management courses when they become available, or from relevant reading. For the rest, it is a matter of learning by trial and error.

The purpose of this book is to to pass on some of the experience gained by the author over the years. The skills to be covered will include such things as a knowledge of the management structure in different types of hospital, and what to look for in a hospital constitution; how to chair a committee or write up the minutes of a hospital board; how to handle public money, and understand accounts and budgeting; the importance of advertising for new staff, preparing clear contracts for those appointed, and helping new staff to settle in. Then there are the difficult problems of staff discipline, and how to cope with conflict. Maintaining good morale throughout the whole hospital community is so vital.

The buildings, equipment and infra-structure of the hospital need skilled maintenance. Extensions may have to be planned. Drugs and supplies have to be ordered in good time. Patient records may need updating. Training facilities for nurses, midwives, laboratory assistants or other staff may need support. The growing complexity of medical administration may seem without end.

And on top of it all will come increasing responsibilities to community and professional associations, and maybe to the State or nation as a whole. Keeping enough time for one's home and family may need fairly strict self-discipline. The doctor who makes a success of administering the hospital and associated primary health care services, for which he is given responsibility, will make a powerful contribution to the welfare and morale of the whole community. The immediate skills he must develop will vary according to the management structure within which he has to work.

CHAPTER 2

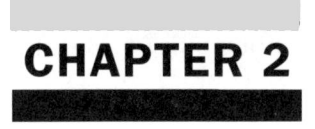

Management Structures

When a doctor is appointed to a general hospital, particularly if he finds himself the most senior doctor there, principal medical officer (PMO) or medical superintendent, he will naturally want to ask questions to ascertain the nature of his responsibilities.

'Is there a job description for this post? What are my administrative duties? To whom am I responsible? Who is responsible to me?'

In particular he needs to know his standing in relation to other senior staff, the matron (or nursing officer in charge), the pharmacist and the administrator (warden or hospital secretary); and also to the district health staff at work in the community.

It is surprising how often knowledge of actual administrative duties is left vague, and experience has to be picked up as one goes along. It is better to ask questions at the beginning, and to look for an authoritative written reply. The answers will of course vary with the type of employer, whether Government, private sector or voluntary agency. Each has its own management structure and ways of doing things.

Public service management

The government system
Most governments have essentially a civil service system for running the state health services. The government management structure, often inherited from a former colonial regime, has proved remarkably durable. The details vary from country to country, but a typical system will be described.

Control from the centre
All countries accept that health services are the responsibility of the state. The state government therefore has a ministry of health responsible for health policy, training programmes and major construction projects. For the day-to-day running of the state hospitals, health centres and other

health-related activities, responsibility is devolved upon the State Health Management Board (SHMB) (see figure 2.1).

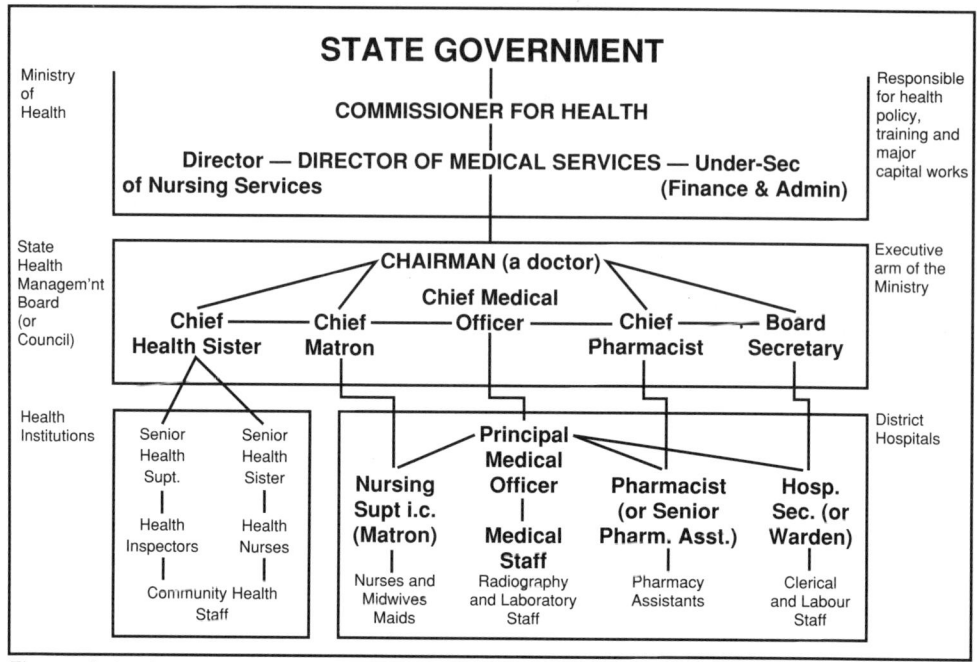

Figure 2.1: *Government administrative structure.*

The ministry will have a director of medical services, and maybe also directors of nursing and pharmacy, all responsible to the government through a commissioner for health. The SHMB usually has a doctor as chairman, and then chief medical officer, chief matron, chief pharmacist, chief health sister, and board secretary responsible to him. All public service staff are employed by this board, but the terms and conditions of service are virtually the same as for other civil servants employed by the state public service commission.

If the doctor wants to know to whom he is responsible, the answer for him, in the system illustrated, is the chairman of the SHMB, through the chief medical officer. In other systems the titles may vary, but the principle will be much the same.

Secondly the doctor may wish to know who is responsible to him, and through him to the board. Theoretically, if he is the most senior member of staff (in terms of salary and grade level), then all other staff in the hospital are responsible to him, and through him to the board. This may or may not work in practice, because each type of staff also has their own chief on the board. The nursing officer in charge has access to the chief matron, the pharmacist has access to chief pharmacist, and the administrative officer or hospital secretary has access to the board secretary. They do not necessarily go through the doctor in charge. If this is the situation, coordination can be very difficult.

Administration is done according to civil service regulations known as general orders (GO). To ask to see the full GO is probably to ask for the impossible. It is voluminous, and subject to change by further regulations from time to time. Only the civil servants at the ministry are likely to have access to it, and understand it. Those at the periphery learn the bits that apply to them as time goes on. For example, all revenue, from fees paid by patients, has to be remitted to the board. Only certain officers are authorised to handle cash, and issue receipts. No money can be retained for local use, such as buying emergency drugs or expediting repairs. An authority to incur expenditure (AIE) can be issued from the board, work carried out at the hospital, completed satisfactorily as certified by the doctor, and then the contractor paid by the board. There is usually no local money for such transactions. At hospital level it is all done by paperwork.

All staff are employed by the board, and are paid from the state capital. Junior staff are generally recruited from near the hospital, and are not subject to transfer. Senior staff are recruited to serve the state as a whole, and are not appointed for any particular post. They are therefore subject to transfer anywhere within the state on the orders of the board.

Advantages and disadvantages

The advantages of the system are that the state government can take full responsibility for finance, and all money is handled by trained accounts staff in the centre (see p.28) where it can be easily audited. If, as tends to happen, most of the professional staff prefer to work in the city, they have to accept transfer to the peripheral hospitals for agreed periods. Each has to take his share of the unpopular posts. No hospital or health centre then goes without staff.

The disadvantages are more obvious to the doctor trying to administer his peripheral hospital than they are to the authorities in the city. First, he has no money, no physical cash which he can use, in order to be responsive to locally perceived needs for improving service to his patients. The paperwork system beloved of headquarters is just too slow. Frequently he is driven to paying for urgent life-saving items from his own pocket, knowing it may not be repaid for three months or more. The small amount of cash sent down from above for day-to-day needs, perhaps equal to about $100, the so-called imprest, is invariably spent before it is received, and de-facto regulation generally forbids it being renewed more often than once a month. Frustration is unavoidable.

Furthermore, since many of the senior staff are there by direction from the board, and not by choice (see p.52), their level of commitment to the hospital and local community may not be very high. They tend to be 'doing their time', and counting the days till they can move back to the city. The doctor in charge, however well intentioned, may have little success in promoting good team work, the first essential of an effective hospital. Key staff in the theatre or maternity department, for example, may be moved at any time without consultation, and new staff sent in.

As senior staff can bypass him – the nursing superintendent to the chief matron, or the hospital secretary to the board secretary, or the pharmacist to the chief pharmacist – his authority is limited. He may wonder how he can raise standards.

Making the best of it
In these circumstances the doctor in charge has a difficult task, but he should not despair. He can exert a leadership role, firstly by doing his own job well, by his punctuality in attendance at clinics, by his attitude to patients and staff, and by his willingness to 'go the extra mile' in dealing with emergencies. He can also press for better medical record keeping, better maintenance of equipment, and more effective use of the limited drugs which may be available. He can mobilise the community to support the hospital, and the other health services in the district, and community leaders can put pressure on the state government for further improvements. Dogged persistence will gradually have some effect. It is only when nobody cares that standards decline so badly.

Can the system change?
When morale is low and frustrations mount, what can be done? Most feel trapped by the system, and do nothing – but not all. Here is a true story.

> Dr A found himself put in charge of small district hospital. The equipment was very run down. There was no money for repairs, no imprest from headquarters, and a desperate shortage of drugs, surgical supplies and X-ray film. Such fees as were taken were all sent up to the state capital.
>
> Dr A's wife was trained as a radiographer. She was put in charge of the X-ray. The machine did work but, without films, was lying idle. The Ministry of Health authorised her to make a charge for X-rays, to keep the money, and use it to buy film. She did, and the little department became busy again.
>
> Dr A said to himself: 'If my wife can have a revolving fund for X-rays, why cannot I have one for surgery?
>
> The following week he kept the fees for the six hernia cases listed, then used the money to buy at a cheap price the surgical supplies which the patients were having to purchase expensively outside, because the hospital had none

– rubber gloves, catgut, syringes, needles etc. Meticulous accounts were kept. He asked his pharmacist to sell supplies to the following week's patients at cost-price. The pharmacist said 'Yes, doctor,' but, out of fear, went at once to report him to the Ministry in the state capital. Dr A took on the sales himself, again with strict accounting. The whole hospital began to feel the difference. Beds were full. The community was happy. The people were getting good service.

After two weeks a letter arrived from headquarters saying: 'It is hereby alleged that you are keeping government revenue, and using it for your own purposes. What have you to say?'

Dr A at once took up pen and paper and wrote in reply: 'The allegations you have made against me are *entirely true*, but I shall go on using the revenue raised in the hospital for the patients' benefit until you supply me with what I need.'

Since it was public knowledge that the hospital was running well, and that every penny was accounted for, the Ministry was reluctant to act. However, after many months a letter was finally sent quoting General Orders 'section 206, para 1108', declaring that 'direct spending of government revenue before payment into the treasury is irregular'. Dr A was asked to desist, or resign. He resigned, and shortly after was providing at least some of the same service as a private doctor from premises loaned to him by the community. Fees remained the same. Most patients deserted the district hospital and followed him.

One doctor showed what could be done, but he acted without official approval.

Permanent change can only come from the top

In 1981 one of the many 'states' in Nigeria modified its management structure and financial arrangements. The state had eight districts, with one or two hospitals in each. For their running costs a bank account was opened in each district's main town, with the PMO and hospital secretary as signatories. A cheque, and authority to incur expenditure, were sent quarterly to each district. Running costs were defined as including:

1. Food for patients, where supplied.

2. Repairs to the fabric, up to N2000 per quarter. (One naira = US$1 at that time).

3. Fuel and oil for the standby generator.

4. Care and replacement of diagnostic instruments etc.

5. Emergency drugs and dressings, up to N1000 per 100 beds per quarter.

6. Petrol for the ambulance, and vehicle repairs.

The system worked well. For instance, when the water pump serving one hospital broke down, the doctor did not have to send all the way to headquarters 100 miles away to ask for a maintenance team. He was able to engage a local engineer to effect the repair on the same day, and pay him by cheque. The service to patients was not interrupted.

The usual centralised system would have taken weeks. If such a point seems minor to the authorities at the top, it is not so to the doctor on the spot. To be able to ensure quick action in response to patient need contributes so much to job satisfaction.

Board management as it can be
A more radical modification of the civil service system is beginning to appear. In this the SHMB is given full and statutory powers to manage the state's health facilities, with general policy directives only from the ministry of health. It has its own budget, and its own administration and audit service. The board, in turn, has the power to decentralise further and set up a hospital management committee for each district general hospital, or a district management committee which administers both the hospital and district health services.

These district management committees are likely to have representation from the local community, as well as from the board, thus ensuring community concern for the government health facilities. The chairman may be appointed by government, the owner of the hospital and related health centres. Preferably he or she should be someone who lives near, and constantly accessible to the hospital and health care staff, with power to act for the committee, in conjunction with the PMO between meetings. The basic leadership team, doctor, nurse and administrator may, with advantage, be made full members of the committee, but be required to withdraw whenever matters personal to them are discussed.

Powers devolved to district level
The district management committees *should not just be advisory*. They must have defined executive powers. These should ideally include:

1. Power to retain revenue from fees, together with supplementary grants from the board. Responsibility for certain heads of expenditure, for example for food, fuel, emergency drugs and hospital maintenance, as in the scheme above. To do this the administrative officer should have a small accounts department, with proper cross checks so as to ensure honest administration of income and expenditure.

2. Power to appoint junior staff, according to an agreed level of establishment, with authority for promotion, discipline and dismissal, with due

safeguards. For senior staff the board should make appointments to specific posts, and not just to a general pool of senior staff. The management committee should have the power to make recommendations for promotion or discipline.

Under such a system the public service doctor really would have the opportunity to administer effectively, maintain the hospital and related health facilities well, ensure high staff morale, and give the patients and the community good service.

World Health Organisation recommendations

This type of management structure with executive power devolved to district hospital level is now being recommended by WHO in its booklet on *The Hospital in Rural and Urban Districts*, 1992 (Technical Report Series 819). This sets out clearly, for the first time at such a high level, the essential services which should be offered in a district hospital, the staff, buildings and equipment required, and the best form of management. On the subject of 'Financial resources' the report notes that:

> 'If fees are charged, the basic levels are usually set by the government, but there are many advantages in local cost recovery: if the hospital can benefit locally, more enthusiasm will be shown for collecting fees . . . In some countries, all fees and donations collected by a first referral hospital are retained in the district. In some instances, 75% is kept by the hospital for its own work, while 25% goes to the district health council for the support of other health services.'

Zambia, Nigeria and other countries which have centralised systems for managing general hospitals, are now studying these and similar recommendations with a view to implementation. For some Ministries of Health it will be quite a revolution.

Outside the public service

Private practice management

A doctor coming to work with an established private practitioner is likely to be joining as an assistant, though maybe with a view to partnership at a later date. As an assistant his administrative responsibilities will be minimal, unless he is put in charge of a branch clinic. It is in setting up on his own that he is faced with the biggest administrative challenge.

Starting up
The doctor on his own in private practice is his own master, and is free to make his administrative structures as tight and efficient, or as free and easy as he desires. If he has a good business head, he will want to keep day-to-

day accounts, and not just rely on his monthly bank statement. However he has no board to present a statement of accounts to. Financially he is responsible only to himself.

Nevertheless, he may feel a social responsibility to his patients and the community he serves. Not all private doctors enter practice solely to make money, whatever may be the stereotype. Some come in because they are tired of the grey insensitivity and slow inefficiency of centralised bureaucratic control, and they believe they can provide a better service on their own. All credit to them. Many have succeeded in building up excellent practices, and even full scale hospitals.

Some practical advice from those who have entered private practice full time is worth recording here.

1. The work is hard, and the hours may be long. Keep to scheduled clinic times for the sake of the patients. Self-discipline is essential.

2. Stick to high ethical standards from the start. Steer clear of the temptation to issue untrue medical certificates, or do abortions not justified on medical grounds. You may earn less in fees initially, but will certainly gain immeasurably more in reputation and self-respect in the long run.

3. Give other staff a square deal. You have to build up a team, and all staff, high or low, are entitled to the security of a written letter of appointment, agreed conditions of service, and at least a living wage. If staff members cannot be admitted to a pension scheme, then all should be offered some form of 'contract addition in lieu', payable at regular intervals. This can be put into a savings scheme if the currency is stable. Such an addition may not seem necessary at first, but when staff come to leave after many years, its wisdom will be clearly seen.

4. Prepare a booklet setting out the aims and objectives of the centre, and the services on offer. Let key staff be named in this, so that all feel part of the venture.

5. Administer prudently, and keep fees reasonable. Patients are often vulnerable, especially those in emergency situations. It is all too easy to exploit sickness; but when this is done, the doctor may be enriched, but the medical profession is demeaned.

6. Know your community. Be responsive to their needs. Cooperate with other health providers in the area. Take a share in provision of preventive care, and in campaigns of health education.

Partnership agreements, or the formation of a limited liability company
1. If two or more doctors run the practice as a partnership then more stringent articles of agreement will have to be drawn up, with the help of legal advisers.

2. If family members, banks or other businesses have been involved, say, in putting up capital for building a hospital, accountants may advise that it should be constituted a limited liability company, and not be owned by the medical director or the partners alone. In that case the company becomes a 'legal person' entitled to own property, receive revenue, pay out bills – and pay tax. The partners and maybe other investors become directors, with shares in the company, and the company pays them in accordance with agreed formulae.

Should the company run into difficulties, and be unable to meet outstanding bills for drugs or supplies, then it can be declared bankrupt. Official receivers are then brought in to sell assets and recover what they can in order to pay off the creditors. The partners themselves lose their company and property and their jobs as directors, but they are not liable to pay off all the debts. It is in this sense that their liability is limited. An accountant with specialist knowledge in tax affairs in the country is the best person to advise whether a partnership agreement or a limited liability company is the most appropriate management structure.

Voluntary agency administration

Voluntary agency hospitals and health services have grown up in many countries through the pioneer work of missionary doctors and nurses, often in remote rural areas. The valuable contribution of mission hospitals to national health care is readily acknowledged, but many governments now feel strong enough to accept the full responsibility for the provision of health services for all their citizens. In some cases parallel health facilities have been set up so that people have a choice as to which they go to. In other cases mission hospitals have been given government grants-in-aid on condition they work within agreed guidelines. Finally, some states have taken over voluntary agency services completely, not always with the most satisfactory results, and it has been known for such takeovers to be reversed and the hospitals handed back.

A system between public service and private sector
A typical voluntary agency management structure lies somewhere between that of government and the private sector. The doctor in charge is not subject to a vast centralised bureaucracy; but neither is he free to run things entirely at his own whim, as he might in private practice. The hospital belongs to a proprietor, such as the Baptist Convention, an Anglican Diocesan Synod, or one of the Catholic orders represented by the local bishop. The

doctor receives a nominal salary paid by the mission or church if a missionary, or he is paid by the hospital if a national, usually at the government rate for the job.

The hospital will be run on a non-profit basis, fees being taken sufficient only to cover costs, with an orientation towards service to the poor. Revenue in excess of salaries and running costs is all ploughed back into the hospital to finance building extensions, or the replacement of vehicles or equipment. Finance is all dealt with at hospital level. Resources may be limited, but what cash there is is immediately available. Most members of the staff come to their job with a sense of dedication. They are there because they have chosen to be, and not because they have been transferred there by a state authority. They form a team. Morale is generally high.

The administrative structure may be very loose, and depend primarily upon trust between the head of the hospital and the proprietor, and a good relationship between the members of the hospital's own leadership team. Increasingly however, such hospitals are realising the advantages of government by a hospital Board, with church, community and professional representation, to ensure more democratic control.

The hospital constitution

Any doctor taking up employment with a voluntary agency hospital should ask to see the hospital constitution. If there is none he is entitled to ask why. A constitution is simply a document setting out the principles on which the hospital is governed. Bye-laws may be added to this to cover additional detail. Together these should provide a clear guide to the administrative framework within which the doctor will have to work if he is put in charge. These documents will vary according to the size and complexity of the hospital.

The constitution is likely to include the following:

1. The name of the hospital, and the purpose for which it was founded.

2. The controlling bodies under which it operates. For example:

    A. The Hospital Board or Management Committee, which is responsible to B. (Let us continue to call A the Hospital Board.)

    B. The proprietor's top authority, such as a church Synod, Conference or Convention.

3. The membership of the board is then defined, and whether members are to be appointed, elected or to serve *ex-officio*. The latter serve on the

board, not because they have been appointed in person, but by virtue of the offices which they hold.

4. The officers of the board, chairman, secretary (and treasurer, if required) should have their method of appointment and tenure of office set out clearly.

5. The frequency of regular meetings should be laid down, and the means for calling emergency meetings. A quorum is the fixed number of members that must be present to make the proceedings of the board valid. Often this will be about half the total, and certainly not less than one-third.

6. The most important section of the constitution is that which defines the functions of the board, the executive powers which the board may exercise on behalf of the proprietor. These will include powers to control staff and money in such a way as to provide the services, and fulfil the objects for which the hospital was founded. Limits may be placed on those powers, for example the amount which can be spent on a major repair, or a capital project. Beyond the limits matters must be referred to the proprietor.

7. Provision for an executive committee of certain key board officers or hospital staff, which can act for the full board between meetings, may be included. In some this may be called a standing committee, or a general purposes committee. Other committees for special areas of administration, such as finance or personnel, may be required in larger institutions. It is also wise to lay down the duties of a regular staff committee.

8. Finally there has to be the power to amend the constitution. This is usually made quite difficult so as to ensure it is not done lightly, or by an unrepresentative bare quorum. Generally a three-fourths majority is required, and notice given in writing at least two months before. Effectively this means that an amendment tabled at one general meeting will be referred to the next regular meeting when the written minutes are presented. The vote to confirm the amendment then takes place.

Bye-laws, which may be added to a constitution
These are further regulations on matters of detail, not matters of principle, and can generally be amended by a simple majority vote at any general meeting. They include such matters as:

1. *Voting procedures* to be followed when a consensus cannot be reached, and the only way is to vote, and follow the will of the majority. If the members of the committee are split evenly on an issue, the chairman may be given

an extra vote (a 'casting vote'), or a tied vote (equal numbers for and against) may be considered as one where the motion is lost.

2. Another essential feature of most bye-laws is a section listing *the duties and responsibilities of each Hospital Officer*, the medical superintendent, the matron, the hospital administrator and so on. These define, for example, what the medical superintendent should do, and the broad areas he should delegate. The matron is likely to be given full responsibility for the nursing service, including discipline of nurses. Thus if ever a doctor finds a nurse falling short in the performance of her duties, he should not take the matter into his own hands, but report the fault to matron, leaving her to investigate the case, and take what disciplinary measure she thinks fit.

This delineation of the duties and responsibilities enables each hospital officer to 'act executively' on day-to-day matters within his or her field, without fear of treading on the others' toes, and without having to take every decision to a committee.

3. Right of appeal. As an essential 'human right' it is also necessary to include in the bye-laws a method by which both junior and senior staff may appeal against disciplinary decisions taken against them which they feel to be unjust.

When a constitution has still to be written
The best way is to find the constitution written for a similar institution, and then use that as a model.

> The constitution, with bye-laws, for Wesley Guild Hospital, Ilesha was fairly detailed, running to nine foolscap pages. It was originally copied from one drawn up by the Voluntary Hospital Association of India, and adapted for use in Nigeria. It worked very well for 20 years (1955–1975) with amendment from time to time as the hospital grew from 112 to 200 beds, trebled its staff and developed a major training component to the work.
>
> Branch institutions, such as a maternity hospital of 44 beds at Ikole, 80 miles away, and a rural health centre at Irhuekpen 120 miles away, had shorter constitutions of only 2 or 3 pages. They proved fully adequate for 20 years, and it was just as important for the smaller centres to have them as for the main hospital.

Based upon this experience a specimen outline constitution is given (Appendix 1). This could be adapted by any community health centre, or small hospital which is to be run on a non-profit basis, and made accountable to a Board for democratic control.

Democratic procedure

Shared responsibility inevitably means that some decisions have to be taken by several people acting together. Official decisions involve meeting in committee.

Committee work

It is all too easy to consider committees to be burdensome and time-wasting, but they cannot be avoided. They are an essential part of democratic control, and the only alternative to allowing the head of the hospital to run things entirely on his or her personal judgement. Even in private hospitals most Medical Directors have some kind of management committee. In voluntary agency hospitals they are essential. The medical superintendent may find himself having to be secretary to his board, and chairman to his staff committee. He may have previous experience of committee work, for his university or for his church or community. If not, he may just have to learn as he goes along. If his skills in this area are poor, the whole hospital will suffer.

Committees enable things to be done. Committees can help to promote team work. Committees spread responsibility, and can facilitate community participation – *but only if they are run well.*

Committee meetings have to be prepared for
This is the task of the secretary, and his assistant if he has one.
1. The notice of meeting, giving the date, time and venue should go to all members 3 weeks or more in advance, depending on the postal service, or means of dispatch. For board meetings, a second notice of reminder may be advisable. With the notice should go the provisional agenda, listing the items likely to be discussed. A final agenda can still be prepared for the day, including any items previously overlooked.

2. With the agenda should also go the minutes of the last meeting, and any documents for the one to come that are ready, so that members have much of the information enabling decision making already in their hands. Writing good minutes is a skill to be cultivated, and although an assistant secretary may take records during a meeting, if the doctor is actually the secretary of a board, he should prepare the final version. Minutes should not be lengthy or discursive. They should be brief and to the point. Minutes should state the facts of who was at the meeting, and *record decisions taken.* If a matter has been discussed, and no decision reached, some would say there should be no minute. However this may be going too far. A short note to say a matter was considered and a decision deferred is in order. No attempt should be made to record all

the arguments advanced from every side. Decisions are what should be recorded clearly and precisely, and the exact words of the resolutions passed at the meeting should be put down.

3. The board or committee room should be set out before the meeting, with chairs, and all necessary papers, including the final agenda, distributed round the table. Documents should bear a number, and be referred to on the agenda. Adequate ventilation, and refreshments half way through the meeting, all help to ensure cool and efficient deliberations.

The chairman's task

The chairman, with his secretary beside him, controls the meeting. He welcomes members, calls for a prayer if appropriate, then calls for each item of the agenda in turn. While he is speaking, no one else speaks. If two members wish to speak at the same time, the chairman decides who shall speak first. If a member speaks too often, or for too long, he may be called to order. A good chairman allows all views on a matter to be fairly placed, then offers a summary of what has emerged in such a way as to carry the whole meeting with him. Decision by consensus is worth aiming at.

Voting procedure

Differing ideas, supported by strong feelings, may make agreement difficult, and in such cases decision by majority vote is the only way forward. After preliminary discussion the chairman may call for one protagonist to 'propose a motion'. If a supporter is prepared to 'second the motion', the meeting then has a defined issue to accept or reject. If another person judges that the issue is more likely to carry approval if the wording is altered, he may 'propose an amendment'. If the amendment is also seconded, the chairman may call for a vote by a show of raised hands. If the amendment is supported by a majority the new wording becomes the motion on which a decision has to be made. If the amendment is lost, then the original motion as first proposed remains the agreed wording. The motion is put to the vote.

As long as there is clear majority either for the motion, or against it, the decision of the meeting is unequivocal. Whatever the majority wishes becomes the decision of the meeting. Democratic procedure requires that all then accept the decision, and loyally implement it, even though some may have voted against it. Difficulty arises when a committee is split down the middle, and there are equal numbers voting for and against the motion. In this situation the committee follows the voting procedure as set down in the constitution and bye-laws.

Some bye-laws (see p.19) say that if there is a tied vote, say 5 including the chairman are for, and 5 are against, then the chairman shall be given an additional 'casting vote', by which a 6:5 majority is achieved, and the motion carried. Other bye-laws do not give the chairman this extra power, and simply say that a tied vote is a vote lost, and this may be the fairest way.

Following the agenda

There is usually a set pattern for well-established meetings. The following order is a common one.

1. Opening and welcome.

2. Apologies for absence from members who have sent messages to say they cannot be present. A register for those who are present is then passed round for signing.

3. *Minutes of the last meeting.* These should then be read by the secretary, or, if they have been circulated in advance, it may be proposed by a member that they be 'taken as read'. This may save valuable time. The chairman then calls for members to state any corrections they wish to see made in the written record, and will lead the committee through the clauses one by one. When all corrections have been agreed, the chairman then makes the statement,

   'Is it your wish that I sign these minutes as a true and correct record of the last meeting? All those in favour, please indicate.'

   This may be by raising a hand, or saying 'Aye'. He then calls for all those against, which is usually a formality, since the minutes have already been corrected. A vote that the minutes are a correct record, does not necessarily mean that a member is happy with all that was decided at the previous meeting. When the minutes have been approved, the chairman signs them, and the record then becomes official.

4. *Matters arising from the minutes.* The chairman then leads the committee through the record, clause by clause, with the help of his secretary, and members of the committee who may have been called to undertake certain tasks. Further developments which have occurred, and the outcome of the various decisions taken, are duly noted. The chairman should be careful not to allow this process to take too long, or the committee may never reach new business in the time available. Major matters, listed on the agenda, may be excluded from discussion at this stage, and brought in at the appropriate point.

5. *New business.* The agenda lists matters to be presented and discussed. These may start with reports from the hospital officers, a general one from the medical superintendent, one from the matron on nursing affairs, and a financial report from the hospital secretary or accountant. Each report

is placed before the board, then clarified through questions and discussion, and, if the actions taken are approved, the report is 'received'. Presentation of financial returns, and auditor's report, are particularly important, since it is the board's duty to see that all money passing through the institution has been properly used. The hospital officers are accountable to the board.

Major new project proposals will be listed separately. The secretary and chairman have to exercise skill as to what items are to be included. Many matters are quite properly dealt with by a medical superintendent or a hospital secretary in their executive capacity, within the powers granted to them under the constitution. Matters of policy, new developments or heavy expenditure, must come for approval by the whole board.

6. *Closing.* The chairman should always keep his eye on the time. He should ensure business is dealt with reasonably quickly, and should set a good example by keeping his own interventions brief. When the time has come to close, it should be announced whether unfinished business, if any, should be dealt with by a standing committee or some other body. The date of the next meeting should be fixed.

After the meeting
The minutes of the meeting should be written up within the next week or two. Under no circumstances should they be left until just before the next meeting. When the meeting is in the recent past, memories will be the clearer, and the record less likely to contain inaccuracies. The very writing of the minutes will bring to mind actions that it has agreed should be taken. Letters can then be written to ensure all decisions are followed up by the persons to whom responsibility has been assigned.

Democratic committee procedure may seem elaborate, but it is a well-tried process and, if followed with care, can lead to stability and steady progress. The time spent will be repaid.

The system is part of the framework which ensures the satisfactory care of public funds. Money is handled in a way which is not only honest but which can be seen to be honest in the eyes of the board, and through the board by the community as a whole.

CHAPTER 3

Handling Money

Attitudes to money

Money is an esssential tool, and the medical administrator must be familiar with the techniques for handling it. Its presence, in adequate amounts, can make the wheels turn round as nothing else can. It can also be a danger. Financial corruption can ruin the best administrative systems. It has been argued in the previous chapter that money is needed *at hospital level* in order to ensure an administration responsive to the day-to-day needs of good service to patients. This presupposes a willingness to adopt the simple precautions necessary for the safe handling of money.

Two simple precautions
Private money and public money must never be kept together
The doctor, and all the staff members, have (hopefully) some personal money in their pockets. That must at all times be kept separate from any hospital money entrusted to them. Private money and public money do not mix. Take an everyday example.

In communities which have not yet become accustomed to using banks, or the credit cards ('plastic money') now the fashion in developed countries, a savings group of around six members is a common feature. They club together to save money and take it in turns to draw from the kitty. Let us say that on the monthly pay day, each receives a net wage of $100. They immediately gather around one person selected as treasurer, and both he and the other five pay over an agreed sum, say $10. The treasurer now has $60 of group savings, and $90 of his own. The savings are public money, the $90 is personal. If the $60 is immediately paid out to the one whose turn it is that month, he has no problem; but if he keeps the $150 together in the same pocket or box at home, what chance is there that, with the next family crisis, or unexpected demand for cash, he will remember exactly how much is his own to use? Memory is fallible, and his only chance is to keep the group savings separately. Private and public money must never be kept together.

Responsibility for public money must be shared

Anyone who handles public money is advised to share the responsibility. The holder of money in quantity can become the object of envy and false rumour from those around however honest he may be. He should never take charge of public money entirely on his own. Two examples from personal experience in China may serve to illustrate the point.

> As a young doctor working in that country in the 1940s the author was assigned to a 100-bed mission hospital where Dr W was the Medical Superintendent. He was a good doctor, and the hospital gave invaluable service, and the community was fortunate to have him. However there was constant back-chat among the junior staff that Dr W was making money for himself out of the hospital. One could not know if this were true or not. Dr W took the patients' fees, and did all the financial transactions himself. He shared the responsibilities with no one. So the suspicions grew, and much of the good work the hospital was doing was undermined. Then came the communist revolution of 1949, when Chairman Mao Tse Tung came to power. The suspicions surfaced into open hostility. Dr W was given a very hard time indeed.

> At another 100-bed mission hospital that the author visited the doctor in charge operated a system of 'open accounting'. Every Friday all the salaried staff, plus representatives of the nursing students and the labour staff, were invited to an accounts meeting. The accounts for the week, signed by two staff members, were passed round the group. The supporting cash books for in-patient and out-patient fees revenue, and for outgoings on purchases of drugs and sundries, were on the table for inspection. Questions were invited, and only when everyone was satisfied were the accounts signed by the Medical Superintendent as correct. Open accounting dispelled rumours, and this led to a happy relationship amongst all the staff. When the revolution came no flaw could be found by the new authorities in that hospital's administration.

Responsibility for handling public money should always be shared. No one individual should go it alone. Inevitably doubts will enter into the minds of some, and before long doubts become suspicions, and staff relationships become poisoned. To avoid this *every transaction should be written down and cross-checked by a second person.* It is surprising how many people fail to realise the importance of this. Having two signatures on cheques for institutional bank accounts is generally accepted. The same procedure should apply to cash payments. They must always be supported by a written document signed by two people. If a staff member takes money from the cashier or accountant to make a purchase for the hospital, then the transaction must be written on a petty cash voucher, authorised by the clerk or accountant, and signed for by the staff member. Memory must not be relied on. It is also wise to have two people initial the figure for a cash balance in the cash book after a weekly or monthly counting of the actual money in hand.

Precautions like these, maintained with conscientious discipline, can ensure that public money is handled safely and effectively. *The people in charge are not only honest, but seen to be honest.* Proper cross-checking is the key.

Alternative approaches
Private practice accounting
It can be argued that the doctor in private practice is accountable to no one but himself. So long as he pays his staff according to their agreed contracts, and settles his bills for drugs and other running costs reasonably promptly, then the finances are his own business. The money is personal. All profit is legitimately his own. True. However, apart from the need to satisfy the income tax authorities, a doctor who runs his practice from his pocket is likely to have only a pocket-sized practice. If the practice is to grow, and additional staff employed to look after finance and administration, the recognised procedures for handling money safely will have to be introduced. The sooner they are begun the better.

A young surgeon recently set up a private practice in a rural township of Nigeria, and adopted a form of 'open accounting'. He called it 'a private medical practice in the public service'.

> 'In our establishment there is no employer or employee. We owe allegiance to our patients who receive the best we can offer, and in return sustain us within their resources. Ours is a cooperative of professionals and non-professionals offering service in the health sector of the economy and in so doing we earn our means of livelihood.
>
> Everybody is placed on a salary agreed by all. These salaries are 20% to 50% above comparative levels in the public service. Every month a meeting of all workers is convened during which all financial returns of the month are tendered and decisions taken on payment of salaries, and what to do with profit or loss.'

Inefficient public accounting – 'fudging'
Many will have encountered situations in public service where there is some local cash to be administered, but the need for the essential precautions is not appreciated. The administrative officer or accounts clerk lack the discipline to ensure that private and public money are never mixed, and that there are two signatories for every transaction. The cash books are never up to date. Money may have been advanced from cash, but nothing written down. Memory is relied on pending the arrival of a receipt. Maybe one item of revenue is kept separate in a drawer in case payment has to be made from it – and then it is forgotten. At the time of the regular weekly or monthly check by a superior officer, the one caring for the money has 'had to travel' and is not available, so the checking is postponed to the following week, by which time the sorting out of discrepancies becomes even more difficult. The

accounts are kept only approximately correct. *This is fudging.* There may be no dishonest intention whatever, but then again, who knows? Good administration is undermined. Before long even the little cash available for local use is liable to be withdrawn by higher authority, and centralised accounting, with all its limitations, enforced as the only option.

Centralised accounting

This is the system adopted by most government administrations. They believe that virtually all money should be handled centrally, where financial discipline can be enforced. Therefore all district health service and hospital revenues have to be forwarded to the state capital. Necessary expenditure at the periphery is facilitated through the 'invisible money' obtained through the granting of an AIE – an Authority to Incur Expenditure – for each particular item. This form, when obtained and not before, allows the doctor to engage a local contractor, for example, to do some repairs which may be necessary. On satisfactory completion the appropriate line on the form is signed by the doctor, and the contractor can then go to the state capital to collect the money due in payment.

On paper this may sound all right, but in practice it can be very frustrating if the regional capital is 100 miles away. Much time is wasted by senior staff travelling to apply for or collect their AIEs, leaving other local responsibilities unfulfilled. Contractors are not always willing to have their payments delayed 2 or 3 months or longer, and if they are, they are likely to inflate their charges by way of compensation.

The system avoids the dangers of petty corruption through the dishonest handling of money in the district, but it turns a blind eye to the poor service to patients which may result, and the frustration experienced by staff. It also ignores the danger that if corruption does occur at headquarters, it is likely to be on a far larger scale.

The place of an 'imprest account'

There are two situations in which an imprest account is commonly used.

1. *Where it is satisfactory on paper, but rarely works well in practice.* The use of an imprest of cash from headquarters is often put forward as an answer to at least part of the problem. The word 'imprest' simply means 'money advanced', or on loan. The amount is kept low, to minimise temptation. For example, say $100 is advanced to the district hospital administrator. He uses it for approved emergency purposes, and collects receipts for each item of expenditure. As soon as his receipts total around $95 he takes them, plus his $5 balance, up to headquarters, where his expenditure is checked, and the cash made up again to $100. It sounds satisfactory on paper, but it rarely works out so in practice.

Many will have experienced the reality. Time and distance dictate that the journey to get the imprest renewed cannot be more often than once a month. The money is never enough to cover more than a fraction of essential running costs for such a period. An all too familiar situation develops. The hospital generator needs diesel but there is no money to buy it with, so if mains power goes off, operations are postponed; the vaccine refrigerator gets warm, and vaccines lose their potency. Maybe a roof starts leaking, but there is no cash to employ a local carpenter to mend it, and the ceiling beneath it becomes soaked and spoiled to make the damage worse. Out-patient cards get used up, and there is no money to print more locally, so expensive in-patient folders are cut up to provide cards for the interim weeks till more come from the stores in the capital. A conscientious doctor or nursing officer in charge will often pay for items from his or her own pocket, so that service will not suffer. They accumulate receipts in the hope of repayment from the next renewal of imprest. Invariably the cash is actually spent even before it has been received. And a further month has to go by before more can be applied for. Sometimes many months go by before renewal.

2. *Where it does work well.* The only situation in which an imprest works as it should is in a self-accounting institution where the money is granted by the accountant to an accounts clerk *working in the same place.* He is authorised for example to collect in-patient fees, and at the beginning of the day he may need coins for change. He may also be expected to pay local market women arriving early to supply small items of food for the hospital kitchen, or brooms for sweeping. At the end of the day he submits his receipts, petty cash vouchers and cash balance to the accountant, note being taken of the advance received at the beginning of the day. The box is emptied, and then a fresh imprest put back for the beginning of the next day. There is no problem with an imprest used in this way.

Efficient handling of money
A summary of the points made so far
- Adequate visible money at hospital level is essential.

- Precautions in handling cash must be insisted on:
  - Private and public money to be kept quite separate
  - Responsibility for all transactions to be shared between at least two people.
  - No fudging to be allowed.

- The imprest system for petty cash to be used only within one institution or in the same town not between headquarters and district, where distance makes effective operation of it impossible.

- Some measure of open accounting should be included so that staff and public may be reassured that funds are being used honestly.

Handled in this way money becomes a blessing. It gives the power to get things done. Good service becomes possible, and the patients feel the difference.

The need for change

For the doctor in private practice, or in a self-accounting voluntary agency hospital, this need for money at hospital level is so obvious it is taken for granted. It is only when he moves to work in a government hospital that he realises there are other ways of looking at it. He may feel that the civil service centralised accounting system is so fixed and immutable, that there is no alternative. This is not necessarily so. The changes made in one state in Nigeria have already been mentioned (see p.13). Modification is possible. In another state, voluntary agency hospitals were 'integrated' into the state system, but management responsibilities were retained by the proprietor. Staff salaries were paid centrally, and a substantial cheque was sent each month to cover running costs on condition that all children were treated free. Accounts were subject to audit. The system worked satisfactorily while the government had sufficient funds.

A similar system is used in other parts of the world, for example in Hong Kong. There the Kwun Tong United Christian Hospital operates with independent management, despite the fact that the government supplies 90% of the revenue. Honest administration and efficient accounting give the government sufficient feed-back to satisfy its auditors.

Basic requirements for a good accounting system

Let us look at the situation in which a regional health management board decides to introduce a measure of self-accounting to one of its district hospitals; or in which a private or voluntary agency hospital decides to improve its accounting system to give greater public accountability. What are the basic requirements of a good system?

A responsible leadership team

The key members of the basic leadership team are:

- the doctor in charge, or medical superintendent,
- the nursing officer in charge, or matron,
- the administrator in charge, hospital secretary or hospital manager (see Chapter 1, p.4).

Training and experience are needed

If the hospital is to be self-accounting then it is important that the hospital secretary should either be an accountant himself, or that he should have a person well trained and experienced in accounts on his staff. The medical superintendent should have a sufficient knowledge of accounts to be able to understand all statements laid before him for approval, and all essential accounting procedures. He will thus want to keep them simple.

At a pinch he should be able to take over the accounting himself should there be a period when the hospital secretary and accountant have to be away. In the last resort, as executive head, he is in charge of finance. The medical superintendent should have a deputy medical superintendent who is competent to stand in for him when on leave; or the matron should be able to fulfill that administrative role.

A bank account

Signatories

Self accounting is greatly facilitated if a bank has been opened in the township where the hospital is, or within a reasonable distance down a passable road, not more than an hour away. A current account should be opened on the authority of the board or proprietor. The signatories should be the medical superintendent and the hospital secretary, with two alternatives to cover leave periods, for example the deputy medical superintendent and the matron, any two to sign.

In some cases the board or proprietor may wish to have a third signatory who is not on the hospital staff, say the chairman of the board, or a community leader appointed as treasurer. This can lead to administrative delays and frustration unless he or she lives near to the hospital, and is accessible at most times. Two hospital signatories from the leadership team should be sufficient. The board will receive the annual statement of account, and the report of the auditors appointed by them.

Use of cheques

It is understood of course that hospital cheques can only be used for the payment of bona-fide hospital expenses, according to an agreed budget. In a regional system the management board specifies the heads of expenditure for which cheques may be issued, and may give a general AIE to cover these. The bank will only honour cheques so long as there is sufficient balance in the account. An overdraft will not normally be allowed, except perhaps by agreement for short periods, and in the presence of other hospital securities, such as a deposit account or savings account in the same bank. The bank may make a charge for its services, and these will appear on the monthly bank statement which the hospital should always insist on receiving.

Security for cash kept on the premises
A wall safe, and insurance against loss

A strong safe, built into the office wall, is essential, in order to ensure safety of cash between visits to the bank. If, of course, there is no accessible bank, the safe may have to take its place. The accountant or hospital secretary should be in charge of the safe, and its key. The safe should be used only for hospital money and not for any other purpose. On the principle that every phase of handling public money requires two people to verify, the safe too should be subject to cross-check by the medical superintendent or auditor, if they so wish, even if only once a year.

A limit should be placed on the amount of cash which may be retained in the safe, and this sum should be insured against loss. Routines will vary as to how often money is taken to the bank. Once a week may be sufficient. Some administrations do it daily. It depends on the cash flow, and the convenience or otherwise of getting to the bank. Cash in transit can also be insured against loss.

Cash boxes

One or more metal cash boxes for the accounts clerks taking fees, or making petty payments, will also be necessary. The contents of these will normally be brought to the accountant before the close of each day's duty, together with supporting receipts and petty cash payment vouchers.

Computerisation – yes or no?

A computer can be of great assistance to good accounting, but it does not take the place of a sound basic system in the first place. A computer is relatively expensive, and should only be considered where the accountant has received the necessary training, and is willing to train the other members of the accounts department. The medical superintendent should also understand the essentials. The change to computerisation, where finance, know-how and good infrastructure are available, is nevertheless occurring quite rapidly. A survey in Zambia in 1993 showed that practically all church-related hospitals of over 100 beds or over, had put their accounts on to a computer, with some advantages (see p.45).

The major drawback is that a steady supply of electric power, with only minimal breaks, *must be guaranteed*. If the power supply is broken while accounts are being prepared on the computer, any figures or details not previously committed to the computer's memory will be lost. A sudden increase in voltage, or surge, may cause serious damage to the machine. Gradual lowering of voltage, due to overloading of the hospital system, may also cause failure to function. An automatic voltage regulator will help compensate for this, but the problem of power failure is still there.

Precautions

The essential piece of equipment, which must be bought with the computer is the *Uninterrupted Power Supply (UPS) unit*. This provides the necessary voltage regulation, from up to 260 or down to 180 for a 220 volt supply. Above or below these levels the unit acts as if the power has gone off. In this event, or in the event of mains failure, an alarm is sounded, and there is immediate and automatic transfer to a battery source of power. The computer is safely protected. The alarm gives warning that all material on the computer must be stored at once. The lead-acetate (or nickel-cadmium) batteries, which stay on continuous trickle charge while mains power is available, provide power *for a limited time*. The more one is prepared to pay for the UPS the longer that time, for example, about $225 for 5 minutes, $900 for 15 minutes or $3000 for 5 hours. The 15 minute UPS is sufficient for most purposes, giving time to store material, and switch on the hospital's standby diesel generator (see p.102).

One other possibility is to run the computer through an *'invertor'* from batteries charged on solar panels if such specialised equipment can be found. In the absence of this, and should there be the danger of very long periods of mains failure – say a week or more – or breakdown of the standby generators, or even shortage of funds to buy fuel for them, computerised accounting should be ruled out, or there may be no accounts at all.

Understanding what is needed

Anyone contemplating computerisation of their accounts needs to know that computers comprise two parts usually called 'hardware' and 'software'. The *hardware* is the actual machinery of the computer and needs to include the following:

- the computer and keyboard – the brain of the machine.

- the visual display unit (VDU) – the television monitor which enables you to see what you are doing.

- the printer – which converts the information in the computer onto paper for record and audit purposes.

The *software* also comes in two main parts, depending on what one wants the computer to do. These are called:

- the 'operating system', often labelled 'DOS', which is usually included in the purchase price of the computer – but make sure it is.

- the 'functional systems', or software programmes, which need to be chosen and purchased at the same time as the hardware. Otherwise the computer is useless.

Software programmes
Many simple programmes prepared for small businesses are available. These are constantly being updated, and if purchased from one of the bigger companies, will generally be replaced (often free of charge) if damaged. Programmes which have been found useful include:

    SAGE ACCOUNTANT,
    SAGE FINANCIAL CONTROLLER 2, and
    PEGASUS BUSINESS MANAGER

These all enable one to have ledger accounts, stock control account, and a report facility which can prepare financial reports such as bank reconciliations, trial balances, debtor and creditor reports etc.

To accompany the chosen accounts programme, one also needs a spread-sheet package such as:

    LOTUS PLUS or
    SUPER CALC – the latter being much cheaper, and just as good.

A spread-sheet is like an analysis book (see p.47) but it can be up to 256 columns in width! The computer can be programmed automatically, for example, to make columns A, B and C to equal column D, and columns D and E to equal column F.

Staff records for pay-roll purposes can also be kept on computer with a programme such as:

    DATA BASE

This can include personal information such as salary grade, annual promotion date or retirement year.

    LOTUS SYMPHONY and SMART

are packages which combine Database with spread-sheet and word processor functions, but not an accounts programme.

The initial outlay on computerisation is very heavy, and one should not be tempted into this expenditure until one is quite sure the system can be efficiently used. Nothing is lost by waiting. The conventional methods of accounting are perfectly good, even if some functions, like the posting of ledgers, take longer.

These will now be described.

A cash book for the year

This is the daily record of all incoming revenue or outgoing expenditure. The hospital should have one main cash book for each financial year. Cashiers or accounts clerks may keep subsidiary small cash books for special purposes, such as in-patient or out-patient fees, and the totals from these are transferred to the main cash book as single entries for each day.

How to keep the book

In the cash book it is customary to place *income on the left hand page, and expenditure on the right hand page.* At regular intervals, daily or weekly, the two sides are added up, and the total expenditure deducted from the total income to find the balance of money still unspent. *This figure must then be checked physically by counting the money in the safe.* Notes, coins, cheques, and debit notes for loans, are added up together. The total should equal the balance in the cash book. Should there be any discrepancy, the reason must be found immediately, that very day. It may be an arithmetical error in the cash book, or in the counting of the cash; or it may be a receipt mislaid, or money advanced from cash and not written down.

It must be an inflexible rule that all money taken out of cash for a hospital purchase, or for a loan to a member of staff, *must be written down* on a petty cash voucher, signed for by the receiver, and placed in the cash box or safe. *Such a voucher is then the equivalent of cash.* It should be counted as such until the purchaser comes with the receipt for the item, together with any cash in change. The slip is then removed, the change put into the cash box or safe, and the expenditure entered into the cash book.

Loans to staff

Requests by staff for money to be advanced before pay-day should be resisted if possible. If an interest free loan has to be given on compassionate grounds the total should not exceed a month's salary, and the repayments should be completed in four or five monthly instalments. Record of the loan may be kept on a petty cash voucher in the safe (see figure 3.1).

The voucher acts as an IOU. Repayments are entered on it as they come in. The balance remaining is then treated as cash. When the whole loan has been refunded, the voucher is removed. No entries are made in the cash book.

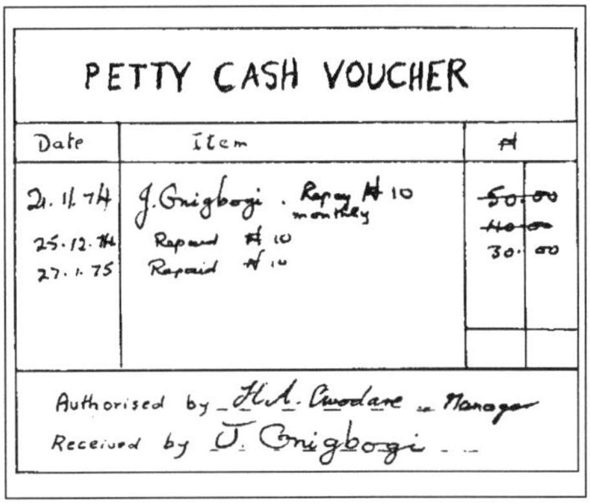
PETTY CASH VOUCHER

Date	Item	N
21.11.74	J. Grigbogi . Repay N 10 monthly	~~50.00~~
25.12.74	Repaid N 10	~~40.00~~
27.1.75	Repaid N 10	30.00

Authorised by H.A. Cwodare – Manager

Received by J. Grigbogi

Figure 3.1. *Petty cash voucher used for a staff loan*

When the figures for the cash balance in the safe and in the cash book have been reconciled (made the same), the balance should be entered, and the book ruled off with the same gross total on each side. The balance is then 'brought forward' ('b/f') on the income side (see figure 3.2).

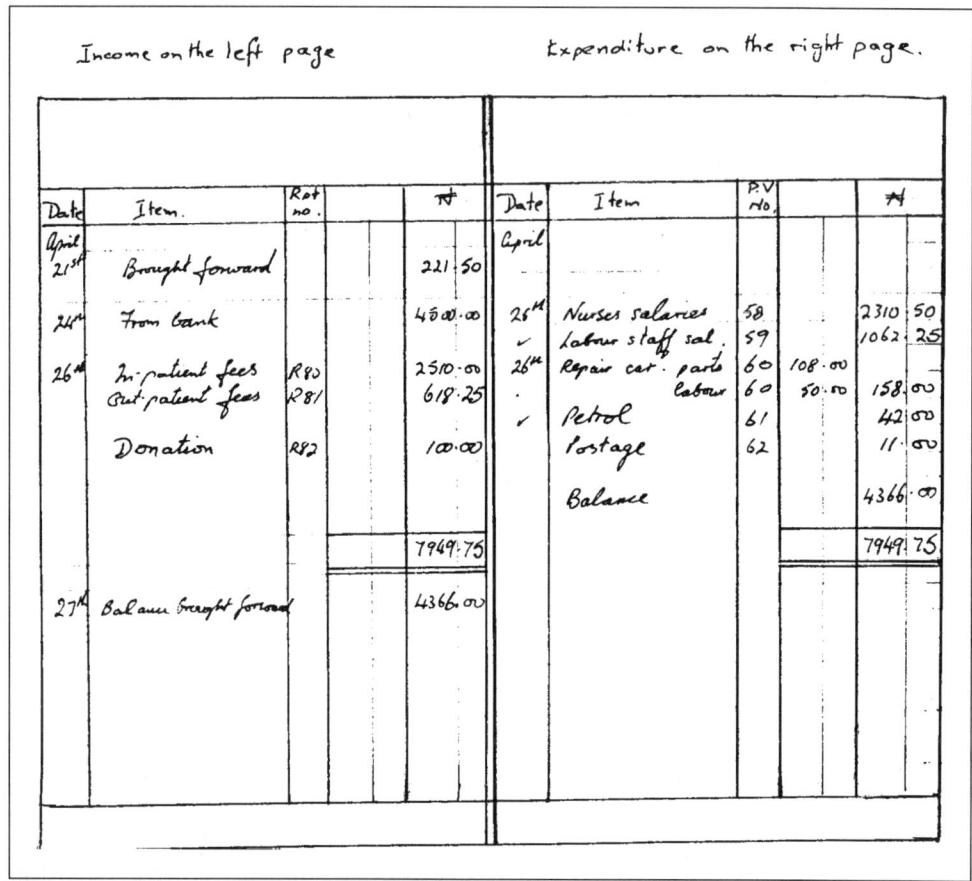

Date	Item	R.ct no.	₦	Date	Item	P.V no.		₦
April 21st	Brought forward		221 50	April				—
24th	From bank		4500 00	25th	Nurses salaries	58		2310 50
				✓	Labour staff sal.	59		1062 25
26th	In-patient fees	R80	2510 00	26th	Repair car. parts	60	108 00	
	Out-patient fees	R81	618 25	.	labour	60	50 00	158 00
	Donation	R82	100 00	✓	Petrol	61		42 00
					Postage	62		11 50
					Balance			4366 00
			7949 75					7949 75
27th	Balance brought forward		4366 00					

Figure 3.2. *Cash book page ruled off and balance brought forward.*

Record of bank transactions

Bank transactions may be given a separate page near the back of the cash book. A transfer to the bank from cash is entered as an expense in the cash section, and as revenue in the bank account section. Otherwise the account is kept in the same way as above. Cheques received as revenue are entered on the income side, and cheques paid out for goods or services entered on the expenditure side. When bank statements come, any bank charge can be entered as an expense. The bank balance can be compared with the hospital's own reckoning, and differences reconciled.

An alternative way is to keep the bank and cash transactions in parallel columns. In countries where the banking system is very well developed, and convenient to use, the bank section of the accounts becomes the main one. The limited number of actual cash transactions are recorded in a petty cash book.

Receipt books and payment vouchers
Giving a receipt is an obligation
Every person who pays money to the hospital is entitled to a receipt. The receipt should have a serial number. Books of receipts are therefore printed and numbered, say 1 to 100. Sometimes books have two receipts side by side, one to be torn off and given to the payer, and the other kept as a record. The better system is to have receipts numbered in pairs, with a carbon paper between; then as one is made out, a carbon copy is made on the paired receipt behind for record purposes.

1. In-patient payments, which only amount to a few each day, can be dealt with in this way without difficulty. When the cashier pays them in at the end of the day, the accountant issues him with a numbered receipt from his office for the total day's fees. The accountant enters this figure in his hospital cash book, and puts the receipt number against it in the small column provided.

2. Out-patient payments, which may run into hundreds each day, are another problem. The use of a cash register machine can be the best answer.

Use of a cash register machine
The system at Wesley Guild Hospital, Ilesha worked as follows:

- The doctor seeing the patient calculated the fee to be charged, and noted the amount on the out-patient (OP) card.
- The patient took the card to the OP cashier, and paid the fee.
- The cashier punched up the figure on the machine, took the ticket receipt, entered the OP number on that, and the receipt number on the OP card as cross reference.
- The patient went with the receipt and card to the pharmacy to obtain drugs ordered. The pharmacy assistant checked that the receipt rendered corresponded with the card.

The method was both quick and fool-proof. The machine kept its own copy of all receipts, and at the end of the day the OP cashier closed with a final total, took out the long paper from the machine, and submitted that with the day's takings to the accountant. He verified the amount against the total recorded by the machine. The cashier was then given a written receipt which he could stick into his OP cash book. The accountant entered the day's out-patient takings in the hospital cash book, with the receipt number beside it.

Payment vouchers (PVs), to be signed by two people

Expenditure, too, has its paper work, though it need not be complicated. All outgoings should have an authorising document which can be used by the auditors for verification. This is the payment voucher (PV). On this document the purpose for which the money is to be used is written by one person, such as the accountant, and authorised by a second person, usually the hospital secretary or medical superintendent.

If the payment is to be made by cheque, the accountant makes it out, signs it himself, and sends it with the payment voucher to the medical superintendent, or whoever is the second signatory. At the bottom of the sheet there is a space to attach the receipt for the payment when it arrives by post, or for the receiver to sign if payment is made to him direct.

Petty cash vouchers for multiple small payments

Many hospitals find it is convenient to use petty cash vouchers for minor items of expenditure which recur frequently. For example the matron or caterer may sign vouchers for the food-sellers who bring tomatoes, onions, meat or whatever to the hospital kitchen. The food-sellers take their vouchers to the cashier who is authorised to pay, and append their own signature or thumb-print when the money has been received. Once a week the accountant totals the receipted petty cash vouchers for each type of payment, and prepares a single payment voucher, say for hospital food, and attaches the pile of supporting slips to it as the collective receipt.

PV numbers

Payment vouchers are numbered serially by hand once a week before the routine completion of cash book entries, and checking of the cash balance. The PV numbers are entered in a small column in the cash book beside the item of expenditure concerned.

A weekly summary statement
Review of money in, money spent, and the balance left over

> It was the custom at WGH Ilesha, and the procedure worked well, for the accountant, or hospital secretary/manager to prepare a weekly statement of account after the 'cashing up' and checking of the balance each Wednesday. A cash-box with the balance of the week's takings, together with the week's receipts and payment vouchers, were sent to the office of the medical superintendent. It was his first duty on Thursday morning to check the weekly statement against the receipts and vouchers, re-count the money in the box, and when satisfied sign the statement as correct, and return all to the accountant. This gave the medical superintendent the opportunity to review the level of fee income, and all hospital expenditure, and thus have direct knowledge of the financial state of the hospital.

Review of money owing, and money due

In times of financial austerity, and irregular arrival of grants and payments, some hospitals have found it advisable to also have a weekly summary of creditors and debtors.

> List of creditors: sums owed for payment for drugs, electricity supply, provident fund contributions etc.
>
> List of debtors: sums owed by individuals, schools, companies, or the government, if the hospital is eligible for grants.

Much depends upon the cash flow for the payment of the most urgent bills. The medical superintendent should share with the hospital secretary or accountant at such times the necessary decisions on priorities, in order to ensure that the needs of the patients are given primary consideration.

However, if the hospital has accepted drugs or other goods on the understanding that payment will be made within a month of the time being supplied, the hospital's good name depends upon honouring that agreement. Every effort should be made to sustain good business practice.

The human problem of unpaid fees

No hospital dependent on fees for services can expect all bills to be paid. Within the budget, allowance must be made for defaulters. A sliding scale of fees, graded according to salary or ability to pay cannot be operated when, for example, the majority of patients are self-employed traders or subsistence farmers. Accurate means-testing is impossible. So how can one be sure of sufficient fee revenue without showing an inhuman disregard for those desperately ill arriving on the hospital doorstep? Experience has shown that the following type of policy is best. Each hospital will have its own variation.

1. *Have a reasonable single scale of fees for everybody.* Wealthier patients who might pay more can be charged extra for an 'amenity bed' in a side-room if admitted, or seen at an afternoon clinic by appointment, with a higher consultation fee. The additional revenue can go to the support of the very poor.

2. *Out-patients who cannot pay,* for whom treatment is urgent, may be referred to an *assessment officer* for fee reduction. In some cultures it is possible to allow the patient to bring the fee at the next visit. A note of the amount owing is written in red on the card. Some will 'lose' their card or go elsewhere, but the majority will try to fulfil the trust placed in them.

3. *In-patients, at the time of admission, should be required to pay a deposit* based on the average fee for the type of illness. Compassion must be exercised for patients *in extremis,* for example a woman with ante-partum

haemorrhage. Should the deposit prove too much, a refund is given on discharge. More commonly, it is too little and more is required. On the discharge day, the relatives are informed of the bill, and given the opportunity to go and collect the money. If, by the end of the day or the next, it is apparent that they are not able to pay, the hospital assessment officer, almoner, manager or medical superintendent may *authorise a rebate,* and list the sum in a book of unpaid bills. The total at the end of the year provides a useful figure on the amount of work done free.

4. *A special fund for the poor.* Some hospitals may solicit help from overseas donors, local industry or individuals, or a 'friends of the hospital' community support organisation, or a 'samaritan fund' (or whatever name is chosen) set up to help less well-off patients, particularly those brought in as a result of accidents. The medical superintendent, or designated person, may authorise a credit note from the fund, to be given discreetly to the patient in need, to cover the shortfall. The patient's dignity is preserved, enabling a return home without a burden of debt which may demorialise and delay return to full health. Such funds may not be big enough to meet the whole need, but they are a great help.

A ledger for the year
Analysis by heads of expenditure, and sources of income
A ledger account book is simply one which enables all items of income and expenditure in the cash book to be classified by type. There is a page or pages for each source of income — in-patient fees, out-patient fees, grants-in-aid, donations etc — and pages for each of the heads of expenditure — drugs,

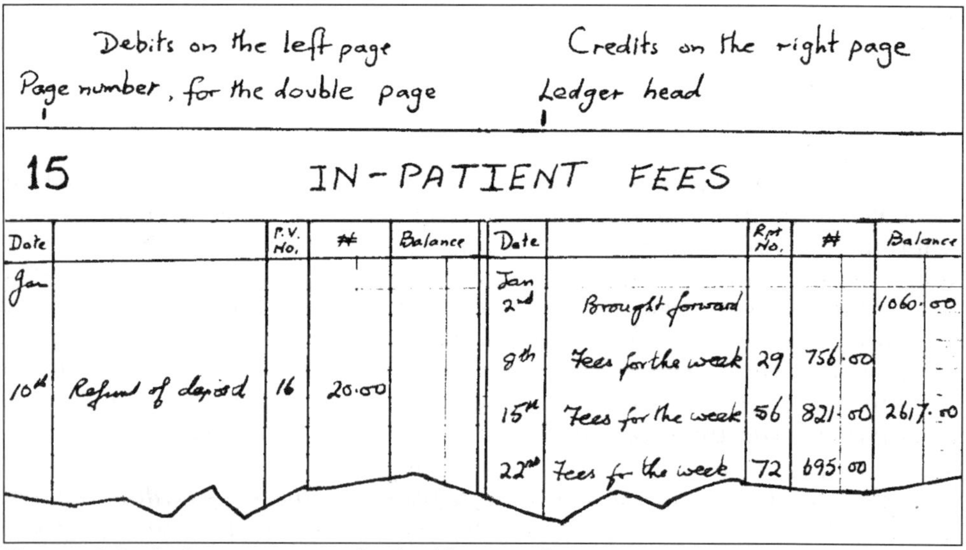

Debits on the left page					Credits on the right page				
Page number, for the double page					Ledger head				
15					IN-PATIENT FEES				
Date		P.V. No.	#	Balance	Date		Rpt No.	#	Balance
Jan					Jan 2nd	Brought forward			1060.00
					8th	Fees for the week	29	756.00	
10th	Refund of deposit	16	20.00		15th	Fees for the week	56	821.00	2617.00
					22nd	Fees for the week	72	695.00	

Figure 3.3. *Ledger pages on the double spread*

maintenance, salaries and so on. Ledger pages are usually numbered for use on the double spread, with a numeral on the left hand page only. In the ledger it is the convention for *credits to be on the right, and debits on the left* – the opposite way round from the cash book. There is a second column on each page for a running balance to be totalled and carried forward.

An index is made of ledger head titles and the page numbers on which each can be found. This may be placed on the inside front cover for easy reference. Once a week, after the summary statement has been checked, and the cash book brought up to date, the accountant 'posts' every item of income and expenditure from the cash book into the appropriate page in the ledger (see figure 3.3).

Each 'ledger head' has a debit and a credit side
Most ledger accounts will be primarily for either income or expenditure, but there should be space for both debit and credit for all ledger heads. Even with in-patient fees – primarily revenue – there may be occasional refunds, for example when a patient who made a deposit on admission dies, and the relatives claim the unused portion as a refund. This appears as a debit to the hospital on the in-patient fee page (see the figure). Likewise on pages which are primarily expenditure, there will be occasional entries on the credit side, as when there has been an overpayment in error, and money is returned, or when some goods supplied wrongly are sent back and the cost refunded to the hospital.

Items from the bank account pages in the cash book will be posted to the ledger, just the same as items from the main cash section of the cash book. Transfers from cash to bank, or vice versa, are not ledgered.

An annual statement of income and expenditure
Close the account once a year
On the same day each year there should be a 'closing of the accounts', and a summary of all income and expenditure items produced and set out in the annual statement. This is an essential element of public accountability, whereby those responsible for handling hospital money may show to their staff, and to their proprietor, how much money they have had and what they have used it for. The hospital authorities in turn can show the statement of account to the public as evidence that the financial administration has been honest and efficient.

Find out the balance of income in hand, if any
The statement will set out all items of expenditure in their appropriate groupings – salaries, hospital running expenses, administration costs etc – and also all items of revenue – fees, donations, grants etc. If there is a balance of income in hand, this figure will be placed under the expenditure column

as 'Excess of income over expenditure', so that when the total is added up it will equal the total for income (see Figure 3.4).

ERIN IGBO HOSPITAL

Income and expenditure account for the year ending 31st December 1979

Expenditure		Income	
Salaries	56 265.00	Fees	44 004.50
Hospital running expenses	37 031.25	Grants	51 637.00
Administration	2 850.00	Donations	4 455.00
Other items	4 459.00	Miscellaneous	1 214.50
Excess of income over expenditure carried to balance sheet	2 205.00		
	101 811.00		101 811.00

Figure 3.4: *Annual statement showing a credit balance for the year.*

Figure 3.5. *A statement showing a debit balance*

ERIN IGBO HOSPITAL

Income and expenditure account for the year ending 31st December 1985

Expenditure		Income	
Salaries	499 834.00	Fees	297 448.00
Hospital running expenses	151 529.00	Grants	239 648.00
Administration	13 756.00	Donations	19 876.00
Other items	12 610.00	Miscellaneous	29 749.00
		Excess of expenditure over income carried to balance sheet	91 749.00
	677 729.00		677 729.00

If, on the other hand, there has been overspending in relation to revenue, and there is a debit balance on the year, the figure for 'excess of expenditure over income' will be placed at the bottom of the income column, so that the total, when added up, will equal the total for expenditure (see figure 3.5). Obviously, when such a situation with overspending is found, the finances of the hospital are distinctly unhealthy, and a remedy should be found to put things right in the following year.

Compare the year just past with the previous year
It is a helpful practice, when presenting the income and expenditure account for the year just passed, to place the equivalent figures for the year before in a column alongside. Comparison can then be made to show trends up or down.

A balance sheet

Following the statement of income and expenditure a balance sheet is then set out. This will show the complete overall financial position of the hospital, including any savings accounts or funds kept in the bank for specific purposes, but not part of the general account. To obtain it a trial balance will have to be drawn.

The trial balance
In this all ledger-head totals in the ledger account are listed, credits on one side and debits on the other. To the credits are added all money held, but owed for specific purposes, such as a building fund waiting to be used, or the outstanding bills for goods or services received by the hospital but not yet paid for. To the debits are added the total of any loans given out by the hospital, say to staff members, and not yet repaid, and also the balances held by the bank on behalf of the hospital. The two sides should add up to the same figure, that is to say credits should equal debits. If they do not the mistake has to be found. It may be due to a mis-posting from cash book to ledger, or the carrying forward of a wrong balance figure from one page to another, or forgetting to record a sum of money advanced. A long search is sometimes required, and this must continue till the discrepancy is located.

Liabilities and assets
The balance sheet has two sides, the credits, usually called liabilities, and the debit side, which are the assets (see Figure 3.6).

1. Liabilities

    On the liabilities side the following are included.

    - *Accumulated fund*
      The balance with which the year was started.

Add the balance with which the year ended (that is, the excess of income over expenditure shown in the statement of account).
- *Other funds*
  Funds held by the hospital as retirement fund, research fund, building fund etc, which are not available for general day-to-day use in the hospital.
- *Sundry creditors*
  Bills awaiting payment.

2. Assets

On the assets side the following are included.

- *Sundry debtors and advances*
  Money owed to the hospital by those who have received loans, or money advanced and receipts not yet obtained.

Figure 3.6: *Balance sheet showing liabilities and assets.*

ERIN IGBO HOSPITAL
Balance sheet for the year ending 31st December 1985

Liabilities

Accumulated fund		
Balance brought forward from 1978	1 087.25	
Add balance from 1979	2 205.00	
		3 292.25
Other funds		
Staff retirement fund	5 178.00	
IPPF research	400.00	
Maternity building fund	4 158.00	
		9 736.00
Current liabilities		
Sundry creditors awaiting payment		2 010.00
		15 038.25

Assets

Current assets		
Sundry debtors		
Staff loans	415.00	
Advance on drugs for 1980	2 300.00	
		2 715.00
Balances at bank and in hand		
Current account	1 790.00	
Deposit account	8 000.00	
Cash in hand	2 533.25	
		12323.25
		15 038.25

- *Bank and cash balances at the end of the year*
  Deposit accounts, if any.
  Current bank account – balance certified by the bank
  Cash in hand – the balance with which the cash book for the year was closed.

Including the value of stock and capital assets is optional
Private hospitals, run for profit, will have to add to the liabilities the value of stocks held in the hospital drug and general store at the beginning of the year, and on the assets side their value at the end of the year. The value of major items of equipment like generators or X-ray machines, at the beginning of the year, less the depreciation over the year, may also be included. The value of buildings may be brought in too. The balance sheet, with these capital assets, does give a better reflection of the net worth of the institution.

Some large voluntary agency institutions may prepare a similar balance sheet. Smaller institutions concerned simply to demonstrate financial viability, and proper accountability for funds used, are advised to be content with the simpler form of balance sheet shown above.

Computerised accounting

All the above functions of conventional accounting are still necessary, but much of it can be done by machine, rather than by hand. All items of income and expenditure are punched into the computer each day, together with an appropriate ledger code so that each item is 'posted' automatically. It is no longer essential for manual entries to be made into cashbook and ledger for the year, though it is advisable to continue using these for cross-check purposes.

'Spread-sheets' can be produced by the computer every month showing the overall income, expenditure and balance in hand. Accounts on the display screen can be consulted at any time. Analysis of each ledger item is instantly available. Any double entries, or errors made in coding can be detected, often by the computer itself, through obvious deviations or failure to balance. Interim statements can be prepared as required, and the Annual Statement of Accounts and Balance Sheet produced by the computer at the end of the financial year.

Manual functions that remain
The use of Payment Vouchers (with space for two signatures) to authorise payments from the hospital, and Receipts for those making payments to the hospital, e.g. for in-patient fees, are, of course, still essential, and have to be produced for the auditor as proof of expenditure and income. Such forms as these can easily be printed out by the computer, and retained in its memory for reprinting as and when required.

Audit
An independent detailed examination, or audit, of the year's accounts, by anyone acceptable to the proprietor, is the best means of proving to the public that all funds have been honestly and effectively used. The board usually appoints the auditor, preferably a qualified accountant who specialises in audit work, if the fees can be met.

Prepare for the auditor
Before the auditor comes it is important to have at least a provisional statement of account and balance sheet for the year prepared by the hospital accountant. If there is still a discrepancy on the balance sheet which has not been traced, an explanation can be given to the auditor, and he will assist in finding it. The cash book, ledger, and the piles of receipt books and payment vouchers (tied up in bundles) are then handed over, together with any other supporting documents which may be requested, such as bank statements. The auditor's team gets down to work. It may take them days or weeks, according to the complexity of the accounts, and it may take several weeks more before the formal audited statement of account for the year, and the auditor's report are presented – together with the bill.

A budget, or estimates, for the coming year
Look ahead in good time
Preparing an estimate of the expected revenue and likely expenditure in the year to come should be done about three months before the end of the current year. Use has to be made of the audited statement of the previous year, and an interim statement for nine months of the current year. With these, one then has to project likely expenditure to the end of the current year, and the probable income and expenditure for the year to come. Inevitably there is much guess-work in making a budget, especially in times of inflation, shortages and unreliability of grants, but the exercise of looking ahead is absolutely vital. Only when this has been done can one know whether it will be possible to employ additional staff, or whether fees may have to be increased or alternative additional revenue sought. The future of the hospital and security of the staff depend on good budgeting.

An important role for the medical administrator
The hospital secretary and medical superintendent will be mainly responsible, with participation from other senior staff as required. The doctor in charge should have a leading role in the determination of priorities, so that the development of the hospital to give better care to the patients and service to the community can be kept paramount. It may be necessary at times to resist pressure for more spending on administration, or highly paid senior staff, unless it can be shown that the additions will greatly improve service, without becoming an undue burden on the patients who pay the fees.

Securing budgetary approval

The budget, and the calculations underlying it, have to be approved by the hospital board. If the hospital uses the calendar year as its financial year, with the accounts being closed on 31st December, then a board may be called for at the end of January, or in February, to receive the provisional statement of accounts for the year passed and the proposed budget for the year just starting. (The auditor's report will come later.) Questions will be asked, and the calculations used will have to be justified, or modified as directed. After approval, the actions proposed, such as increasing fees, or employing more nurses, can be implemented forthwith.

Self-accounting makes budgeting realistic

In the public service there is a tendency for administrators in district hospitals to submit inflated estimates for their needs for the coming year, often double what is really required. They know the state health management board will cut their estimates by half. This is one of the anomalies caused by centralised accounting. The district hospital does not have to balance its expenditure with local revenue. Any fees taken are sent up to the capital. Hence, budgeting at hospital level is unrealistic, and the state board knows it.

Leaders of self-accounting institutions, on the other hand, know that the only money they can spend is the money that they generate. Estimates have to be realistic from the start. The hospital board is in control of its own destiny.

Accounting in branch centres delivering primary health care

The advantages of self-accounting at district hospital level are clear. What happens when that same hospital develops primary health care outstations? How should they be administered? Should they also be allowed to retain revenue and be given the power to spend? The answer depends upon the size and nature of the unit, and the ability of the staff member in charge, but the same principle still applies. The maximum possible self-accounting should be encouraged. The exercise of trust, with the normal precautions and financial cross-checking already outlined, will promote responsible service by staff at the periphery, and give them job satisfaction. Simplification of the accounting system outlined is possible.

An analysis book

This combines the function of a cash book, and a simplified ledger. The book is wide, with up to 20 columns on the double spread. The date and all items of expenditure are written in the first column. Then comes a series of narrower columns for expenditure analysis. Each of the main heads of expenditure is given a column — salaries, petrol, general maintenance etc — and the figure from the first column is written again in the appropriate analysis column. Towards the right of the page all items of income can be put in one column, leaving the final column for the balance (see Figure 3.7).

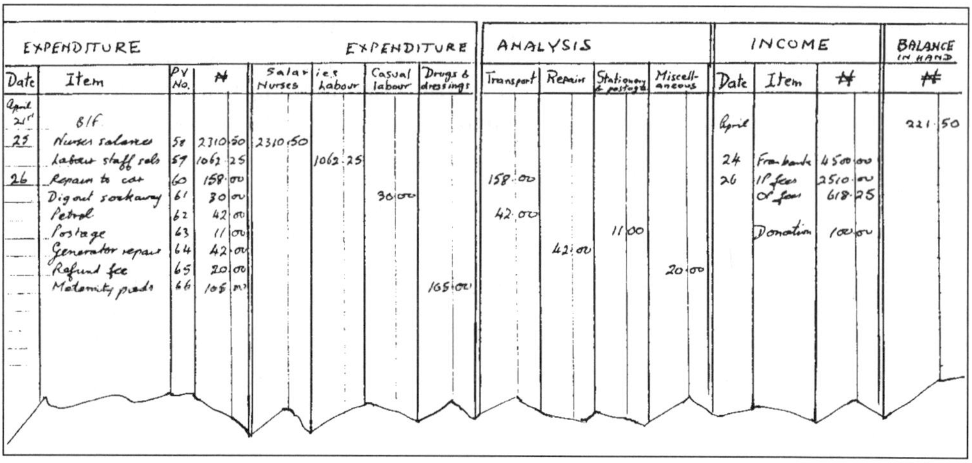

EXPENDITURE				EXPENDITURE			ANALYSIS				INCOME			BALANCE IN HAND
Date	Item	PV No.	₦	Salaries Nurses	Casual labour	Drugs & dressings	Transport	Repair	Stationery & postage	Miscellaneous	Date	Item	₦	₦
April 21st	B/F										April			221 50
25	Nurses salaries	58	2310 50	2310 50										
	Labour staff sals	57	1062 25		1062 25						24	From bank	4500 00	
26	Repairs to car	60	158 00				158 00				26	IP fees	2510 00	
	Dig out soakaway	61	30 00		30 00							OP fees	618 25	
	Petrol	62	42 00				42 00							
	Postage	63	11 00						11 00					
	Generator repair	64	42 00					42 00				Donation	100 00	
	Refund fee	65	20 00							20 00				
	Maternity pads	66	165 00			165 00								

Figure 3.7. *Analysis book page.*

If the figures for income and expenditure are put in at the end of each working day, the analysis columns can be filled in and totalled, and the balance checked, at the end of each month. It is then not difficult to produce a simple statement at the end of the year.

How it may work in practice

The examples which follow illustrate the variety of accounting procedures which may be used at peripheral centres. Three are from the author's experience of voluntary agency rural health work in Nigeria, and a fourth from government experience in Senegal. In each case the emphasis is on allowing the maximum of financial responsibility at the periphery, in relation to the ability of the health workers in charge.

1. *Ilesha district dispensaries.*

Around the town of Ilesha were seven 'dispensaries' at 9 to 30 miles distance. They were staffed by midwives and helpers, and visited fortnightly by a health sister based at Ilesha. The dispensaries functioned as maternity centres, delivering up to 30 babies monthly, and as child welfare centres, using growth-charts, and giving simple medical care and immunisations as required. First aid was given to adults.

Fees were charged for delivery and services to adults, and out of the money taken purchases of kerosene, cleaning materials etc were made, and payment was made for local labour to clean the compound and carry water. Once a month the visiting sister would check the attendance register, the fee book, and the small cash book in which expenditure was recorded. The balance in the book was checked against the balance of cash in the cash-box. Sums were small so there was no safe. The sister brought with her the salary packets for the midwives and helpers, prepared by the hospital accountant. She also brought a supply of drugs for the month from the hospital pharmacy, prepared in accordance with a requisition made earlier by the midwife in charge. The sister noted any larger items required, such as a new well or a reserve water tank, and these requests were passed on to the hospital manager at Ilesha, who provided them from hospital funds. The balance of cash from the dispensaries was brought in by the sister after her visits, and credited as income from dispensaries by the hospital accountant.

2. *Maternity Hospital, Ikole-Ekiti.*

80 miles north-east of Ilesha was the 44-bed Ikole Maternity Hospital, with one or two resident nursing sisters, and visited monthly by a doctor from Ilesha. Much of its emphasis was curative, and until a state hospital was built 3 miles away it was the only source of medical care in the district. The general out-patient department was busy, as were the maternity and children's wards. Preventive work centred on the antenatal clinic, under-five's clinic and an immunisation programme in the district.

The senior nursing sister ran the administration with the help of one clerical assistant. The hospital had its own constitution and management committee, with local community and church representatives, and the medical superintendent from Ilesha. All staff were recruited locally by the sister, and the hospital successfully trained Grade II midwives, until that grade was discontinued.

Fee revenue was collected by the clerk, and he and the sister made all necessary purchases, and prepared the salary packets for all staff and student midwives each month. Drugs came from Ilesha and were debited to Ikole's account. Accounts were kept by the sister in an analysis book, and the accountant from Ilesha visited once a month to complete and total the analysis columns and check the balance. The system worked well.

3. *Wesley Rural Health Centre, Irhuekpen, Bendel State.*

When this 20-bed centre was opened, 120 miles from Ilesha in buildings provided by the community, it was decided from the beginning that it could only be viable if it was not only self-accounting, but self-governing. It was too far from Ilesha for monthly doctor's visits as at Ikole. Medical supervision from a state hospital 20 miles distant was negotiated. A responsible male nurse with out-patient clinical experience at Ilesha, with his wife, a qualified Grade I midwife, together with one hospital clerk who was native of Irhuekpen as Executive Officer, volunteered to leave Ilesha and be the pioneer core staff. Other staff were recruited locally. The centre was given its own Constitution and Board of Management. The Medical Superintendent from

WGH Ilesha came to this twice a year, but was otherwise available in Ilesha for advice if this was sought.

A local headmaster on the Board was elected Treasurer, and the Nursing Superintendent and Executive Officer kept the accounts between them under his supervision. The nearest bank at that time was in Benin City, 45 miles away, but the road there was good and a weekly visit quite practicable. WGH Ilesha provided the initial stock of equipment and drugs, and used its good offices with local firms to ensure they would open accounts for the health centre and provide further supplies. The Annual Statement of Accounts and Budget were brought to the Board each year by the Nursing Superintendent who was Secretary to the Board.

This system of administration worked remarkably well. There were ups and downs, partly because of divisions in the local community, but the centre survived even the upsets of the Nigerian civil war which raged over the area. Good service was maintained by the original core staff for over 20 years.

4. *Local government health service, Pikine, Senegal.*

In 1985 Jancloes (5) described an experimental initiative aimed at finding the right balance between community and government in the sharing of financial responsibility. Local health committees (LHC) were set up in an urban area and allowed to supervise revenue retained at their health centres. As a free health service was not possible treatment fees for children and adults were agreed, and these were paid as the patient entered, receiving a numbered ticket in return. Medical care was provided by the nurses, with doctors visiting on a consultant basis. Each day the nurse in-charge cross-checked the amount of cash collected, and he and the ticket seller initialled the daily record. The cash was then handed over to the LHC treasurer, who banked it twice a week. The nurse looked after the cheque book, and used cheques (after obtaining signatures from LHC president and treasurer) to purchase local supplies. Community participation and staff satisfaction were assured. Further research on the respective roles of government and community in self-accounting health services is being carried out.

The illustrations given show ways in which primary care units, whether rural or urban, can successfully be allowed to be self-accounting in varying degrees, and when adequately prepared for it. The examples are mainly from the non-governmental sector, but show also that in local government community responsibility can be greatly increased. Another example of a State Ministry of Health devolving responsibility on to its districts was given in Chapter 2 (see p.13).

The virtue of 'self reliance' in community health services is often extolled, but not always allowed in practice, yet money handled wisely at local level contributes to high morale and the effectiveness of the health centre or hospital as a 'therapeutic community'.

CHAPTER 4

A Therapeutic Community

The mother of a very sick child once arrived at a hospital over 100 miles from her home. The child was febrile, anaemic and almost at its last gasp. As the doctor hurried to provide emergency care he asked the mother why she had come to this place, so far from her village, passing a health centre and two other hospitals on the way. She could have got help so much more quickly close at hand.

'Yes, but they smile at you here' she said.

Her reply was naive perhaps, but she knew what she was looking for. A smile conveys sympathy, and hence the possibility of understanding.

The very atmosphere which patients find as they enter the hospital can be an important part of the treatment. If the place is well run, with a caring spirit, and with sympathetic dedicated staff at all levels – from the man at the gate to the doctor in charge – the patients know the difference. Such a hospital can be a 'therapeutic community', genuinely appreciated by the people from a wide area around. As a source of hope and improved morale the effects are immeasurable.

A hospital in which this kind of spirit is found may not have ultra modern buildings or the latest in technology. If there is any secret it lies with its staff, their good relationships with each other, and their concern for the people all around. Much depends on good leadership, and corruption-free administration, but there are many simple elements of personnel management which can contribute. The medical administrator should introduce these where he can.

Personnel management

Staff appointments
Let us consider this from the point of view of filling a vacancy, and bringing in a new member of staff. How you begin can determine how you go on.

Staff should be in a particular place by their own choice.
Attention has already been drawn (Chapter 2, p.12) to the problem of staff being recruited centrally, and then transferred to peripheral centres for service. Many state health services have been unable to break away from this pattern. Since it often leads to separation of husbands, wives and families, and much frustration and resentment, it should be reconsidered. Rural postings should never be looked at, whether consciously or subconsciously, as a punishment. Staff must be in a place by their own choice, if they are to settle down and be happy. Yes, city posts will doubtless be snapped up first. Few want to go to the country. But there is a limit to the number of city posts, and some people are ready for the challenge of a more rural station. If they choose to go, they are more likely to stay, and two who are glad to be there are worth ten of those who are not.

Advertising vacancies
Private hospitals, and voluntary agencies, normally advertise for specific posts in a particular hospital or health centre. An adequate description of the job is given, and the pay and conditions stated. Incentives, such as free housing,

Figure 4.1: Advertising posts
Advertisement for a specific post – from the *Lancet*.

Northland's Area Health Board
SURGEON SUPERINTENDENT
Bay of Islands Hospital, Kawakawa, Northland, New Zealand

Applications are invited for the above position.

Bay of Islands Hospital has 79 beds which include medical, surgical, paediatric and maternity beds. Major cases may be transferred to Northland Base Hospital, 54 kilometres away.

Kawakawa is adjacent to the internationally famous tourist area of the Bay of Islands. The population of the region is rapidly growing and is currently 25 000.

Preference will be given to applicants with specialist qualifications in obstetrics and gynaecology who are able to continue the present service offered in that specialty, and to share general surgical duties with a part-time surgeon. The post also carries administrative responsibility for Kaikohje Geriatric Hospital of 25 beds, which is 20 kilometres distant.

The present automatic specialist salary scale is from NZ$52 600...*(details given)*. Housing is available.

Applications must be made... *(address and details follow)*.

or addition to salary, may be added if there is need to attract applicants away from more popular urban centres.

If no suitable applications come from the first insertion, the hospital should by no means give up. It is always worth spending money on additional insertions in the same, or another, paper or journal. If the advertisement finally comes to the eye of the right person, the cost has been amply repaid. Advertising is not cheap, but it is vital to allow money to be spent on it, if one wants to have staff serving where they choose to go.

Technically there is no reason why a regional health management board should not follow precisely the same strategy, when looking for staff midwives, nursing officers, health sisters, MOs, PMOs or any other category of staff. Specific posts should be advertised (see Figure 4.1), whether in the city, or in the rural townships. Attraction to the latter should, if possible, be enhanced by incentives not available to those who work in the city.

Developed countries do it this way. Why not the world over? Staff taken on then go to their post by choice. If, after a few years, they want a change or accelerated promotion, they apply for another post at the appropriate level. Arrangements for continuation or transfer of pension eligibility are possible, if the policy has been approved.

Personnel specifications

These will be made known in the advertisement, and will include the basic qualification and the type of previous experience preferred. Specifications should be in realistic terms, such that some suitable applications will be received. The advertisement may be posted on the board of the hospital concerned, should there be existing staff eligible for promotion, as well as going to the daily papers or professional journals. Letters from two or three referees are usually requested, though these may be of less value than the actual interview on which choice for the job is made.

Letters of appointment

These should be routine for all staff appointments whether junior or senior. Junior staff may receive theirs on the day they start work, after a full explanation of all the conditions of service involved. Clarification can be given in answer to questions. The worker signs the hospital copy, and takes his own away. Senior staff will normally receive two copies of the proposed letter of appointment by post. If accepted, one copy will be signed and returned to the administrator.

The letter will generally include:

1. The name of the post, or designation

2. A brief description of duties and hours

3. The starting salary, and any incremental allowances

4. Fringe benefits, such as housing provided, car allowance, or free medical attention for self plus family

5. Length of appointment, in the first place, and the means for extending it

6. Probation period, if any

7. Annual leave period, and any leave allowance, or provision for fares

8. Arrangements for pension or retirement gratuity

9. Means for terminating the appointment by either the employer, or the employee.

Termination of appointment is normally possible by giving one month's notice from either side. For the most senior staff, the period may be three months. Should there be need for the break to be immediate, then the employer can pay a month of salary in lieu of notice. It is a human right that no worker should be cast adrift without something to live on, especially if he has served the employer for many years. This also works the other way, and no employee should leave his employer in the lurch without giving the due period of notice. If he fails to, he should forfeit a month of pay. However, since abrupt departures usually occur just after a pay day, this is not always observed.

It is worth writing into the appointment letter a short period of three months' probation during which either side may terminate without any notice or payment in lieu. This allows for the occasional case where the new employee finds the job is not what he or she wanted after all, or where the employer notices there is a serious personality clash between the new person and other senior staff which time seems unlikely to resolve. It is better to cut losses and let the person go sooner rather than later. Three months is usually sufficient to reveal such problems.

In the public service the word probation carries a different meaning from the above, and refers to the period, usually three years, after which a person's performance is reviewed. If this has in all ways been satisfactory, then probation is deemed to have been passed, and the temporary appointment of the first three years is turned into a permanent appointment. This carries the promise of security of tenure, and a pension on retirement.

Job description

In Chapter 2 reference was made to the hospital bye-laws setting out the duties and responsibilities of each hospital officer, the medical superintendent, matron and administrator (see also Appendix 1). These are job descriptions for the administrative functions of these posts. They set out clearly their relation to each other within the basic leadership team.

Some sort of job description should be available for every staff member. This may be found in the handover notes from a predecessor in the post, or from one's immediate supervisor. The job description should clarify details of the work to be done, the person to whom one is accountable, and the junior staff for whom one is responsible.

Such clear definition of duties can promote better work all round, and a better team spirit. Where work is done well approval should be shown. *A word of praise can be very important.* Where there is failure to do the job properly, this can then be pointed out firmly but kindly, and the criticism is more likely to be accepted without resentment.

Eligibility for pension or retirement gratuity

This is built into the civil service employment system, and is a major attraction to many who enter it. Such an arrangement can equally be made, at least in a small way, in private or voluntary agency service. It does mean that the institution will have to build up its own retirement fund, and out of this retirement gratuities or pensions can be paid when staff reach retirement age. Staff may be required to contribute a portion of their salary each month, say five per cent, while the hospital puts in an equal or higher share; or the scheme may be 'non-contributory' by the staff member, and all costs met by the hospital. The latter is unusual in developed countries.

In some countries there is a national provident fund, or a national insurance, to which all employers and employees have to contribute. The returns from these do not occur till retirement age (55, 60 or 65 years, according to the country) and may not be substantial even then. Many employers supplement national insurance with private schemes run by the institution, or by an insurance company acting on their behalf. Benefit may be claimed after a given period of service, 10 or 15 years say, or on retirement at 60 years of age. Making provision for employee pensions or retirement gratuities is always expensive, and a long-term option, but this is not a reason for ignoring the issue. Long-serving staff will ultimately demand what they feel to be, with justification, their right. It is better to be prepared.

For short-term benefits employers, in the private or the public sector, may offer *contract appointments,* where an additional percentage of salary (15 or 25 per cent) is paid each year, for each year (or quarter) of the agreed period of time that has been completed. The 'contract addition' is given in lieu of eligibility for pension. In times of uncertainty, and much job mobility, some staff may prefer such an option, if it is offered. However, unless the contract addition goes into a savings account which offsets inflation, or into property, it provides no long-term security.

Housing and caring for staff
Junior staff are likely to be recruited from the immediate neighbourhood, and can therefore live at home. Senior staff are more likely to have to come from further afield, another state, or even from overseas. If the hospital is close to, or in, a major urban centre, then they may only need help in locating accommodation for rent reasonably near the hospital. In smaller townships, or rural areas, there is often no choice but to provide housing. In fact, this has advantages, since staff housed at the hospital provide a natural core for the hospital community.

A nominal rent may be charged for hospital housing, and the amount deducted from salary. Rent-free accommodation may be provided to certain senior staff as an inducement, and in return for taking on-call duties in the hospital, or general responsibilities for the hospital community.

One section of the hospital grounds, or compound, may be set aside for staff residences (see Figure 4.2). The houses should have at least two, and preferably three, bedrooms, with basic hard furniture provided. This will

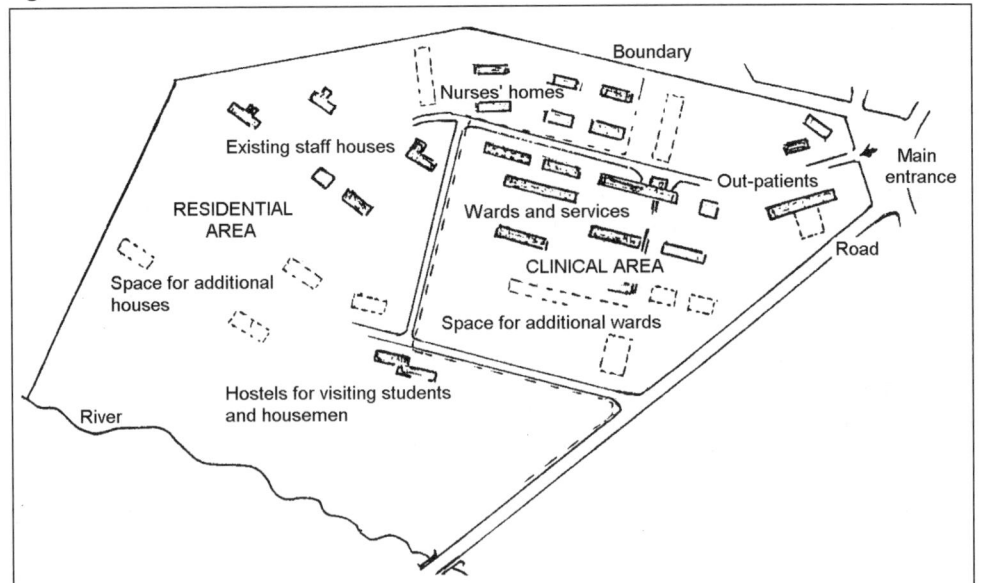

Figure 4.2: *Staff residential area on 36-acre site, WGH, Ilesha. 1960.*

include beds and mattresses, but not sheets; it may include, for example, armchairs and settees with cushions, but not cushion covers. The windows may have curtain rails or fittings, but not curtains. In such a case, sheets, cushion covers and curtains are said to be 'soft furnishings', and to be the responsibility of the staff member. A kerosene or gas stove should be provided for cooking. If it is the latter, then one full bottle of gas should be provided, and perhaps a spare empty bottle. Further refills of gas will be the responsibility of the staff member. A refrigerator may be provided, preferably electric and compression operated (it hums when switched on) if power supplies are sufficiently constant. The alternative, a kerosene fridge, is not so easy to operate, but better than nothing. Houses that are at one end of a hospital compound can be given access to emergency supplies of electric power from the hospital's plant without difficulty, and emergency water supplies too.

The welcome to new staff

Staff should be made to feel welcome when they first arrive. The medical superintendent, or his wife, or another resident member of staff, may be asked to take responsibility for this, and call in others to assist. When somebody new is left to move in by him or herself, without any help, it can be difficult, it can be lonely; it can even be traumatic (see Figure 4.3). For

Figure 4.3: *How many faults can you find that need repair?*

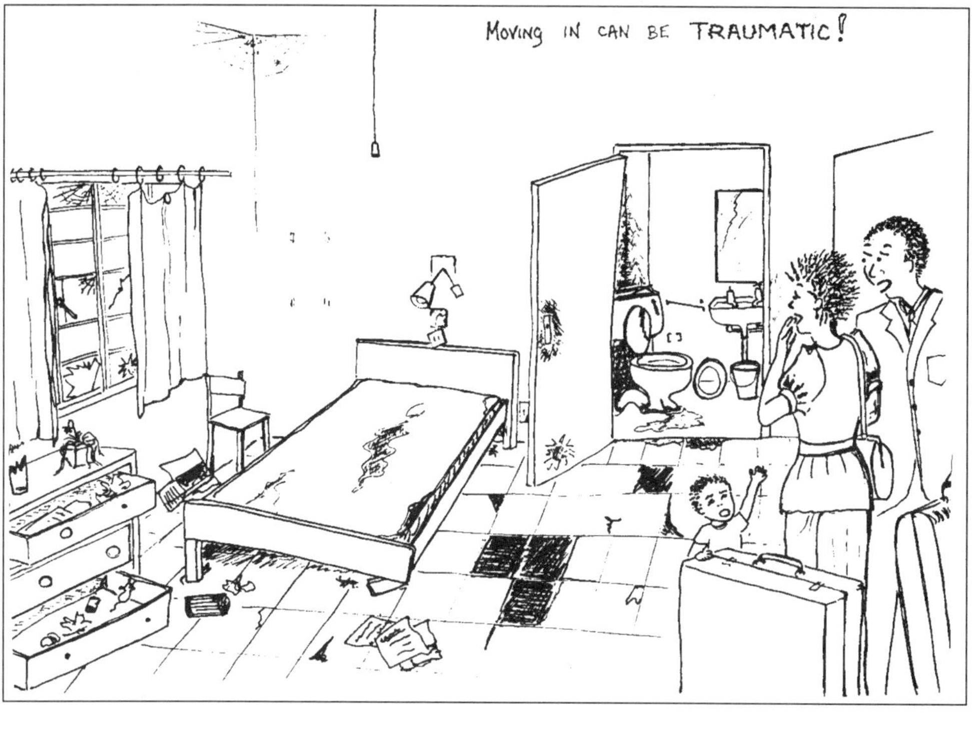

the sake of a good team spirit, and good future relationships, helping hands will be appreciated.

The house should be clean
This is really the responsibility of the outgoing householder, but it is surprisingly often neglected. Not only should all the rubbish have been collected and disposed of, all the drawers and cupboards emptied, but the floors should have been swept and wiped over, and cobwebs removed from the ceilings and corners. It should be possible to call in hospital labour to assist in giving a thorough spring-clean. Dirty walls should be washed, and if still bad be repainted, particularly in places like bathrooms and kitchens.

Checking the inventory
Before the former occupier goes, the hospital administrator should check with him the house inventory, that is the list of furniture and equipment provided with the house. Items missing, or broken, should be noted for replacement or repair. When the new householder comes in, he should be shown the inventory, and allowed to check that it is complete.

Redecoration
Repair of plumbing and sanitary fittings, and external redecoration, are usually the responsibility of the hospital. Internal redecoration may be the responsibility of the householder, but help from the hospital may be appreciated at the start. If particular colours are requested, this should be welcomed. It shows that the new member of staff is keen to make the house 'look like home', which is evidence he is happy and wants to settle down.

Personal introductions
In addition to a warm welcome from other residents, it will be a help if the new person can be introduced to nearby markets, post-office, churches and other community facilities. The hospital may need to provide an introduction to a local bank. An initial small cash loan from the hospital to cover the first month should be given if requested.

A few essential items of food in the house – eggs, vegetables, tinned milk or bread – can be a friendly gesture from neighbours. An invitation to eat out with another family for the first couple of days may be of the greatest help, allowing the newcomer to unpack and set up house without having to cook meals him or herself.

Formal meetings for welcome and introduction to the hospital staff will naturally be arranged as appropriate.

Community activities
Social and religious
Resident staff may develop social activities among themselves, or they may look for friendships outside. There is need for both. Where appropriate a weekly evening meeting for informal discussion and prayer can do much to promote happy relationships. This was a feature at WGH Ilesha. People's ideas and background differed greatly, but the fellowship enjoyed led to tolerance and a sense of common purpose.

Some voluntary agency hospitals, and private hospitals too, in areas where Christians predominate, have a purpose-built hospital chapel or a room set aside for worship, open to both staff and patients. A morning assembly of some sort can be a useful uniting point for the hospital community each day. Where Muslims predominate a room, or open space, set aside as a mosque or prayer ground may also serve to promote social cohesion.

Recreational and educational
Recreation facilities for both staff and their young families should be considered if not otherwise available. Senior staff members may be ready to contribute to the cost themselves.

> When WGH Ilesha was rebuilt on a new site in the 1950s, there was a debate as to whether to provide a tennis court or a small swimming pool. When a good water supply from the town became available the choice went to a pool. This was only 15 feet x 30 feet, and 6 feet deep, and with senior staff providing much of the labour, cost only £200 ($300) to build. Never was a better investment made. Children learned to swim as soon as they learned to walk, and adults got their exercise. The tennis court came later.

Note should be taken as to the availability of schools for staff children. If there are no pre-school facilities it may be possible to help a group of mothers to start a play-group or nursery school themselves. The hospital may be able to help by allocating a room for the purpose which is not otherwise required.

Landscaping the hospital and residential area
The environment is worth caring for and the senior staff may themselves have a considerable part to play in this. Hospitals which make some effort to keep the hospital grounds beautiful find that it adds a great deal to the general well-being, with benefit both to staff and patients. In a voluntary agency or private hospital it is possible to give attention to all the ground between the hospital buildings and staff residences together, using hospital labour. A resident should be encouraged to beautify the area immediately around the house, planting flowers, hedges or flowering bushes, and growing fruit trees and food crops in designated areas. It all adds to contentment and the sense of being at home.

In government (or university) campuses the area around staff residences is generally left entirely to the householders, whether they are interested or not. If they do not have the time or inclination to give essential care the area soon becomes untidy and overgrown. The grass may not be cut and all but the area very close to the house reverts to 'bush'.

This is a pity, because with just a little care, and with cooperation between the hospital administration and the residents, it is possible to produce a beautiful environment.

1. *Grass.* Some are afraid of grass growing too close to buildings in case it provides a cover for snakes. If grass is kept cut short this should be no danger. Its appearance is pleasant, and it keeps down dust and erosion. The ground should be levelled reasonably smooth to facilitate grass cutting by machine. It is an advantage to the householders and everybody when the hospital takes care of this. One machine with an engine run on petrol/oil mixture can easily do the work of 20 men cutting grass by hand, and soon pays for the outlay. However, such machines are very noisy, and on grass close to wards or nurses' lecture rooms it is better to have a machine run by electricity, with a long lead which can be plugged in at any convenient point. There is rarely need to plant bahama or any other special grass. One type of carpet grass may prove native to the area, and will grow uniformly well simply with frequent cutting and removal of competing growth. However, if a very hard 'wire grass' becomes ubiquitous, this may need removal by hand.

2. *Rock.* Some surface rock may be retained as part of the landscape design. Other boulders may need breaking up and removing. In Zambia this is done by digging away the earth around the boulder, heating it with burning sticks or old tyres, then throwing water on the hot rock to crack it.

3. *Flowering bushes.* If a compound is fenced, and goats excluded, then a wide variety of flowers and bushes can be grown in most tropical countries. If goats are a problem then one is limited to the species they do not favour, such as the thorny-stemmed bougainvillea. The many colours of hibiscus, or the red or green leaved acalypha, are much too tempting to goats and sheep. Alongside covered ways, or where rain pours down from a roof, one can combat erosion by planting a hedge of ice-plant (*Phyllanthus nivosus*) or red ixora. Hedge cutters have then to be provided to keep the hedge trimmed.

4. *Trees.* Beside the roads, or at suitable points with space to spare, trees can be planted which add greatly to the scenic beauty of the hospital grounds and house gardens. Pink cassia, peltophorum, flamboyant, or bauhinia –

all grow very easily where rainfall is adequate, but need protection with wire-netting and stakes while young, and watering in the dry season. As soon as their roots get down to the water-table they can look after themselves. The common mistake is to allow them insufficient room. A flamboyant tree spreads to a radius of 6 to 10 metres (20 or 30 feet) when full grown.

Most trees or bushes will grow from cuttings taken from established plants. These can be obtained from commercial or government botanical centres, or may be begged from those in charge of neighbouring compounds or personal gardens. Planting in the wet season and daily watering through the first dry season will be essential. A beautiful environment does not come without labour and loving effort.

Staff health

A hospital will naturally wish to provide good health care for its staff. Applicants for new posts will generally be required to bring a medical certificate of fitness, together with a chest X-ray. Hospitals may wish to supplement this with their own check-up.

Preventive care

Staff should be protected against infectious diseases with which they may come in contact; so all should be offered Mantoux or Heaf test, and BCG if negative. Yellow fever immunisation is advised in some countries. Good hygiene, and normal barrier nursing methods, should be sufficient to protect from such conditions as typhoid, cholera, and even Lassa fever and HIV disease, should they occur. Where tuberculosis is common, chest X-ray should be offered to any member of staff who is worried by cough or weight loss. Female staff with pregnancy should be given free ante-natal care and tetanus immunisation. Staff families should have the benefit of the normal hospital welfare service and childhood immunisations.

Curative care

Regular clinics, arranged for the convenience of nurses and other staff, and organised by the matron or one of the nursing sisters, should be held. The medical superintendent, or his deputy, should be available for this. The health of staff is a prime responsibility. Complaints may be minor, but they need dealing with sympathetically. If at times the number reporting sick appears to be larger than usual, it is worth enquiring gently from the supervising sister whether there is any source of tension in the nursing service or wider hospital community – examinations due, or perhaps some disciplinary dispute. Such episodes commonly lead to an increased reporting of ill-health owing to heightened anxiety and feelings of insecurity. Patience and sensitivity will be needed in dealing with such situations.

If nurses are sent off duty because of sickness, the matron or sister on duty should always be informed. In the case of other staff the hospital secretary should be informed. Interim replacements can then be arranged if necessary.

A small sick bay, or side room, for sick nurses needing in-patient care, is usually advisable. Other staff may be accommodated on the wards or amenity-bed side rooms as appropriate.

Staff consultation

If the staff are to be happy they need to be kept 'in the know' as to what is going on day by day, and to be allowed to participate in decision making wherever possible. Good communication between all sides of the hospital staff is essential, otherwise misunderstandings arise all too easily, and rumours abound. The informal occasions for a word in the corridor, or a chat over coffee have their place, but formal meetings are also necessary.

Staff committee

The regular staff committee is an indispensable part of hospital organisation. Its size, frequency of meeting, and its membership will vary according to the size and complexity of the hospital.

> The membership of the WGH Ilesha Staff Committee was set out in the hospital constitution. Of the 18 members, half were on by virtue of their office: the basic leadership team, plus pharmacist, accountant, laboratory superintendent, principal nurse tutor and chaplain.

> The other half were elected, and included other doctors, sisters and representatives of the staff-nurses and workers. It met on the first Wednesday of every month, and the staff felt it was sufficiently important to give up an evening for it. It sat from 8.00 to 9.30 pm, or later if the business went on. Discussions were at times very lively, and decisions had to be settled by a vote. The basic leadership team did not always get its way.

Departmental meetings

In larger hospitals each department, for example the maternity department, or the nursing school, will need its regular administrative meeting. Clinical meetings and journal clubs, to promote the training of housemen and registrars, may be organised by the doctors.

Coping with conflict
Disciplinary procedure

Within every institution there will be times when personalities clash and conflict occurs; or when individuals offend against the accepted regulations which operate within the hospital, and a case is brought against them. Hospitals need to have an understood procedure to deal with such matters.

The immediate supervisor of a staff member should be the first to try and settle the matter. The staff member should be asked to see him in a side-room, away from other members of staff. Correction should never be done in front of patients, or more junior staff. If two people are involved the supervisor should always hear both sides before advising on a solution. The blame is generally due to 'six of one and half a dozen of the other'. Apologies made and accepted, and a word of caution to those involved may be sufficient.

However, if one side is found to be involved in a serious misdemeanour which the supervisor feels requires punishment, he should refer the case through to his superior. It would be his reponsibility to hear the allegations, and the staff member's defence, and decide if punishment is necessary. The principle of punishment from two levels above, and never from the immediate supervisor, should be adhered to.

Matters of nursing discipline should never be dealt with directly by doctors on a ward, but always referred to the nursing supervisor – and to the matron if need be.

Junior staff
Matters from the clerical and labour staff will generally be dealt with by the hospital administrator with a system of written warnings. Offences involving misappropriation or dishonest handling of hospital money should generally be dealt with by termination of appointment forthwith. No compromise should be tolerated if an incorrupt hospital is to be maintained. However, it should be remembered that right of appeal, to the staff committee or executive, for junior staff, and to the board for senior staff, may be written in to the constitution. This should be respected.

Senior staff
Discipline of senior professional staff is always difficult. In government it is handled by civil service procedures in the state capital. Owing to the security of tenure guaranteed to confirmed public servants the offender may simply be transferred to another hospital, often in a more rural area, as the punishment. His or her attitude and behaviour may continue to be an embarrassment in the place to which he/she is sent, but he/she will be on parole.

In a voluntary agency hospital the medical superintendent should have machinery for handling professional staff discipline, or any challenge to his own authority. On the principle already given, he should not deal with it himself, but pass it on to the level above him, that is to the board. This may involve setting up a disciplinary committee under the chairman, and a few local board members from the community.

Negotiation with unions
Group action by a staff union generally takes place within the trade union legislation current in the country at large. If it is part of regional or nationwide conflict there is little the hospital authorities can do, apart from try to limit the damage done to patient services. If it is due to a dispute within the hospital, then the procedures for negotiation should be followed. Representatives from the union, usually the president and secretary, should be invited to meet the hospital secretary and medical superintendent to state their case, and to hear the hospital's case. It may be possible to reach a compromise solution. Strikes should not normally be called, or threatened, without due notice, and without exhausting all efforts at conciliation. Irresponsible calling of strikes, particularly in an institution like a hospital where lives may be at risk, is against trade union law in many countries. The professional feelings of nurses and health workers generally ensure that care for serious emergency cases is maintained.

The settlement of such union disputes, when they occur, will again involve the board. An emergency meeting, called without prior notice, by phone or direct messenger, may have to be convened immediately at the request of the medical superintendent. Action taken to settle the dispute will then be reported to a subsequent general meeting for approval.

At times of tension or rapid social change it may be wise to have a regular negotiating committee, with equal members of management and union, say three of each. Matters likely to lead to misunderstanding can then be raised, from either side, and discussed coolly and dispassionately before feelings have been aroused. Agreements reached should be written down in brief sentences as the discussion proceeds. These are read out at the end. All members of the negotiating committee then initial the page on which the agreements have been written before the meeting adjourns. Full committee procedure for the approval of minutes is not necessary at the next meeting. The record has already been signed and accepted. Further negotiation can commence at once.

Handling oneself
Getting feedback
As much of the overall happiness of a hospital community depends upon leadership, the doctor in charge should also seek to get some feedback from those around him. An immediate colleague with whom he has good rapport can be an immense asset. Perceptive comments may come in such relaxed moments as the morning coffee-break.

The one in charge is always in danger of pride, which can lead to arrogance and impatience with criticism, or with those who fail to come up to expectation. The doctor who has the reputation of 'biting people's heads off', or who throws instruments around the theatre, will find that most people are afraid to speak to him. Conversely, if he is ready with his greetings, and has a smile and a word of appreciation for any member of staff when he sees work well done, then relationships will be easy. Feed-back will come.

Setting standards

Leadership is most effective from the centre of the team, rather than from a remote position at the top, aloof from open criticism. The senior doctor should accept the same discipline which he expects from his staff. If the hospital's 8-hour working day runs from 8.00 to 4.00 p.m., the doctor should not work less. If a clinic is scheduled to begin at 9.00 a.m. he should be as prompt as he expects other staff to be. If hospital transport cannot be used by senior staff for personal journeys he should accept the same restriction. Precautions already mentioned for the handling of hospital money should be most carefully observed by the medical superintendent/PMO, who is ultimately in charge.

Such leadership will filter down to staff at all levels, and be a major factor in securing the happy hospital atmosphere which patients appreciate. The hospital becomes the therapeutic community.

CHAPTER 5

Medical Records

A good hospital can be judged by its records
If the registration desk, which is the patient's first port of call, is filled with irregular piles of unfiled documents from previous days; if old file jackets are being cut up to provide temporary cards because proper ones are out of stock; or if the patient's out-patient record, used three days – or three years – ago, cannot be found for a re-visit; or if the card, when finally found, fails to give the doctor a quick and full appraisal of what happened last time – then such a hospital is failing to provide good care at the most elementary level. The medical records system is poor.

No system is perfect and even a good one can be spoiled by careless use, and slack maintenance. However, there are some systems which discourage even those with the best of intentions.

Yardsticks for evaluation

There are three principles, or yardsticks, by which the records system may be evaluated.

Good medical records should be . . .
- economical – and within the hospital budget to maintain

- concise, but clear – and not too bulky for easy filing

- easily retrievable – being filed in such a way that old records can be quickly traced, and thus promote satisfactory continuity of care.

Sometimes doctors, and medical records officers, dream up complicated cards and charts for out-patient and in-patient services, and they are pained when they find the system proves highly expensive to maintain, and the folders bulky and untidy to file.

After a few years an old record becomes next to impossible to retrieve except after a lengthy search, so all too often when a patient returns he or she is issued with a new card or chart 'to save time'. This overburdens the bulging shelves even more, and continuity of care goes out of the window.

Look before you leap
When the author first arrived at WGH Ilesha he was appalled to find that the out-patient (OP) records were just plain, lined, index cards the size of a post-card. On this everything had to be written: name, age, sex, town, registration number, complaint, history, clinical findings, investigations, orders, diagnosis, drugs to be supplied, amount to be paid and receipt number. Impossible, was the first thought. Let us design a bigger card, with room on it for all we need.

In addition to the OP card, patients were issued with a small registration card, nicely printed, with the hospital's name and badge, and on this the patient's name, town, and registration number were written. This small card was held by the patient. The OP card was filed in a bank of card-index drawers. The system had been in operation since the 1920s, from not long after the date when the hospital first opened. Yes, time for an update.

But second thoughts prevailed. It was noticed that when some elderly patients returned 30 years later bringing their original small card, which had been carefully kept in a cigarette tin at home, the clerk at the registration desk was able to find the matching OP card within half a minute. With such excellent continuity would it have been wise to make a change? So the system remained, and the doctors adapted by writing with a small hand, and making their notes neat and concise. Frequent attenders did have a lot of cards clipped together, but for most adult patients one or two cards were sufficient. For children, with even more frequent attendance during their first five years, additional home-based cards were developed which did not require filing.

Changing the records system is difficult

Once hospital staff, and the community served, get used to one system of records, it is not at all easy to introduce changes. Sometimes it has to be done. The doctor in charge of a hospital, who wants the best for his patients, should look at the system in use, and, in consultation with his staff, consider where improvements could be made. All proposed changes should however be checked against the yardsticks of a good system:

Is the change within the hospital's economy to maintain?
The answer to this question can cut both ways. It is a mistake to try to be too economical. Many hospitals fail to budget properly for records, or fail to realise the true quantity required. Stocks of important cards or case sheets are allowed to go out of stock before more are ordered, so the whole system may be thrown into confusion. There must be realistic estimates for reprinting, and orders placed in good time before stocks fall too low.

On the other hand, before introducing new documents the initial cost, and continued annual expenditure, should be looked at carefully, and weighed against the benefits which may accrue in better patient care. In some cases it may be wise to run a pilot trial for a period with documents produced on paper with a duplicating machine, before running to the expense of printing on card enough to meet the needs of all patients, say for the first two years.

Will the records be concise, clear, and not too bulky to store in future years? There is always a temptation to make bigger cards, or cards with many prepared spaces on for each category of information. Regrettably many doctors respond by writing very large, each line sprawling over three or four lines on the form. The prepared information boxes may be ignored. The space is just wasted.

In Britain the National Health Service cards for general practice patients were originally all designed to fit into 7 x 5 inches (180mm x 130mm) envelopes. The shelf storage space required was minimal. Many GPs are now moving to use the A4 size, 11 x 8 inches (300mm x 200mm), but with a great increase required in storage space.

One reason advanced in favour of the bigger size is that in-patient and out-patient documents can be stored together. This generally involves providing a relatively expensive folder for each patient into which all the charts, cards and letters can be placed. At first sight this appears to have great advantages, until the problem of storage presents itself.

Then, where previously one small shelf per year was sufficient for out-patient cards, and another shelf for in-patient charts, now the combined system may require ten large shelves per year, and after five years the records room is full. In most hospitals only one patient in ten is admitted, so only one-tenth of the folders will contain in-patient charts. Nine-tenths will contain purely out-patient records, and often a medley of notes, lab reports and letters in no particular order, and in such confusion as to be of little use in reviewing a case anyway.

Smaller cards are quite adequate for the fairly brief notes required in primary and secondary care, where doctors are generally hard-pressed for time, with many patients awaiting their attention every day. They should be encouraged to write concise, clear notes on the patient's complaints, with their significant positive clinical findings, and important negative ones. The Provisional Diagnosis should be underlined, and a brief indication given as to the proposed management. When a patient attends frequently for a variety of complaints, he will need several cards clipped together. The use of a Problem Summary Card (see p76), clipped on top of the OP cards, can provide an instant aide-memoire as to the current problem, and any previous diagnoses which may be relevant.

Will records be easily retrievable, and provide the continuity of care, which every hospital or health facility should aim to give?
Retrievability means the ability to find old records when the patient comes again. In a busy hospital, with perhaps a long queue at the registration desk, this means that it must be possible to locate a record within half a minute, or even a few seconds. This means the documents should be filed neatly, with the index number, or letter, seen easily, and the shelves or drawers conveniently accessible to the registration clerk. Any system, where the stored records take up a lot of space, are difficult to file tidily, or where the index number cannot be seen until the file is pulled out from the shelf – all these make retrieval difficult. Clerks do not have the time to spend ten or twenty minutes finding just one former record; so a temporary new one is issued, and all too often the old one is never found again.

One seemingly simple solution is to allow patients, adults as well as children, to take their out-patient record home. Much administrative time searching for records may be saved on return visits. However, *home-based records for adults* have both advantages and disadvantages. A hospital in Malawi with this system found that 95% of the patients retained their cards and did not lose them. A hospital in Nepal reckoned that two-thirds of patients on repeat visits came back with their old card, at least within the first two years, but cards tended to get creased and greasy and difficult to write on. *Few were retained for up to 5 years.*

Every patient has a right to continuity of care – for life, if possible. Retrievability of records, by one means or another, is therefore essential. A medical records system may look impressive, and claim to be very comprehensive, but if old charts cannot be found quickly when wanted, the system is defective, because continuity is threatened.

In the light of these principles the patient registration procedure, and the various essential records, will be looked at in turn. Where appropriate the system developed at WGH Ilesha will be used as an example. There is nothing unique about the Ilesha records, but they worked reasonably well, and continuity was good. Every hospital has its own way of doing things. A medical administrator should look closely at his records.

Out-patient records

The main out-patient register
All out-patients should go through one registration system for their first attendance, so that they can be given an out-patient registration number, which they will retain and use whichever clinic or service they attend, and whenever they re-attend in subsequent years. Other clinics, such as the ante-

natal, may keep subsidiary registers for their own repeat attendances, but initially every patient must come through the main desk to get their registration number, or 'hospital number'.

Attendance statistics

The registers must be kept in such a way as to provide, with the minimum of trouble, certain essential attendance statistics. These are, for each year:

- the number of new patients,
- the number of first attendances, and
- the total of all patient attendances.

New patients

This figure is quite easily obtained from the final figure on the year's registrations. However, this figure does not tell you how many individual patients made use of the hospital in the year, apart, that is, from the very first year of a hospital's existence. In all subsequent years many old patients will have attended again. On their first attendance in the year they are, in a sense, 'new' for that year.

First attendances

Some way must be found for recording the first attendance of old patients in each year. Adding that figure to the new patients for the year will give the figure for the total number of individual patients who have been served. Some hospitals have separate registration books for new patients and old patients, but this is not the answer, unless some means of indicating and counting up the first attendance of old patients is included.

Total attendances

The total number of out-patient attendances for the year will give some idea of the work-load of the staff. It will be a composite figure from the main out-patient register and from all the secondary registers at the various clinics around the hospital recording repeat visits – ante-natal, under-fives, dressings, injections, and special clinics for patients with tuberculosis, leprosy, or diabetes. To get the total out-patient attendances in the year, all these figures must be added together. This may be done monthly, and then the monthly figures added up for the annual total.

One way of doing it

At WGH Ilesha the general out-patients department had two clerks on duty at the registration desk each day, one for men and one for women, and each kept a register ruled as follows (see Figure 5.1):

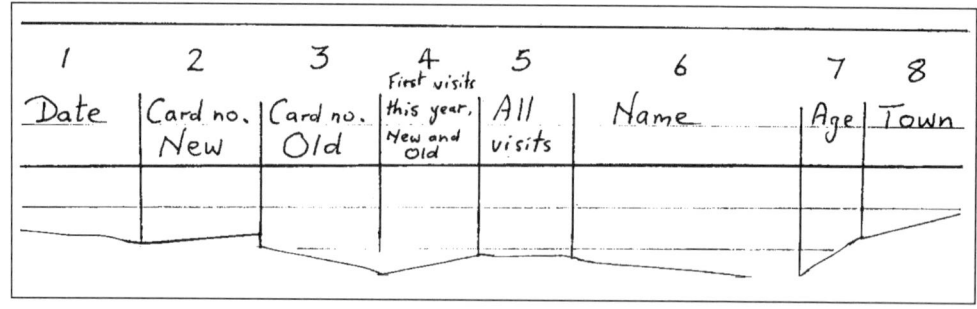

1	2	3	4	5	6	7	8
Date	Card no. New	Card no. Old	First visit this year, New and Old	All visits	Name	Age	Town

Figure 5.1.

Totals from the two registers, for men and for women, had to be added together at the end of the year.

Column 2 started at 1 on 1st January with new index letters for the year, a pair of letters for men and a pair for women. The two running totals together gave the total new cases attending for the first time in that year.

Column 3 recorded patients coming on a repeat visit, whether from previous years, or within the same year. The registration numbers here would all be for previous years, recognisable from the index letters.

Column 4 was a special one for counting all first attendances in the year. It was simply a running total, starting at 1 each 1st January, and a digit was added for all new patients, and for all old patients *coming for their first visit in that particular year*. The registration clerks had to scrutinise each old card as it was found to see which ones were first visits for the year. During January, of course, nearly every old patient was also a first visit in the new year. As the months went by, fewer were first visits, and towards the end of the year they were uncommon.

Column 5 was also a running total, starting from 1 on each 1st January, and a digit was added for all new patients (Column 1) and all old patients (Column 2). The final figure at the end of the year gave the total of all attendances at the general out-patient department. To this would be added the attendance figures from the other clinics to find the grand total of all attendances for the whole hospital.

Columns 6 and onwards recorded the patient's name, town etc.

A portion of page completed would look as follows (see Figure 5.2):

General out-patient cards and forms
In one style or another, the following are all needed.

The registration card
This is the small card given to the patient when he first attends as a new patient and is given his personal registration number.

1	2	3	4	5	6	7	8
Date 1974	Card no New	Card no Old	First visits this year New & Old	All visits	Name	Age	Town
12th April	FG 641		4153	44646	Isaac Okeke	24	Ndubo
✓		FE 3645		44647	Akin Olaniyan	41	Oro
✓ *		FE 9532	4154	44648	Gbadomosi Onu	19	Ilare-odo
✓	FG 642		4155	44649	John Ajayi	3	Ilesha
✓		EW 52		44650	Akintunde Jimo	64	Ilesha
✓ *		EU 6186	4156	44651	Peter Ogunsanmi	33	Oshu
✓		FE 1011		44652	Ola Ayeni	10	Ilesha
✓	FG 643		4157	44653	William Nwoeze	30	Oru
✓		CD 5415		44654	Patrick Mewoyeka	77	Okitipupa
✓ *		CX 651	4158	44655	Vincent Ejwola	29	Iwaraje

* Indicates old patients on first attendance in the current year; hence counted in Column 3

Figure 5.2.

He takes the card home, and brings it on each subsequent visit.

1. *Design of the card.* Since it has to last the patient for his lifetime, the card should be well produced, printed on firm card (or plastic), with the hospital's name and insignia on one side, and on the other, room to write the patient's name, registration number, sex, age and town of origin (see Figure 5.3).

It is worth spending money on the card, and a small extra charge may be made for it, so that the patient will value it, and preserve it carefully. He should be advised to bring it whenever he attends again. Some centres provide a small polythene envelope in which to keep the card at home.

2. *The card in use.* The registration clerks should ask every patient if they already have a registration card, however many years earlier it may have been issued. If patients can be saved a further card fee, and the out-patient card can be found quickly, the patients will be glad to cooperate. If patients forget to bring their small card, they may, if living fairly near, be sent home to bring it. Naturally this would not be done in cases of severe illness or emergency.

Occasionally patients conceal the fact that they have been before, perhaps because they want to see a different doctor, or because they know their OP card contains a diagnosis they want to hide, or maybe the note of a debt owed to the hospital.

If a card is genuinely lost, but the date of the last attendance is known, the clerk may be able to trace the name of the patient in the attendance register, and find the registration number from that. He can then pick the out-patient card.

Figure 5.3: *Registration card 2 x 3 inches folded for storage at home.*

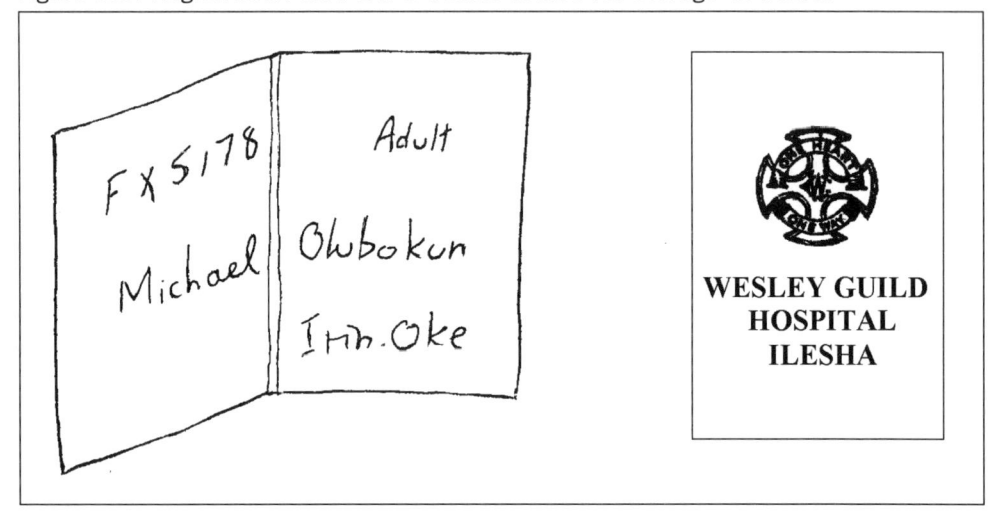

The registration card may be adapted for other purposes:
- Date of next appointment

- Record of tetanus immunisation

- Medical diagnoses for which the patient should have his or her own record. These include such things as: penicillin allergy, sickle-cell haemoglobinopathy, diabetes mellitus, and certain operations such as gastrectomy or hysterectomy.

Should the patient attend any other centre in an emergency, such items of information could be vital.

The out-patient card (OP card)
1. *Design of the card.* The card should not be large. 4 x 6in (100 x 150mm) should be sufficient. The WGH Ilesha card was only 3 x 5 inches (see Figure 5.4).

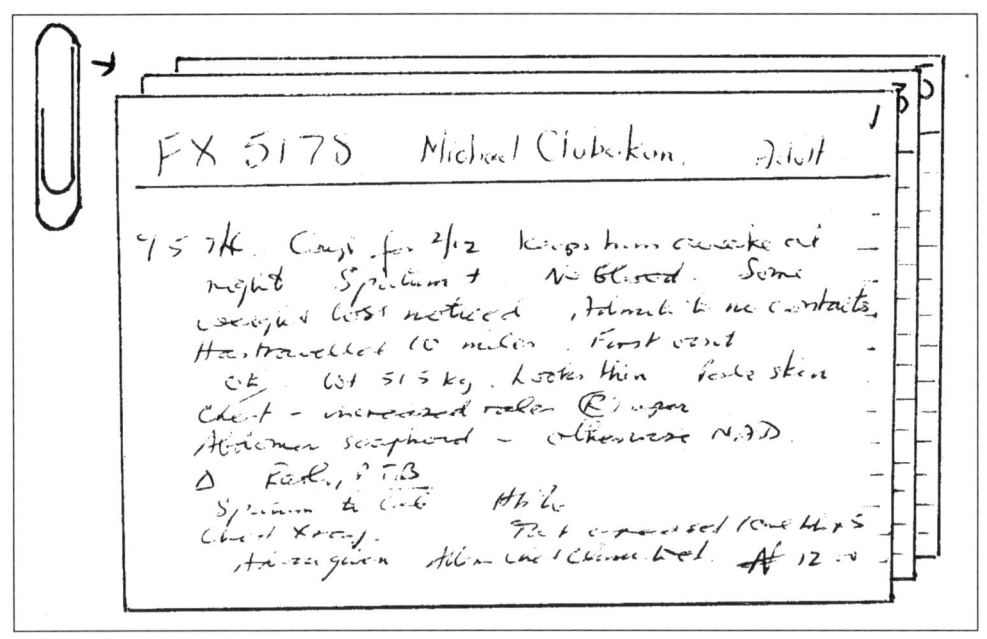

Figure 5.4: *A simple out-patient card – use both sides. Fix continuation cards with clip in page order like a book, page one remaining at the front.*

The card should be simple, with room at the top for essential clerical details, the OP registration number, name, age, sex and town, and lined space for writing on both sides. Many patients will attend rarely, and for them one card will be sufficient. When the front side is full, the reverse side may be used. Other patients will attend quite frequently, and a second card will have to be clipped to the first.

Multiple cards should always be clipped together in book order, with page 1 remaining on the top and new cards clipped behind. Sometimes a clerk likes to put the fresh new card on top, because page 1 looks grubby, but if he does so, the record will be out of sequence and therefore confusing – like trying to read a book where the page numbers go 3, 4, 1, 2! For the few very frequent attenders, with a bunch of cards clipped together, it is particularly important that the cards be in the proper order.

2. *Use of the card.* If doctors write neatly, and concisely, it should be possible to compress the essential record of each consultation into a relatively small space. All positive findings, essential negative findings, a provisional diagnosis – underlined – and a note of tests ordered, with a summary of results, should be included. The treatment plan should be itemised, and the names of drugs ordered, with the number of days for which each is to be supplied.

Problem summary card

A problem summary card of a different colour but the same size as the general OP card, can be a very important clinical aide. It may be used as a routine for all patients, or kept for those who attend more frequently. It should be placed in front of the other cards for quick reference as each consultation begins. All significant diagnoses should be transferred from the OP cards to the summary card as the clinical conditions become clear. Important points of family or social history may also be included (see Figure 5.5).

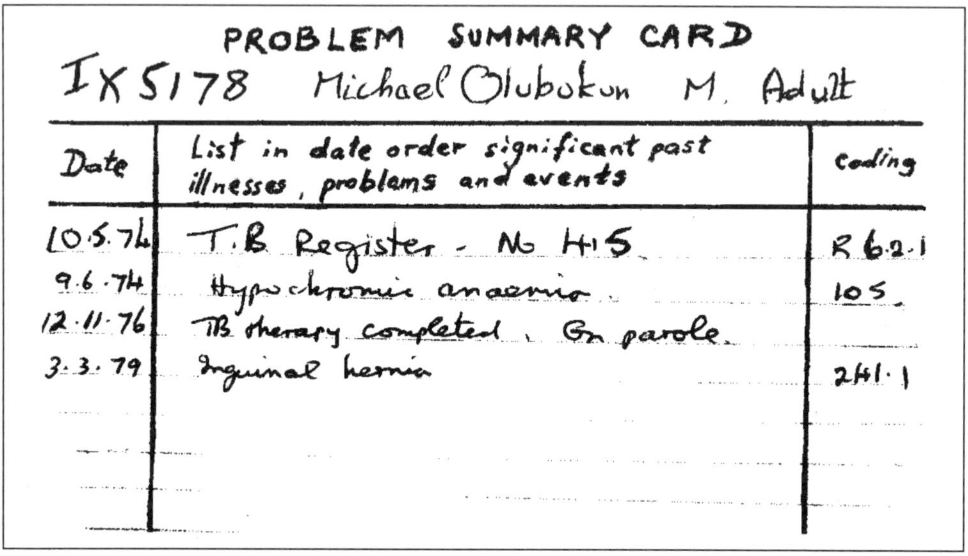

\<PROBLEM SUMMARY CARD\> IX 5178 Michael Olubokun M. Adult		
Date	List in date order significant past illnesses, problems and events	Coding
10.5.74	T.B. Register - No HiS	R 6.2.1
9.6.74	Hypochromic anaemia	105
12.11.76	TB therapy completed. On parole	
3.3.79	Inguinal hernia	241.1

Figure 5.5: *Problem summary card.*

Request forms for investigations

For many simple tests, done perhaps in an out-patient branch laboratory, the requests may be written by the doctor direct on to the OP card – blood for malaria parasites, or haemoglobin, stool for parasites, urine for albumin and sugar, sputum for AAFB, and so on – and the laboratory assistant can record the result on the card, in answer to the request. However, if the main laboratory handles all requests for bacteriology or biochemistry, then special request forms are likely to be required. So, also, will request forms to the radiology department for X-ray.

Prescriptions

Prescriptions for drugs may be written in full on small prescription forms in pads, indicating the name of the drug, dose, frequency of administration, and number of days for the course. It is important for the doctor to write the total number of tablets to be dispensed. This provides a clear instruction to the dispensing assistant, and also makes sure the doctor is aware as to how much he is prescribing.

Admitted patients, and the OP record
When a patient is admitted in the ward, a set of charts for in-patient use is available on the ward this summary can go directly on to it, and the final diagnosis can also go on to the problem summary card if such is used. Some hospitals use a special discharge summary card.

1. *Admission from regular clinics.* In this case there is no problem. The doctor in the OP department writes 'Admit' on the OP card, and the patient takes it to the admission room, where it can be clipped together with the in-patient chart.

2. *Admission as an emergency.* Patients presenting as casualties or emergency admissions may have to go direct to the admission room or wards, and bypass the OP department. Some kind of temporary OP card will have to be given until the next week-day morning when the OP department is open again. Any previous OP card the patient may have can then be collected.

Discharge summaries
When the admitted patient is ready to go home the doctor should make a summary of what has been done in the ward, noting any medicines given on discharge, and plans for subsequent management. If the OP card is available on the ward this summary can go directly on to it, and the final diagnosis can also go on to the problem summary card if such is used. Some hospitals use a special discharge summary card.

Making a discharge summary serves two purposes. It ensures that the doctor looks through the in-patient record thoroughly to make a clinical review before the patient goes home. Points that might have been overlooked for follow-up are sometimes brought to mind; and secondly, when the patient returns to the OP department for a further visit, the essential features of the period spent in hospital are immediately available.

Hospitals which maintain a single folder for in-patient and out-patient records may feel they have some advantage, since the doctor in the OP department will have all the in-patient charts to hand. However, there is a danger that too much paper is retained.

The ante-natal clinic (ANC) cards
Most hospitals and maternity centres have their own ANC card. For the most part these are filled in by midwives, and the doctors pay them too little attention, until patients are referred to them with obstetric problems.

Two cards are really needed.

Many women in tropical countries aim to have a child every two years, and for each pregnancy a new ANC card is issued. Much of the information on the card, such as maternal height, blood group and past obstetric history, has to be laboriously re-written every time. It is better to divide the information into two, with one card for the relatively permanent features specific to the woman, and another for the features specific only to that pregnancy. This was done at Ilesha, and the cards used there will be described.

Maternity record card

This was the first card that contained all the more permanent items of information, such as maternal height and genotype. It was retained by the mother between pregnancies, and brought with her when coming to register for a subsequent pregnancy (see Figure 5.6).

The obstetric history allowed room for two pregnancies on the front, and eight more on the reverse side, ten in all – whether as abortions or going

Figure 5.6: *Maternity record card.*

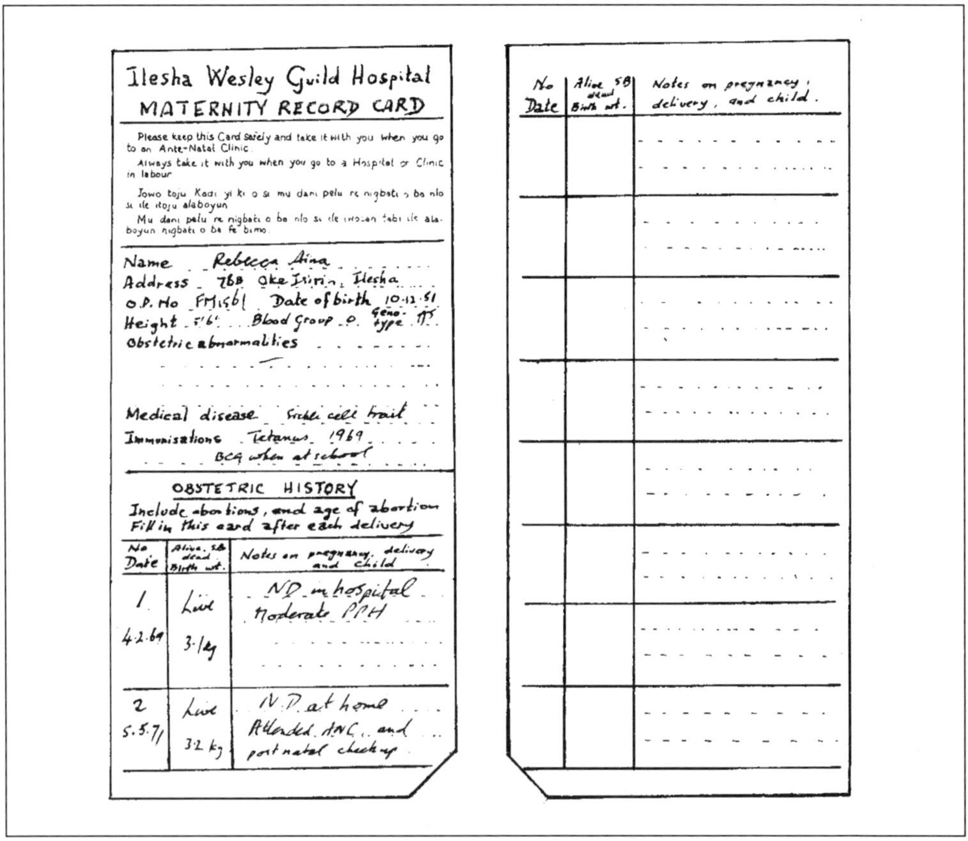
Ilesha Wesley Guild Hospital
MATERNITY RECORD CARD

Please keep this Card safely and take it with you when you go to an Ante-Natal Clinic.
Always take it with you when you go to a Hospital or Clinic in labour

Jowo toju Kadi yi ki o si mu dani pelu re nigbati o ba nlo si ile itoju alaboyun
Mu dani pelu re nigbati o ba nlo si ile iwosan tabi ile alaboyun nigbati o ba fe bimo.

Name Rebecca Aina
Address 78B Oke Isirin, Ilesha
O.P. No FM1561 Date of birth 10.12.51
Height 5'6" Blood Group O Genotype AS
Obstetric abnormalities —

Medical disease Sickle cell trait
Immunisations Tetanus 1969
BCG when at school

OBSTETRIC HISTORY
Include abortions, and age of abortion
Fill in this card after each delivery

No. Date	Alive, SB dead Birth wt.	Notes on pregnancy, delivery and child
1 4.2.69	Live 3.1kg	ND in hospital Moderate PPH
2 5.5.71	Live 3.2 kg	N.D. at home Attended ANC, and postnatal checkup

No. Date	Alive SB dead Birth wt.	Notes on pregnancy, delivery, and child.

to term. This was filled in on the first visit to the ANC. If the patient delivered in hospital, the outcome for mother and child was filled in on the next space in the obstetric history before the mother's discharge. Should the patient deliver at home, or some other centre, there was just the one space to fill in on her maternity record when she came for a subsequent pregnancy. There was no need to ask for, and write out, the entire history all over again.

Ante-natal card

This was more like the usual ANC card, except for the absence of the obstetric history. Features of the history relating to this pregnancy, and the findings on first examination for booking, were recorded on the front. On the centre spread there was room for the usual parameters of weight, blood pressure, height of fundus etc. The doctor added notes in the right hand column, and any special treatment orders. On the back of the card the midwives ordered routine anti-malarials and folic-acid, and dispensed the tablets from their tables in pre-packed envelopes (see Figure 5.7).

Figure 5.7.

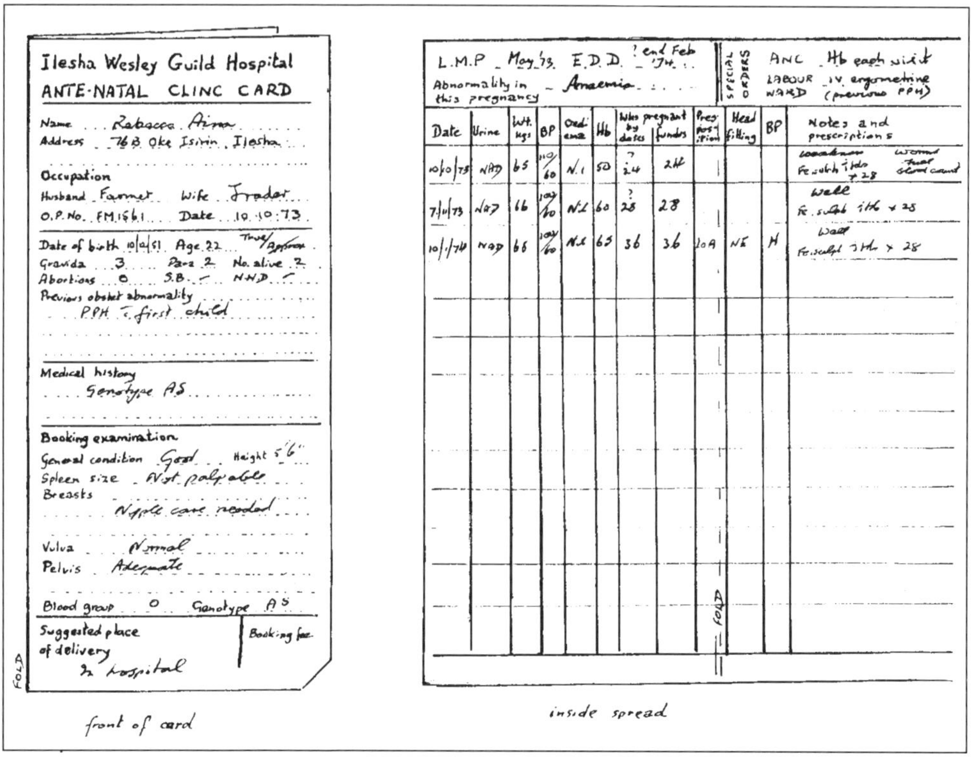

Under-fives clinic cards

Up to 60 per cent of the patients seeking out-patient care in tropical hospitals are likely to be children, so there is much to be said for hospitals providing them with special clinics. Many will have already been through the selective

80 *Medical Administration for Front-line Doctors*

Figure 5.8: *Under-fives Clinic card, growth chart and polythene bag.*

Chart opened up: the first three years.

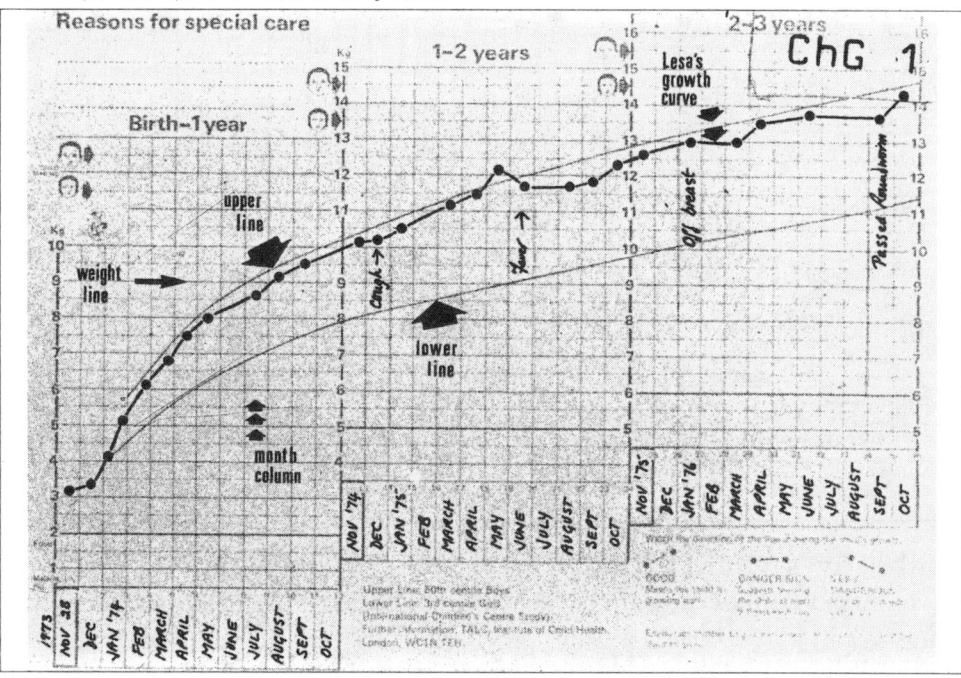

processes of primary care in neighbouring clinics, and be referred because of a serious condition. Childhood illnesses can also change rapidly for the worse. Mothers with small babies or toddlers, waiting in a general queue, may be reluctant to ask for care before their elders, unless they see signs of terminal illness in their children, and become desperate.

Primary health care (PHC) centres are increasingly organising under-fives clinics. They use home-based growth charts and the clinic cards that go with them. If hospitals also organise their OP services in such a way that children under five years are seen separately from the adults, this can greatly improve the services for all. If there is no purpose-built separate clinic, hospitals can sometimes run under-fives services in the area used at other times for ante-natal patients. Hospital records for children should, if possible, be similar to those used in neighbouring PHC centres, and be interchangeable (see also p.219).

First attenders

New patients should register at the main desk, and receive a hospital number and registration card, in the same way as older children and adults. The OP card may be made out, but be put straight into file and not put into service till the child reaches the age of five. For immediate use the clerk would issue a growth chart and under-fives clinic card, together with the polythene bag to keep them clean when taken home (see Figure 5.8). If the mother of the child showed that she already had such a growth chart and card from another centre, the hospital number should simply be added to that, rather than issue another. Continuity of care between primary care clinic and secondary care hospital would thus be maintained.

Repeat visits

To cope with the large numbers there should be a separate registration desk to which mothers coming for follow-up visits can take their children. They already hold their records in their hands, so it is really sufficient for the clerk just to write down the hospital registration number. Fuller details of name, town of origin etc, could be available on the registration card, or from the first attendance in the main register, if required.

> At WGH Ilesha the under-fives clinic register simply recorded hospital registration numbers in this way (see Figure 5.9). No time was wasted. Separate columns were used for:
>
> 1. *New patients.* These were already accounted for in the main register so were excluded when submitting figures for hospital statistics of total attendances.
>
> 2. First attendances in the current calendar year.
>
> 3. All other attendances.

The totals in columns 2 and 5 could be added to the hospital's general totals for first attendances in the year, and the total of all attendances.

The system was very simple, and 500 patients could be registered by one or two clerks every morning. The same clerks would also go on to do the weighing of each child and the graphing of the weight on the growth chart. The patients then waited to be seen by a midwife with additional paediatric experience, of whom there were five. Each saw about 100 children in the morning, giving essential nutritional advice, simple primary care and ordering immunisations as required. About 10 per cent of the patients with more serious problems were referred to the paediatrician.

After the fifth birthday

Another home-based card was issued at WGH Ilesha for schoolchildren (aged 5 to 14) and a separate clinic arranged for them. Other hospitals, with fewer school children attending may treat them with the adults.

Figure 5.9: *Under-fives clinic register.*

Date 4.9.70				
New	**Repeat** First this year	**Attendances** All	other attendances	
FS 3210	FG 616	FS 260	FS 2919	FP 7170
FS 3211	FP 4919	FP 3851	FQ 10	FP 3441
FS 3240	FQ 7618	FQ 10	FS 3100	FQ 5161
FS 3241	FO 589	FO 25	FS 3016	FR 72
FS 3243	FR 4190	FS 2981	FO 515	FS 3058
FS 3255	FQ 1061	FQ 4182	FR 6066	FP 3142
	FP 5381	FQ 4011	FR 821	FP 2511
	FQ 4010	FS 2851	FS 2989	FQ 1099
		FS 2404	FP 8501	FQ 689
		FS 1399	FP 405	
		FS 2950	FS 2851	
		FT 69	FO 618	
		FO 851	FO 6464	
		FR 75	FQ 7919	
		FP 6010	FS 2986	(57)
		FO 731	FR 85	
	(8)	FQ 6051	FT 857	
		FS 2991	FO 6052	
		FS 3001	FO 7776	
		FS 3119	FP 6164	
		FO 6621	FP 759	
		FQ 7180	FQ 81	
		FP 32	FS 3158	
		FS 3035	FP 95	
(6)				

Special disease clinics

When hospitals find they are dealing with substantial numbers of patients with a particular chronic disease requiring long-term management for months or years, then special clinics on regular days should be organised for them. Such clinics may cater for patients with hypertension, epilepsy, diabetes mellitus, tuberculosis or leprosy, according to local need. Such patients need:

- local care – as close to home as possible, to obviate long, frequent journeys, with the expense entailed, and to encourage compliance

- structured care – utilising, where possible, standard management patterns and drug regimes, with evaluation at regular intervals. One doctor should take responsibility for a particular clinic to provide continuity of care.

Special clinics will each need their own disease register, which can provide the statistics for the particular condition; and also special cards. The cards will be designed to fit the structured management regime chosen, and the periodic evaluations agreed to be necessary. The cards may show a whole year's management on one side, and thus provide instant information to the supervising doctor as to the point reached in the treatment, and the patient's response. This is infinitely better than trying to monitor random visits to the general out-patient department, often at irregular intervals, and seen by a variety of doctors, with erratic changes of regime according to their clinical whim. Clinics for two diseases are taken as an example.

The tuberculosis clinic, or chest clinic

The hospital may produce its own special card for this, or make use of the one produced by the World Health Organisation for national tuberculosis programmes, if it is available.

> The essential elements of the chest clinic card used at WGH Ilesha were that it was ruled for visits every two weeks, and lasted for one year. The drugs were given out at the clinic in standard packs, and the streptomycin injections were crossed off each day as given till the course was completed. The patient's weight, progress notes and X-ray findings were entered in the space opposite.
>
> So long as all was going well the patient just saw a doctor after one month, three months, six months and a year. Intermediate visits, weighing and handing out of drugs were dealt with by a clerical assistant. Any problems were, of course, brought to the doctor's notice.

Whatever the treatment protocol in use, the card can be designed to show it for the six months, or the year or more, as required. After the prescribed period the patient should be put 'on parole' for two more years. If he remains fit, he should then be *discharged* from the chest clinic, and not remain for ever as a 'known TB patient' with the stigma often attached to that label.

The tuberculosis card may be stored in the envelope with the patient's chest X-rays. These envelopes should be retained in the chest clinic rather than in the radiology department. Patients with non-pulmonary TB may be issued with an envelope too, and their card stored with the others. These make a neat chest clinic records section.

Leprosy clinic
Leprosy is now treated on an out-patient basis, rather than in closed settlements. Infectivity, contrary to popular assumption, is known to be low, and after a few weeks of treatment even lepromatous patients become unable to pass on the disease. General hospitals may therefore run clinics for treating patients in the area. Such clinics should be held at a time when the pressure from general patients is over, such as in the afternoon. Again, there should be a leprosy register, and a special treatment card.

> At WGH Ilesha this was known as the dapsone card. The card may be similar to the one used for patients with tuberculosis, and allow for a year's regime per side, with a monthly issue of drugs, and routine skin or nasal smears for *M. leprae*, to check for progress. A new card may be issued for each year. Such a card is even more necessary for the correct multi-drug therapy.

In-patient charts and registers

Special attention should be given to the hospital's in-patient records to make them as concise, clear and convenient for clinical use as possible.

Charts – the usual style

Most hospitals have a simple in-patient chart, sometimes called a bed head ticket in government hospitals. This allows space for the clerk to fill in clerical details, and for the doctor to write the present complaint and history, details found on examination, provisional diagnosis and progress notes. Other sheets are then issued for drug and treatment orders, temperature chart (sometimes one for twice daily readings, and another for four or six-hourly), nursing notes and treatments given, plus fluid intake/output charts, and any necessary continuation sheets. To all this paper there may later be added report sheets from the laboratory or X-ray departments. All are placed in a folder and attached to a clip-board at the bed-head. When the doctor wishes to review the information collected, he has to turn over page after page before he can put the whole story together.

In the giving of treatments ordered there is a particular danger in having the doctor's orders on one sheet, and the nurse's response on another.

Changes in treatment easily cause confusion. Treatments may be duplicated, or cancellation of one order may be forgotten, so that a drug is continued long after it should have been stopped. Furthermore correlation between treatments given and the effect on the patient shown by the temperature chart and progress notes is not readily seen. Several hospitals have experimented with ways of improving in-patient charts.

Columnised medical charting

The system used at WGH Ilesha, originally devised by a Dr Willis of Canada, was described fully in Maurice King's *Medical Care in Developing Countries*, OUP 1966 (8). The charts were printed locally, and continued in use for 20 years, proving very successful. Any hospital can adapt the idea for its own use.

Design of the chart

There were two main parts to the chart, the in-patient card and the continuation sheet, both of quarto size. The latter was pasted to the former down one edge. Further continuation sheets could be added as required for however long the patient might remain in bed.

The front of the in-patient card had the necessary space for clerical details, and the doctor's history, examination and operation notes (see Figure 5.10). On the reverse side was the temperature chart, and space for other nursing

Figure 5.10: *Columnised in-patient chart, side 1. See over page for sides 2 and 3.*

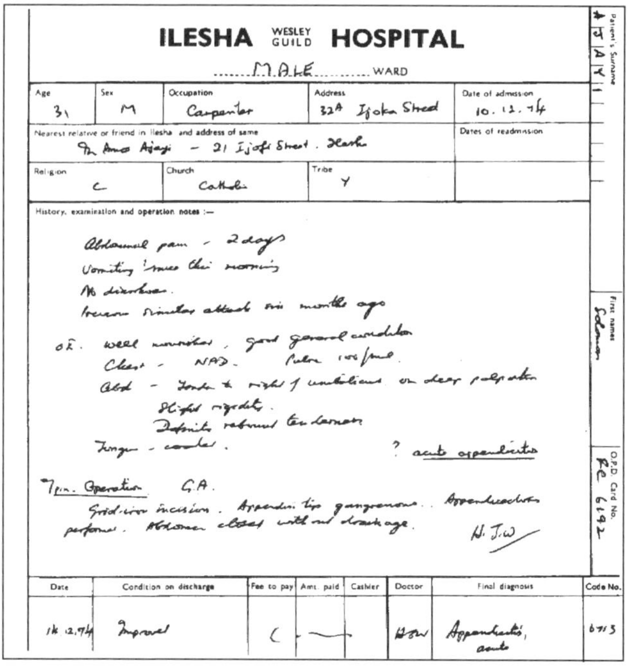
ILESHA WESLEY GUILD HOSPITAL

MALE WARD

Age	Sex	Occupation	Address	Date of admission
31	M	Carpenter	32A Ijoka Street	10.12.74

Nearest relative or friend in Ilesha and address of same — Dates of readmission

Religion: C — Church: Catholic — Tribe: Y

History, examination and operation notes :—

Patient's Surname — First names — O.P.D. Card No.

Date	Condition on discharge	Fee to pay	Amt. paid	Cashier	Doctor	Final diagnosis	Code No.
16.12.74	Improved	C	—			Appendicitis, acute	6713

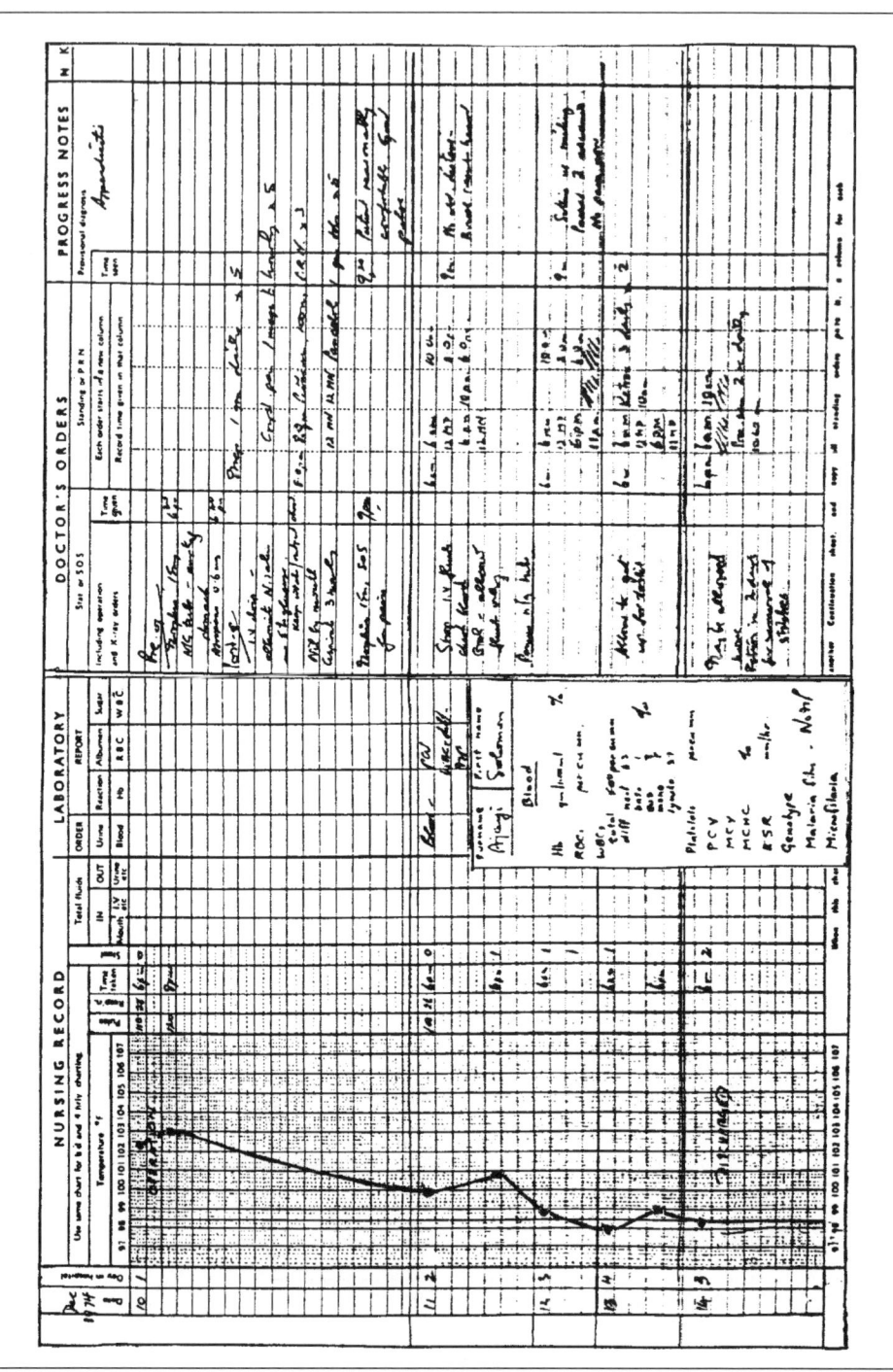

Figure 5.11: *Sides 2 and 3 of columnised in-patient chart.*

observations – pulse, respiration, stool and fluid intake/output totals. An unusual feature was that the temperature chart went down the page, rather than across it. Alongside the temperature chart, in a series of columns going right across both the card and the paper sheet, were spaces to record the patient's pulse, respiration, bowel motions, fluid balance, laboratory reports, doctors orders and the progress notes. *All the vital signs and essential on-going observations were in these parallel columns; hence the name 'columnised charting'.* Doctors and nurses used the same chart as they shared in-patient care.

The chart in use

When the charts were first introduced in 1954 the nurses, though a little doubtful at first, quickly got used to charting the temperature down the chart rather than horizontally across it. The time of observation was left for the nurse to fill in, so, when changing from four hourly to twice daily observations, for example, the same chart could continue to be used. Nurses' observations on the urine were recorded by them in the laboratory column (the blood observations were little used in practice). Laboratory investigations were ordered on small coloured slips, 150mm x 50mm (6in x 2in), with space at the bottom for the result to be written on by the technicians. The slips could then be pasted on to the chart in the laboratory column opposite the day on which the specimens were taken.

The doctor's orders were divided into:

- those given once, and
- standing orders.

The *single orders* included all drug orders to be given 'stat' or once if required (that is 's.o.s'), and also such general management orders concerning diet, insertion of naso-gastric tube, preparation for operation, and date to be allowed up, or be discharged. For drugs there was a column for the nurse to insert the time when the order was fulfilled.

Standing orders were separate because they remained in force until discontinued. This section was divided by dotted lines into several columns. Each standing order, one written under the other, *started in a new column*. The times at which the drug was given could then be written by the nurse *in that column* (look again at Figure 5.11). When the drug order was to be discontinued the doctor simply cross-hatched a square in the column under the last dose given. That column could then be used for another drug order if required. Standing orders for drugs to be given as required ('p.r.n') were also included in this section. For example, in the chart shown, Pethidine 100mg p.r.n. x 3, was discontinued on the third day, and on the fourth day 3 Ketrax tabs daily x 2 was ordered as an anthelmintic. There was room on the chart for five standing orders at any one time, and this was usually sufficient.

The fact that the *time of each drug administration was recorded by the nurse on the same sheet as the doctor's order for the drug* was a major advantage over the usual style of case sheet with separate sheets for nurse and doctor. Any charting system which fails on this score should be questioned.

At the end of each day the night-nurse drew a line across the whole of the double page, below whatever orders or observations may have been made. The first day might take up five lines or even half the page, but subsequent days, with fewer observations and orders, took up progressively less space. Chronic patients would require just two lines per day, so one page would last three weeks. The distortion which this variation in space for each day gave to the temperature graph did not seem to matter in practice.

When the bottom of the first double page was reached, side 3 was folded over, revealing a repetition of side 2. Another continuation sheet was pasted on to the spine of the chart, to provide the spread of sides 2 and 3 together again. All standing orders from the bottom of the first double page were then copied over by the nurse on to the next double page. As many continuation sheets as necessary could be added by pasting on, even if the patient stayed three months. The average stay was, of course, only six or seven days.

Chart boards

Hospitals vary as to where charts are kept while in use on the ward. Some keep them on boards in a special trolley; others hang them at the head or foot of the bed.

At WGH Ilesha the foot of the bed was used, but the columnised charts needed to be kept open at the current day's double page spread for easy review. Quick correlations could be made of temperature, pulse, laboratory findings and the drugs in use. The whole record could be seen at a glance, and progress notes added as desired. Ordinary chart boards for quarto or A4 size would have been too narrow. Wide chart boards were needed, and these were made in the hospital workshop (see Figure 5.12).

Figure 5.12: *Wide chart board for the columnised chart. Six inch (150mm) clip taken from standard 9 x 12 inch chart-board and fixed to piece of plywood 18 x 12 inch with split-rivets. Small wooden ledge on lower border.*

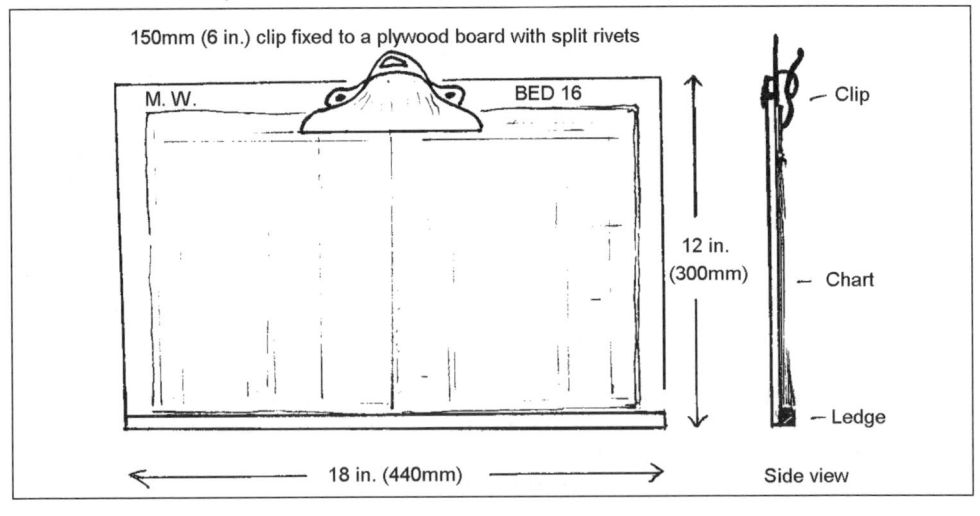

Storage of charts
When a patient was discharged the outcome of treatment, final diagnosis, disease code number and doctor's signature were placed on the front card in the space provided (see Figure 5.10). The discharge summary was written on the OP card by the doctor. Any extraneous sheets of paper that had accumulated were sorted. Some, such as detailed fluid balance sheets, could be discarded. One or two others such as the permission to operate form, signed by the patient, had to be kept for legal purposes. These were pasted in. OP cards were returned to the OP department. In-patient charts were routed via the ward sister and cashier to be stored in the medical records office (see Figure 5.13).

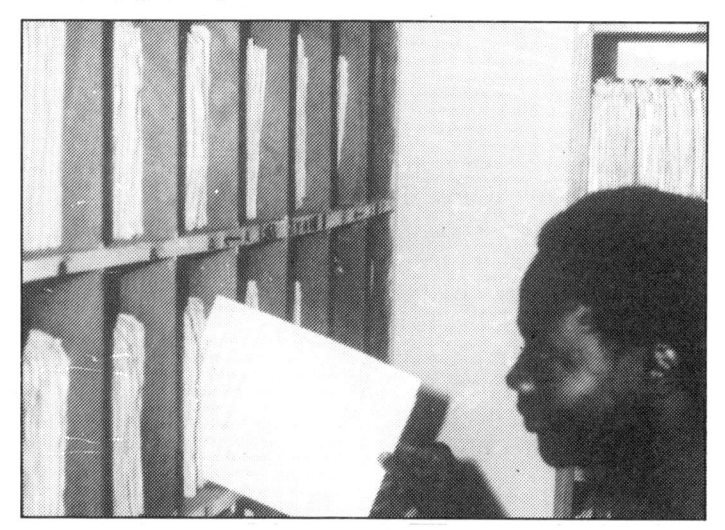

Figure 5.13: *Storage of columnised in-patient charts.*

Because the chart was in one piece, like a book, it could be stored on its side, directly on the shelf without a folder or envelope. Charts were stored in alphabetical order according to the patient's surname, which was written in capital letters along the edge of the card. It was thus immediately visible in the file. In Nigeria, where not all people used family surnames, the hospital had to ask for the husband's surname for married women, and the father's surname for children. All charts from every department were filed together in years. Some hospitals may prefer storage according to an in-patient number.

The in-patient register, or admission book

Although ward sisters may keep their own register of admissions for internal use, it is desirable that the hospital should have a master register for all in-patient admissions (and discharges). This means that there must be one receiving station, or admission room, through which all but the most dire emergencies will pass. Here the essential clerical details will be entered, the in-patient charts issued and an in-patient serial number assigned. Any patients rushed past this station, for example for imminent delivery of a baby, or an emergency with serious haemorrhage, should have their names entered later the same day, or the following morning.

Space for discharge details
If the in-patient register is ruled across a double page there should be room to leave 100mm (4 inches) on the right for details to be filled in when the patient is discharged, the date, the number of days spent in hospital, and, most important of all, the final diagnosis. There is no point in including a provisional diagnosis at the time of admission. It is the final diagnosis, made clear after investigation, observation and treatment, which matters. To make this possible it is necessary to have a system of daily returns from every ward.

Daily returns and in-patient statistics
The form for daily returns must be filled in by the ward sister every morning, detailing all patients admitted the previous day, and all patients discharged – and the number of empty beds, if any. These returns are collected up by the admission room clerk and used to complete the discharge section of the master in-patient register. It may also turn up the occasional patient who bypassed the admission room in an emergency, and where the system for reporting this the following day failed to work.

The in-patient register therefore becomes reasonably reliable, and a good source for drawing up in-patient statistics for the year. An index of diagnoses for patients treated on the wards can also be extracted.

The annual hospital report

Most hospitals produce a record of their activities for the year, the number of in-patients treated, babies delivered, or operations performed and the number of out-patients attending. It is good that these statistics should be duplicated and made available to the public. Government and voluntary agency hospitals have also to make their returns to the ministry of health or proprietor.

There is much to be said for going further and compiling a full hospital report each year, or at intervals. It should include information about achievements and new developments during the year, as well as the bare statistics. The report should list all the staff, both senior and junior. All are equally members of the hospital team.

The list of diagnoses of all in-patients can make interesting reading. Attempting to list out-patient diagnoses is generally less valuable, and very difficult to collect with any accuracy at all. Details of surgical operations performed can be obtained from the operating theatre register, and the maternity department can provide its statistics on all deliveries and related complications. The administration should be ready with a financial report and a statement of income and expenditure and balance sheet for the year.

The booklet may be enlivened with stories of special events and interesting photographs to make the whole document appealing and readable. Such a report, if printed, will not be as cheap as a duplicated news sheet, but should be considered part of a hospital's responsibility to the community it serves.

From records we move on to consider the general maintenance of the hospital, and in particular its supplies of water and power.

CHAPTER 6

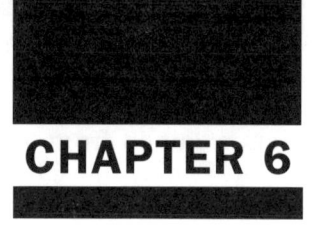

Infrastructure and Maintenance

A general practice registrar going on his first ward round with the medical superintendent of his training hospital received a surprise when they came to use an X-ray viewing box that did not work. Suspecting (correctly) that the plug was faulty, the medical superintendent took out a screwdriver from his pocket, and repaired the plug there and then. The X-ray film was duly looked at, and the ward round continued . . . The registrar had learned an unexpected lesson – that the doctor has a responsibility for his hospital and the equipment with which he works. So he resolved to carry a screwdriver as well as a stethoscope in his pocket, and to learn what he could about maintenance.

A modern hospital is a complex structure, and even a simple district hospital in the bush can present quite a challenge to the doctor who wants to see it work effectively.

> An experienced young local doctor was asked to be PMO of a 36-bed government hospital. Officially it received mains water and power, but he found that water flowed for only a few hours once or twice a week, and the power was off often for days on end. There was a high-level reserve water tank with a faulty valve, but anyway the mains pressure was rarely strong enough to lift the water so high. Of the pair of 70 kva standby diesel generators installed 10 years before, one was broken and had been cannibalised to repair the other; but the diesel consumption of that was so heavy there was rarely enough money to run it; and the starting battery was flat, and no longer retained a charge. Help from the ministry of health in the capital had been requested months before, and was still awaited . . .

The story is all too familiar, and many doctors in such a situation would shrug their shoulders, and feel helpless – but not this one. He sought help from the local community and built a low-level water tank beside the tower, so that when mains water did come it would flow into it. He obtained a small water pump to lift water to the high-level tank, and repaired the valve on that. He used 44-gallon drums to make additional reserve water tanks for the theatre and maternity, and made 6 foot high platforms for them using discarded iron bed frames. For reserve power he managed to obtain a 5 kva generator, which the hospital could afford to run, and arranged for emergency wiring to be run to the theatre and to the wards. The hospital began to function once again.

Not every doctor has experience gained from 'do-it-yourself' maintenance in his own home. What he can do safely himself may be limited. He should take every opportunity to learn what he can. The more he knows and understands about electrical and mechanical equipment, plumbing, building, painting and general repairs, the better. At the very least he should have a lively appreciation of what needs to be done, and what must be done as a priority, to maintain vital services to the patients. The development of a maintenance department, employing experienced artisans, or a hospital engineer, will be seen by him as an essential part of the hospital. Its most vital work will be in relation to the 'infra-structure' provided by water and electricity.

Infrastructure

Water is undoubtedly the most important pre-requisite for running a hospital. There are alternative sources of power for light and heating if electricity is not available, but it is difficult to run anything without water.

Water

A good water supply is the life-line of a hospital or health centre, and it may be a major factor in dictating the site on which it is to be built.

In many parts of the developing world a mains supply is still a luxury, and even if it is available, it cannot always be depended on. A hospital should make it a rule *always to have a second-line reserve water supply* – and even a third-line for the dire emergency when the second-line runs dry. Water is life.

Alternative sources of water
1. *Storage tanks for mains water.* Most hospitals have a water tower storage tank, with a capacity of 10,000 gals or so, which can see them through short breaks in supply. If pressure is frequently poor, then several ground-level, or underground tanks, are better. They can be filled from the mains, when it runs, or with the help of a mobile tanker. All tanks must be covered, to prevent contamination, and growth of algae.

   Construction of a covered underground tank need not be technically difficult, provided the soil structure is compact, and one can dig down six feet without encountering rock (see Figure 6.1). Rain water can be ducted into it and an electric or semi-rotary handpump can be used to raise the water into ceiling-level cisterns to provide gravity feed.

   Very large circular tanks, or reservoirs, of up to 100,000 gallon capacity can only be built under the supervision of a structural engineer. They should, if possible, be sited on a slope, so that they can be drained by gravity through a vent pipe at the bottom for periodic cleaning. Such a tank was built at WGH Ilesha, fairly low on the site because mains pressure was by then so often poor.

Figure 6.1: *Building an underground water tank.*

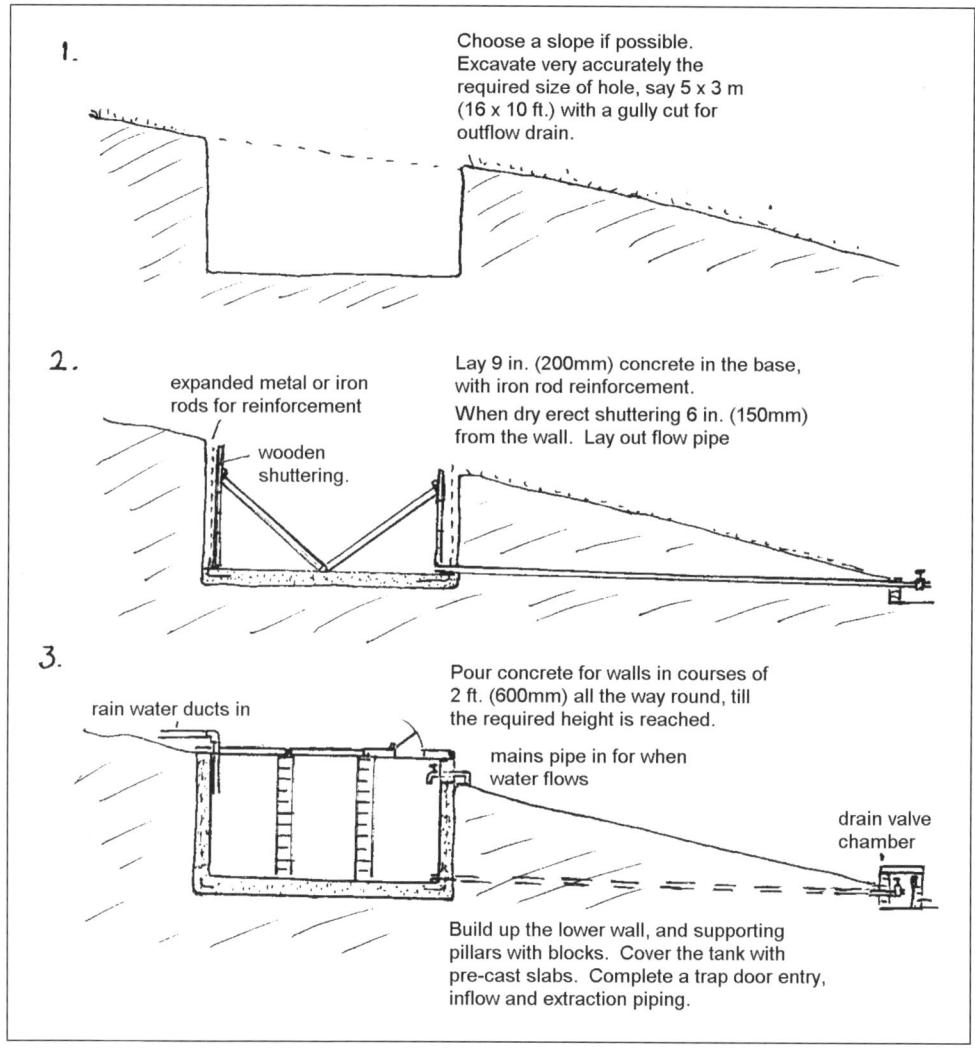

1. Choose a slope if possible. Excavate very accurately the required size of hole, say 5 x 3 m (16 x 10 ft.) with a gully cut for outflow drain.

2. expanded metal or iron rods for reinforcement / wooden shuttering.

Lay 9 in. (200mm) concrete in the base, with iron rod reinforcement.

When dry erect shuttering 6 in. (150mm) from the wall. Lay out flow pipe

3. rain water ducts in

Pour concrete for walls in courses of 2 ft. (600mm) all the way round, till the required height is reached.

mains pipe in for when water flows

drain valve chamber

Build up the lower wall, and supporting pillars with blocks. Cover the tank with pre-cast slabs. Complete a trap door entry, inflow and extraction piping.

2. *Artesian bore-hole.* This is an exciting but very expensive option, and available only in certain geological situations where a boring can reach water trapped deep down over an impermeable rock layer, or where there are fissures in a hard rock structure retaining water in adequate quantities. Most companies insist on charging the full cost of sinking a bore-hole, whether water is located or not. If found, one has a bountiful, clean and

independent source of water, which may last for many years. If not found, the outlay is wasted, so a visit from a geologist is advisable first.

3. *Surface water.* If a small stream can be dammed to create a reservoir adjacent to the site, one may have a copious reserve supply. To be dependent on a well, or wells, or a spring as the sole source, is quite inadequate, except for the smallest health facility.

ECWA Hospital, Egbe, Nigeria, is built on the lower slopes of a high hill. A stream from the hill, dammed at a point above the hospital site, provides adequate water by gravity feed for the hospital and resident community all the year round (see Figure 6.2).

4. *Rain water from roof collection.* Availability is subject to climatic and seasonal variation, but there is often more available than one thinks.

A 10-bed maternity and child-welfare centre was planned for Kaiama, in a savannah area of Nigeria with three months rainfall in the year. The design was compact, and incorporated an underground tank 20 feet by 12 feet in size, and 5 feet deep (see Figure 6.3). Strong gutters were provided for every stretch of roof, and 4-inch soil pipes used to duct the rain water collected into the tank. Water was raised through a 3/4-inch galvanised iron pipe and

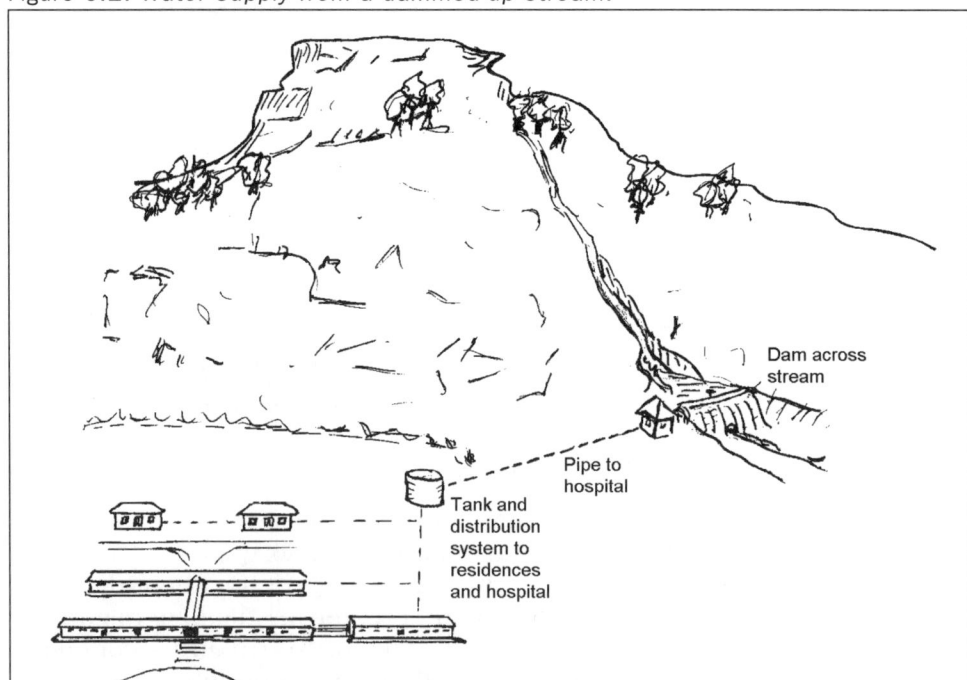

Figure 6.2: *Water supply from a dammed-up stream.*

Infrastructure and Maintenance 97

semi-rotary pump to a cistern in the roof space, to provide a running supply to several sinks. The tank itself was covered, and the inspection hatch kept locked. Supervision was tight. The centre proved popular, with many patients attending, and water was never a problem. The three months of rain provided sufficient to cover even the nine months of dry. However, some years later, when supervision was relaxed, the tank was neglected, and allowed to dry out. It cracked and began to leak, and the centre declined.

Tropical rain-storms are very heavy, and a common mistake is to use materials for guttering and ducts which are far too flimsy. 100mm (4 in) wide guttering, 50mm (2 in) deep, made from flattened out standard (gauge 24, 0.56mm) galvanised iron roofing sheets, will last little more than a season. This sight is all too common (see Figure 6.4).

Figure 6.3: *Roof-ducting to underground tank (as at Kaiama, Nigeria).*

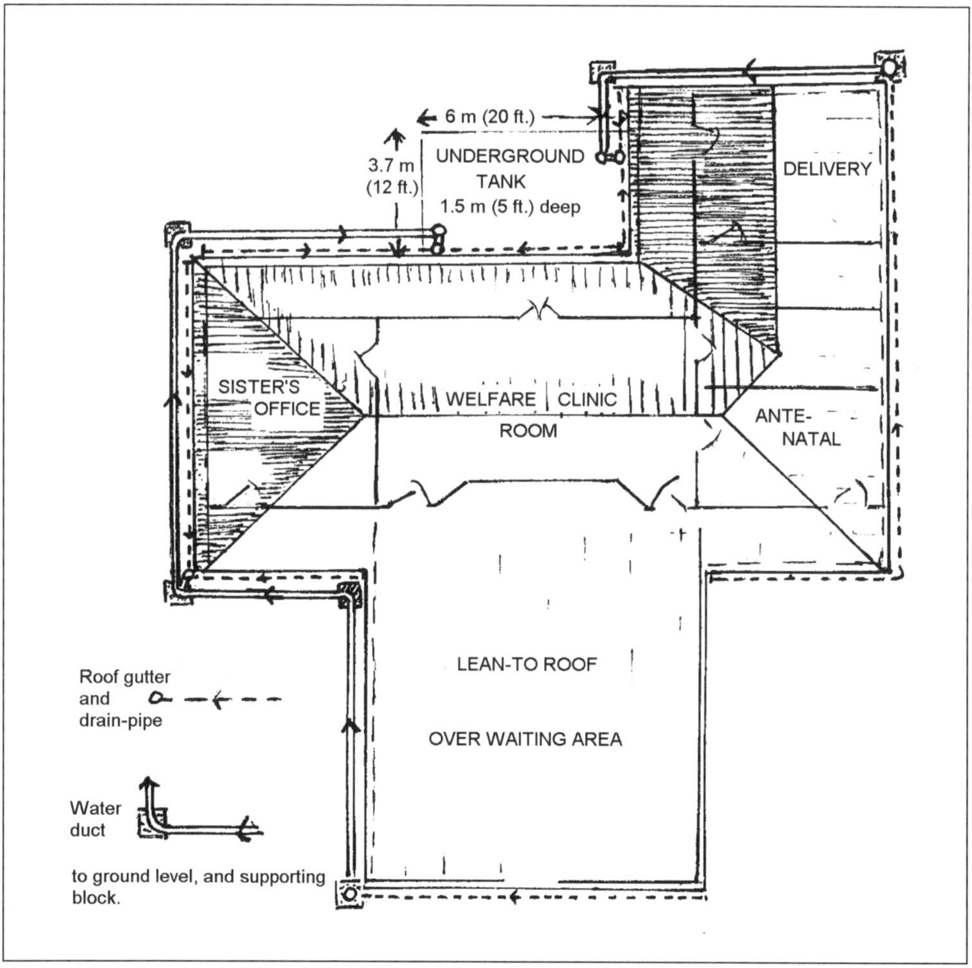

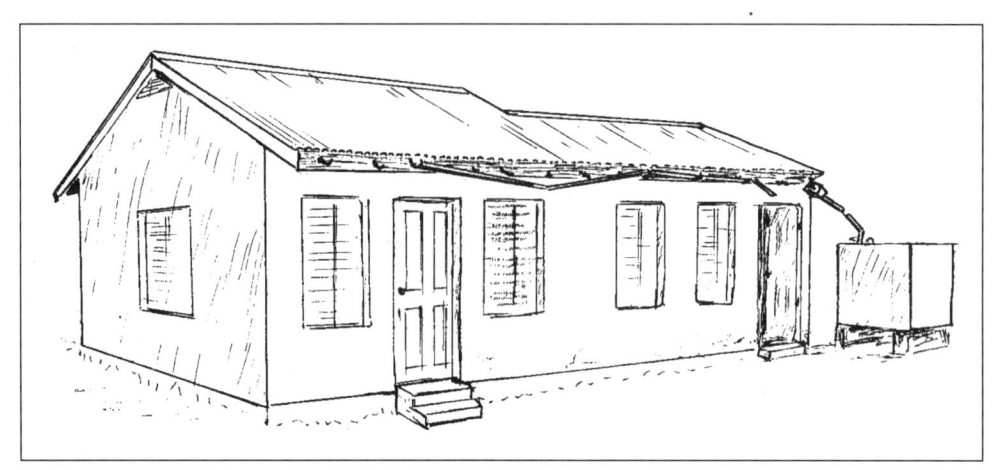

Figure 6.4: *Weak and decrepit roof guttering.*

Figure 6.5: *Strong guttering and down-pipes.*

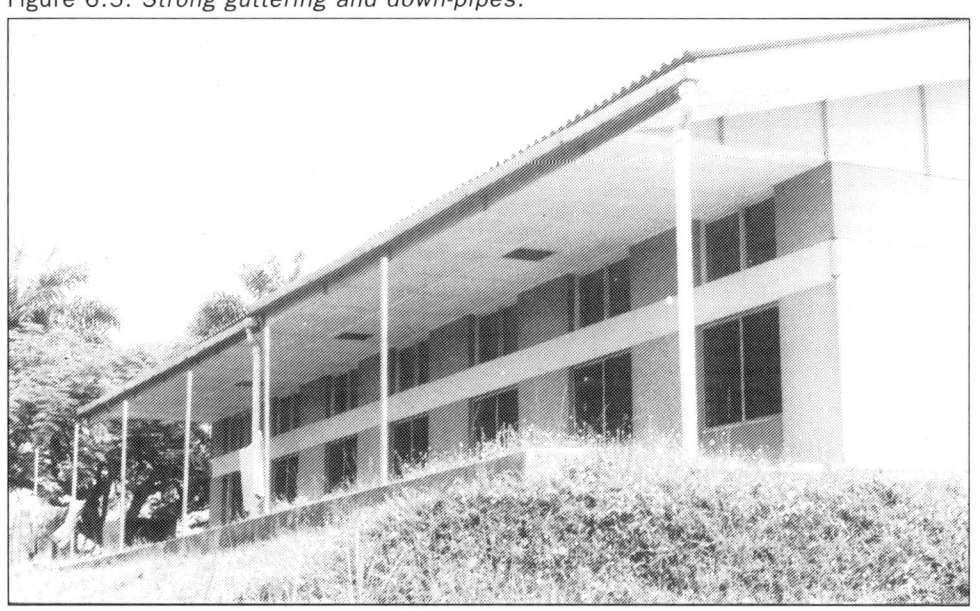

The following specifications for strong guttering should be followed:

- For a long roof the fascia board fixed to the rafters should be strong (25mm, 1 inch thick), and wide enough to allow for an adequate fall in the slope of the gutter down the length of the roof, 200 to 300mm (8 to 12 inches) according to the length of the building.

- If plastic (PVC) guttering is used it should have strengthened supports at not less than 1 metre (3 feet) intervals. Small plastic supports, as generally supplied for use in temperate countries, or rough wooden ones, are likely to be inadequate. Supports prepared from iron rod by a welder will repay their cost.

- Stronger guttering, can be made from flat g.i. sheeting, thicker than the standard 24 gauge. If available use 20 or 16 gauge (the latter 1/16th-inch thick). Successful use was made of this for the main roofs of a new maternity department at WGH Ilesha. The guttering was 150mm (6 in) wide and 100mm (4 in) deep, and fixed with iron brackets every 900mm (3 feet). It proved comparatively expensive, because the items had to be made to order, but has functioned well for 15 years (see Figure 6.5).

- The collecting pipes must also be strong. When asbestos-cement soil pipes were in common use, as when the Kaiama MCH centre was built, they proved excellent for the purpose. Being rigid they could be supported with a short, stout concrete pillar at the bottom, and right-angle bends used at the top for collection from the gutters. PVC piping would need additional support. Remember what force there can be in a tropical storm, and the weight of water in overflowing gutters and ducts.

Quantity and quality of water needed
The most important decision to be made in building, or modernising, a hospital or health centre concerns the extent to which water is to be used for sanitation. If water-closets, leading to septic-tanks, are to be used then 10 gallons (5 buckets) of water per user resident per day should be provided. If pit latrines are to be used, then 3 gallons (1.5 buckets) per person per day should be sufficient.

This matter is discussed in more detail in 'A model health centre' (6). Calculations there show, for example, that a busy 10-bed centre, with 200 out-patients per day, and undertaking surgery and maternity care, would need 3000 gallons per day if water-borne sanitation is to be introduced. Without it, and depending entirely on pit-latrines, 200 to 600 gallons per day should be sufficient, depending on the services given.

Having 'to manage'
Unfortunately many hospitals have been built without making these calculations, and have found the available water supply quite insufficient. WCs, installed in hope, have had to be locked up, and patients asked to use old pit latrines, or even to 'go bush'. In other cases, the water supply which was fine at first, has become woefully inadequate owing to heavier usage by a growing population, or because the dam, or other source of mains supply, and the purification plant, have been poorly maintained. Few developing countries have the money to put towards improvements and expansion at a pace to match growing demand.

People can manage on less water, by flushing toilets just once or twice a day, rather than after every usage, though this is far from ideal. Washing with a shower, or with a half-bucket (1 gallon) of water in a bath, is economical, and the used water can be collected and re-used to flush toilets. Bucket and pit latrines are not popular, because of smell, and the attraction to flies. If water shortage rules out a full water-borne system, modified pit latrines or aqua privies are a possibility (see next chapter).

In a hospital, where water is not only needed for sanitation, washing and drinking, but also, very heavily, for cleaning and sterilisation, the first service to be curtailed when the water supply fails is the performance of elective surgery. Emergency surgery and midwifery are carried on with difficulty.

A sufficient quantity of water is the first consideration in most developing countries. Quality, unfortunately, tends to come second.

Water that has been piped into a house has been shown to be far more effective in combating water-borne disease, than water brought only as far as a stand-pipe in the road outside. Water in the house is used in greater quantity than water which has to be carried.

Purification of water

If mains water has been provided for a township from which the hospital can benefit, one hopes that the authorities have been able to put in a water treatment plant at source. If not, and the hospital has to pump from a polluted source like a river, it may be wise to consider building a sand-filtration plant. Morgan, in his excellent book, *Rural Water Supplies and Sanitation*(13), describes a filter system which can provide 300 people with 20 litres a day, but notes that the process is a slow one, and there needs to be a relatively large pre-treatment reservoir where excess silt can settle, and a storage tank, post-treatment, into which the treated water can flow before being drawn off for use. Maintenance is almost cost free, but must be done with great care. Morgan also describes the alternative method of treatment with chlorine, which costs a little more. For this one must obtain the chloride of lime or alginate. The latter is easier to store without waste. Daily attention to the system is necessary.

Should neither method be possible, water provided in a hospital for drinking may have to be boiled and filtered, or treated by ultra-violet light by placing in clear plastic bags or bottles, and exposing to sunshine for 30–60 minutes. More technical equipment for this is also becoming available.

Power

The energy requirements of a hospital are a major contributor to running costs. Decisions have to be made as to the most cost-effective source in relation to the various purposes for which energy is required. These will be made in the light of the availability of supply, effectiveness, cost per unit, and convenience or suitability. Electricity, bottled gas, kerosene and firewood are still the main sources, but solar power is becoming an increasingly available alternative which some would like to see put first (see p.104).

Choosing the energy source

- For lighting, electricity is undoubtedly to be preferred over kerosene, gas or candles, in terms of effectiveness, cost and convenience, so long as it is available.

- For running motors, such as ceiling fans, water-pumps, centrifuges, suction machines and drills, the amount of electricity used is small, so long as it is available when needed. However, remember that hand-operated semi-rotary pumps, drills or centrifuges may still have a place, and the foot-operated Ambu suction pump is rightly popular.

- For refrigeration, with compressors, the cost of electricity is moderate, and so much more convenient than kerosene refrigeration. Therefore electricity will generally be chosen if it is available on a 24-hour basis, and with a minimum danger of power cuts. If power cuts do become common, it may well be necessary to keep a kerosene refrigerator for use as a back-up, and have a good manual on how to use it (7) in case staff have forgotten. Running a deep-freeze is more expensive, because of the lower temperatures which have to be maintained.

- Air conditioning, though it depends upon a motor to drive the compressor for cooling, and fan for distribution, is nevertheless a heavy user of electricity because of the work which has to be done in cooling entire rooms, (though usually with recirculation of the air), and the length of time units have to be on. Great caution should be exercised before allowing the installation of air-conditioners just for convenience. Essential purposes may include cooling of the operating theatre, X-ray department, or stores used for items spoiled by heat. Improving ventilation and working conditions by ceiling fans, or by design of rooms to secure through ventilation and shade over windows should always be tried first.

> At WGH Ilesha, the only air-conditioning, pre 1975, was a special large unit for the operating theatre, which did not re-circulate any internal air. Apart from that, the climate was such, at 1200 feet above sea level, that, in rooms with good through ventilation, even fans were not essential. We called it 'natural air-conditioning'. In some countries, such as Ghana and parts of India, air conditioning in the offices of public buildings, and in private houses, is forbidden because of the excessive load this places on the mains power supply. Air conditioning is limited to certain essential services, such as those mentioned above.

- Electricity used to generate heat for cooking, autoclaving or boiling water is always expensive, and should only be chosen when the time during which power is required is very limited, or when suitability and convenience outweigh the expense. For example a thermostatically controlled electric kettle uses 1 kw of power, but boils the water in less than 5 minutes and then turns itself off, so the expense of running it is limited, and its convenience very great.

The difference between lighting and heating is not always realised
An electric autoclave, using 12 kilowatts of power, switched on for 1 hour a day, uses as much electricity as the lighting provided by forty 60 watt bulbs left on for 5 hours a day.

Alternative means of cooking in hospital kitchen and staff houses on the hospital compound should be the rule. Firewood, kerosene or bottled gas should be used according to availability, cost and personal preference, but electric cookers should be ruled out.

> At WGH Ilesha, firewood was used in the main stove in the hospital kitchen, preparing food for all patients daily. The stove was built to an Indian design, the Herl stove (see page 126), and worked efficiently for over 30 years.
>
> Firewood was also used to produce steam for sterilising. Small logs were fed into a vertical, 8 foot high, Weldun steam boiler (of 200 pounds per hour output at a pressure of 20 pounds per square inch). The steam was passed through lagged pipes to theatre and central sterile supply department, for the autoclave and boiling sterilisers. Operation was very cost-effective.

Some hospitals have used kerosene burners to heat autoclaves. One has to accept that the containers will become blackened by soot. For cleanness and convenience electricity is ideal for hospital autoclaving and sterilising *as long as sufficient power is available.*

> Our Lady's Hospital at Iseyin, Nigeria, used a small, vertical electric autoclave, run by two nurse aides under the supervision of a nursing sister, and covered all the sterilising needs of the theatre, maternity department and wards. Sterile instrument packs were prepared for all major operations and stored on shelves in a room adjacent to the operating theatre.

Standby generators
If a hospital is dependent on its own generators entirely, or for long periods of time when mains power is off, *then the size of the generator must match the demand.* If it is too small then it will not produce full voltage for lighting, and the lights will be dim. The generator may stop altogether when heavy use equipment items such as sterilisers or air-conditioners are switched on.

If, on the other hand, the generator is too large, though there will be no danger of overload, the fuel consumption and expense will be heavy. A lightly loaded generator also runs less efficiently than one just below maximum load. The generator should be neither too small, nor too large.

> When WGH Ilesha had only 75 beds, and electricity was used mainly for lighting the wards, heating a few boiling sterilisers, and operating a 30 milliamp portable X-ray machine, a 4.5 kva diesel generator was sufficient. When the hospital was rebuilt on a larger site with 120 beds, and with light provided to staff houses, and street lighting for the road network, then a 10 kva generator was provided, with a second beside it for when the first was being serviced.

> As the hospital grew over the years to 200 beds, a larger number of resident staff and nursing students, technical departments with more equipment, and a 400 milliamp X-ray machine, the generators were replaced, first with 25 kva machines, and later with 60 kva machines.

The 70 kva generators supplied as standard to some government 36-bed district hospitals would appear to be far in excess of need, and unduly expensive to run. A 44-gallon drum of diesel fuel would be required every 24 hours. Emergency power for the theatre, maternity and ward lighting can be provided with a 5 kva machine, with a fuel requirement a small fraction of the above.

Doctors, who find themselves without back-up power for their own residence, may find, as the author did at Igbo-Ora, that a 2.5 kva petrol driven Honda generator, was sufficient for all domestic use – lighting, fans, electric iron, refrigerator, small deep freeze, and a second refrigerator for health centre vaccines.

Rationing power supply

Once a hospital becomes dependent on electricity it should be remembered that power is needed by day as well as by night. It is needed for light at night, particularly from 6 pm to 11 pm, but also all through the night for good nursing, and care of emergencies. If economy dictates that the generators should be turned off at 11 pm, emergency lighting, for example with paraffin hurricane lamps, can be provided. Some hospitals have developed small battery-operated systems, whether for the theatre alone, or for wards as well, using 12-volt bulbs as in car headlights, with a trickle charger to recharge the batteries next day.

Power is also needed by day – for the laboratory centrifuge, for the theatre lamp and suction-pump, for the X-ray, and in many cases also for sterilising. All these purposes are as important to the hospital as light at night. If there has to be rationing, let there be five hours by night and five hours by day, and not just the period at night alone.

Light bulbs

Ordinary light bulbs (globes) have a limited life, and lights should be switched off whenever they are not needed. However, bulbs do 'blow' after a few weeks, and often this is first noticed at night, particularly if in a vital position. It is important that the night sister, or the doctor doing the night round, has access to a small supply of replacement bulbs of the various sizes required. He should know how to change the bulb himself, or be able to call someone to help.

Some light bulbs have to be left on all through the night hours, e.g. on corridors, or even for the 24-hour day, e.g. when used for providing slightly warmed, dry air, as in a simple baby-incubator, or linen cupboard, or inside a piano. In such cases it is an advantage to have two bulbs wired in series. At half voltage each bulb will burn at half brightness. Together, warmth and light produced will be the same, but the bulbs will last for a year or more.

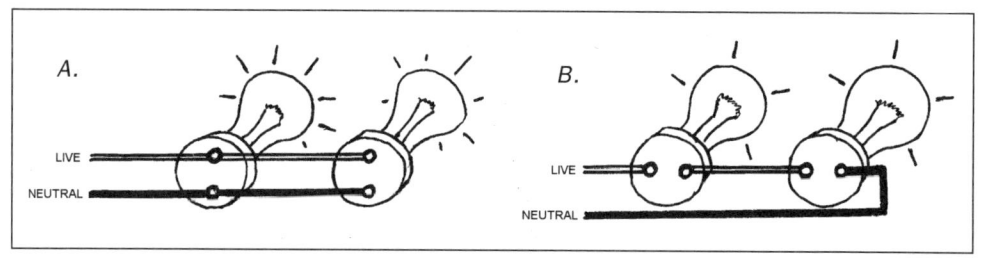

Figure 6.6: *A. Normal wiring of two bulbs in parallel — each gets full voltage. B. Wiring of two bulbs in series — voltage shared.*

Alternatively, a hospital may make use of strip-lights, which cost more to install, but provide bright illumination with low electricity consumption. Intermittent function will often give warning when a strip needs replacement. This can be reported to the maintenance department the following day.

Solar power

Solar power is now used very commonly for water heating in countries such as Israel, Australia and Papua New Guinea. Though running costs are just those of maintenance, capital costs are still relatively high, and solar-powered equipment has yet to be widely adopted in developing countries.

Solar power has been applied in hospitals to the pre-heating of water for laundry services, refrigeration, water pumps and emergency lighting. Maurice King (8) described its use for water heating (see Figure 6.8). The system depends simply on the absorption of heat from the sun's rays by water in a series of pipes under glass in a heat collector. The hot water moves upwards to be stored in an insulated container till needed. Cool water flows from below into the pipes, to be heated in turn.

Direct conversion of the sun's energy into electricity is achieved through the photo-voltaic (PV) cell. Current generated is stored in batteries, from which a continuous DC supply can be obtained to run refrigerators, pumps or lighting systems. Derrick (9) has reported on the extensive trials in Zaïre, where local manufacture has started. Capital installation costs of a PV-powered refrigerator are still about $5000, compared to about $1500 for a kerosene-powered one, but the initial costs may be offset by the free energy supply from the sun, improved reliability and reduced vaccine loss.

Undoubtedly, as costs come down, such equipment will become common-place in tropical countries where solar energy is available in such abundance. Medical administrators should be ready to invest in solar-powered items of equipment as soon as their cost comes within affordable range.

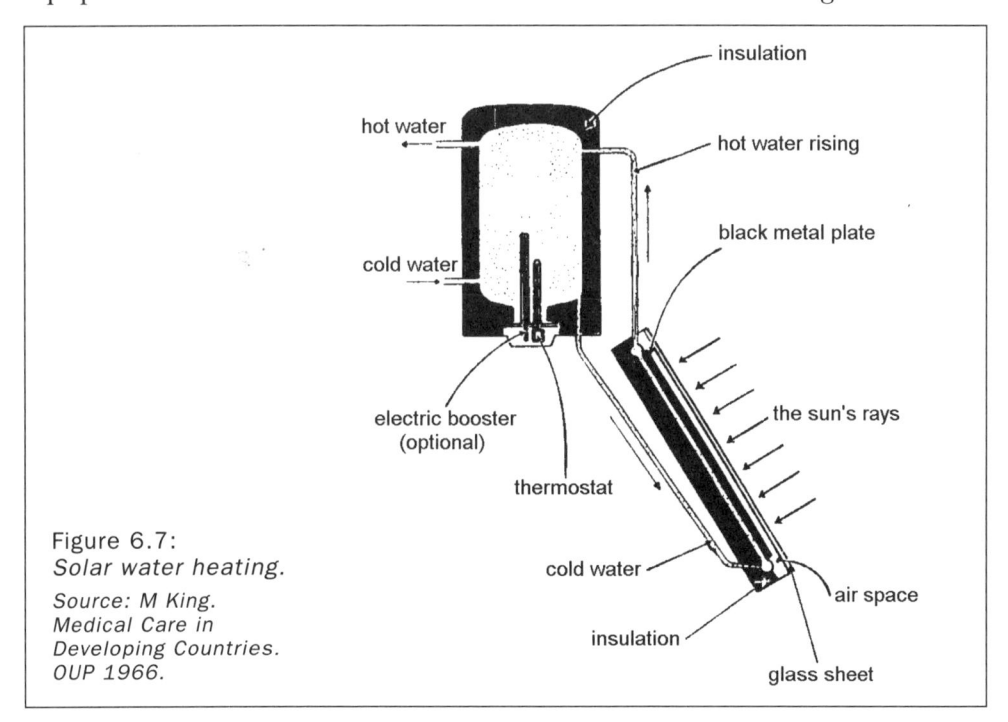

Figure 6.7:
Solar water heating.
Source: M King.
Medical Care in
Developing Countries.
OUP 1966.

Hospital maintenance

The maintenance department
Staff required
Every hospital or health centre needs staff whose responsibility it is to maintain the fabric. In a health centre it may just be a clerk/handyman, or a driver-mechanic. In a well-managed hospital there should be a full team of artisans, and maybe even a hospital engineer. The need for such staff is

frequently not allowed for in the budget, for example in government hospitals, since it is argued that maintenance work can be carried out by a mobile team from a central Works Department, or even by a separate Ministry of Works.

The slow response which this brings to the routine maintenance requirements of these hospitals is unfortunate. There is enough work in each hospital for some staff, though in the smallest centres the multicompetent handyman may be more useful than a fully trained artisan strictly limited to his own trade. The experience gained at WGH Ilesha is now given as one example of how maintenance needs can be met.

> WGH Ilesha in 1952, when only 75 beds in size, employed a driver-mechanic, who looked after vehicles and generator. A carpenter was employed to make furniture for the new hospital when it was being rebuilt in 1953, and he stayed on permanently as hospital carpenter. He was never idle for one day in 20 years. As the hospital grew to 150 and 200 beds the artisan team was gradually extended as the work-load increased. In 1975 it included:
>
> 3 mechanics, 2 electricians, 2 carpenters,
>
> 2 bricklayers, 1 plumber, 1 painter and 3 assorted apprentices.
>
> There was also a visiting consultant engineer, of great all-round competence, who stayed for varying periods and contributed immensely to the relatively high standard of maintenance achieved.
>
> The maintenance department included a mechanic's, electrician's and plumber's workshop, with a store for spare parts, a carpenter's shed and wood store, and a painter's store. For much of the time the artisans were out on jobs around the hospital. Many minor building extensions within the compound were carried out entirely by them.

Provision of tools

Although a carpenter generally has his own set of tools, many essential tools have to be provided by the hospital for the workshops, including workbenches with vices. An electric power drill, with hammer mode and masonry bits, size 12 or 14, and the appropriate plastic or fibre wall-plugs, can revolutionise the carpenter's work in putting up shelves or other wall fittings. Carborundum oil stones for sharpening knives, and necessary tools for car servicing, electrical work, and plumbing, must be included.

Notification of repairs to be done

The hospital manager, matron and medical superintendent should carry maintenance request forms in their pockets, or have them at their respective offices. If any staff member reports an item of equipment in need of repair, or if any defect is noted personally, then the place and item can be written down at once, before it is forgotten, and sent forthwith through the hospital manager to the maintenance department, for the attention of the appropriate artisan. When the artisans are on site there is no great delay between notification and effecting action, so long as a remedy is within their power. Referral by the administration to outside contractors is, of course, necessary for major matters, such as rewinding electric motors or repair of the X-ray.

Preventive maintenance
An effort should be made to see that equipment, once installed, is given the periodic check-ups recommended by the makers, for cleaning, oiling, and replacement of worn parts. The conception of preventive care in relation to machinery and equipment, does not come easily to the average person. Many prefer to use equipment continuously till it breaks down and will not work at all. There is then no alternative to spending money on a major repair. Such people fail to appreciate that spending a little money on routine servicing, while an item of equipment is still working, will improve its efficiency and greatly extend its life. This is preventive maintenance.

Its importance is one major lesson which all those responsible for hospital upkeep should learn, and none more so than the Medical Superintendent himself. A smoothly functioning hospital, with the minimum of frustration due to breakdowns, contributes to good morale, and hence the effectiveness of the 'healing community'. Routine preventive maintenance of hospital vehicles may even prove the saving of lives.

Care of instruments
In this area of maintenance the doctors have an obvious personal interest.

Diagnostic instruments
The stethoscope, sphygmomanometer, auroscope and ophthalmoscope, are extensions of the physician's ears, eyes and hands. They are the everyday tools of his trade. Just as a carpenter keeps his chisels and other tools sharp, so the doctor should take some responsibility for his own diagnostic instruments.

- Stethoscopes are simple enough, but need some care. The ear-pieces need to be unscrewed occasionally, and any aural wax removed. Stethoscopes that are hung up in a consulting room, and not used every day, may be an attraction to mason wasps that can build a mud nest in the tube. One may then be surprised to find that the stethoscope has become mono-aural. Sound is conducted through one side only. This may be confirmed by blowing through one ear piece, with a finger blocking the chest piece opening. If this does not produce a jet of air from the other side, take action to poke out the mud and wash clean.

- Mercury sphygmomanometers are notorious for developing faults in tropical heat. Rubber tubing perishes, particularly near to junctions where stretched. Cutting off an inch of tube and refitting may help for a time. Replacement pressure-tubing should be available.

A leaking pressure release valve can sometimes be repaired, but leaks from the hand bulb, or the cuff and armband, generally mean that replacement is needed. The glass tube for the mercury column needs to be cleaned from time to time, and a pipe-cleaner is usually supplied with each new sphygmomanometer. In doing this, great care should be exercised not to allow any of the mercury to spill out and escape. Use a metal tray to work on, so that, should there be any spill, it is contained (see Figure 6.8). Place the sphygmomanometer in the tray, laying it on its side, with the mercury reservoir downwards. The mercury drains back into the reservoir, leaving the glass tube clear. Get a second person to help. One lifts the cap at the top against the strong spring which holds it, while the other levers out the tube. Moisten the pipe-cleaner with spirit, and thread in from either end to clean. Replace the tube with the '0' at the lower end, and the scale marks at the front.

Sometimes the chamois leather disc in the metal vent cap at the top of the tube becomes clogged with oxidised mercury, causing the pressure to rise or fall sluggishly when the instrument is in use. Replacement of the disc is very easy if the right material is available. A rubber disc is no use. Mercury cannot escape, but neither can air. Filter paper is no use. Air can pass through, but so (surprisingly) can mercury. It must be chamois leather. Spare discs cost next to nothing.

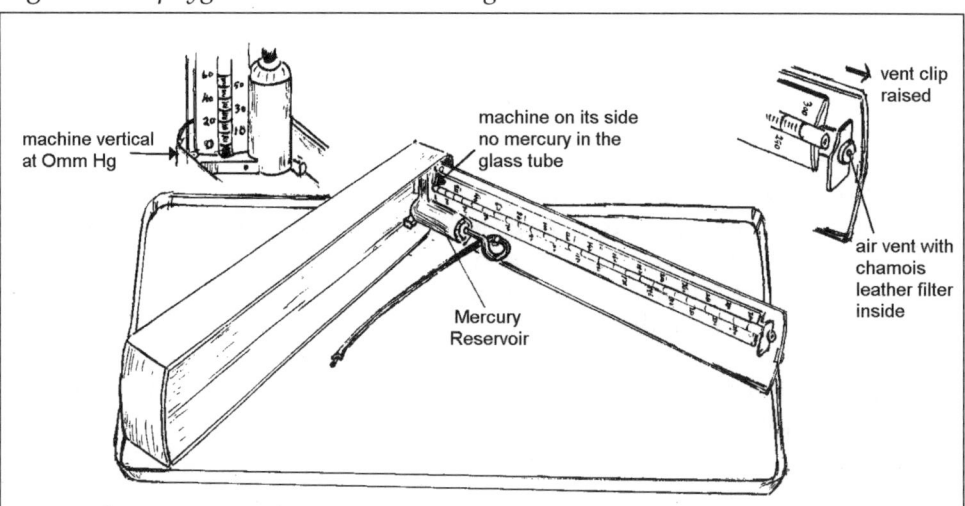

Figure 6.8: *Sphygmomanometer servicing.*

Faulty sphygmomanometers give inaccurate readings – too high or too low. New sphygmomanometers are expensive. It is worth making sure that spare tubing, valves, rubber bulbs, arm-bands and cuffs (adult size 9 x 5 inches), and chamois leather discs are kept in stock.

Aneroid sphygmomanometers tend to have fewer faults, but are considerably less accurate. In one comparison by Burke *et al* (10) fewer than 2 per cent of mercury sphygmomanometers, but 30 per cent of aneroid instruments, had errors greater than 4 mm Hg, when tested at pressures of 90 and 150 mm Hg.

- Auroscope/ophthalmoscope diagnostic sets are often hard to maintain in bulbs and batteries. If a doctor carries his own set, a pair of batteries may last a year. If the hospital supplies a set on a consulting room desk used by various doctors and nurses, the battery tends to last only a week. The switch is so easily left on, or may even get pushed on inadvertently as the instrument is replaced in its box. To prevent the latter it is a good rule to ask staff always to unscrew the head of the 'scope' from the handle, before replacement in the box. This automatically turns it off wherever the switch lever may be. The nurse or aide who checks and tidies up consulting rooms each day, should be taught how to check auroscopes/ophthalmoscopes for functioning batteries, and be advised how to obtain replacements. Some hospitals may prefer doctors to have their own set, or to take personal responsibility for one hospital set and keep it always working.

Sets which still do not work with a new battery, or change of bulb, should be sent to the maintenance department for a check. Faults on the switch rheostat, or due to poor contact with the spring at the base of the handle, can often be corrected.

Surgical and other instruments
1. *Keeping knives and scissors sharp*
   Most hospitals use scalpels with replaceable blades (Bard-Parker), but at times solid scalpel blades, or the blades of a skin-grafting dermatome, may need to be sharpened. If possible, a theatre assistant should be taught the technique, using a carborundum oil stone. To test for sharpness, look first at the edge of the knife. A sharp edge should not be visible to the naked eye. Test it on the back of a finger-nail that has been moistened with saliva (see Figure 6.9). Resting the knife on the nail by its own weight only, then move the blade over the nail. If it slips across the nail easily, it is blunt. If it 'bites' on to the nail, it is sharp.

   Scissors can be greatly improved by simply tightening the axis screw a fraction, and flattening the rivet end on the other side with a light hammer (see Figure 6.10). A grindstone or a fine carborundum held across the blade, and moved longitudinally up and down it, may be used for freshening up the cutting edges (see Figure 6.11).

2. *Needles*

The use of fresh, disposable needles for every injection is an ideal rarely reached, as yet, in developing countries. If as HIV prevalence rises, there is more urgency to achieve it. So-called disposable needles tend to be boiled and reused many times. One can at least eliminate all needles that have become 'hooked', by drawing the needle back through a piece of gauze or cotton wool. The tell-tale wisp of cotton sticking to it indicates the hook. Sharpening of needles on a fine grindstone is possible, but rarely satisfactory.

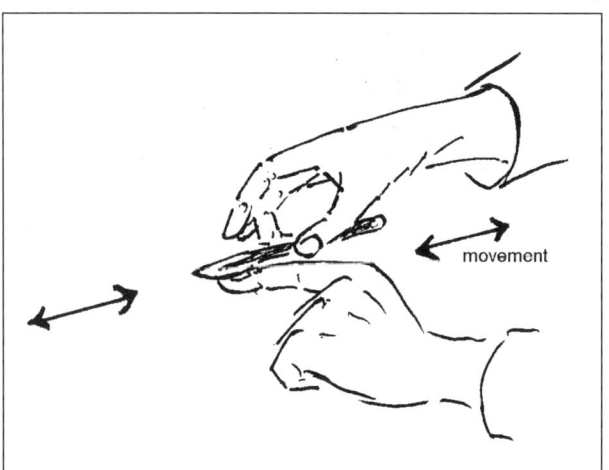

Figure 6.9: *Testing a blade for sharpness.*

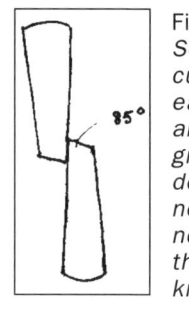

Figure 6.11: *Scissor blades cut against each other, and are therefore ground at 85 degrees (i.e. nearly flat); never sharpen them like a knife blade.*

Figure 6.10a and 6.10b: *Tightening a pair of scissors.*

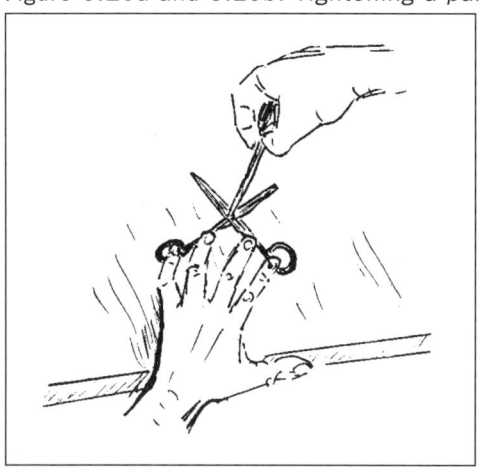

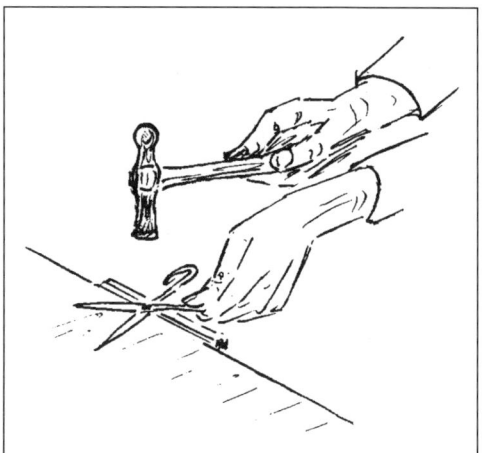

Infrastructure and Maintenance

3. *Suction machines*

   Electric suction machines generally have a long life, and just need care in cleaning. If the glass rim of the bottle becomes chipped, the lid gasket will not seal, and no vacuum can be drawn. After cleaning, nurses are taught to put in about 200 ml of antiseptic fluid to sterilise the mucus or pus which may be next drawn into it (see Figure 6.12).

Figure 6.12: *Care of suction machines.*

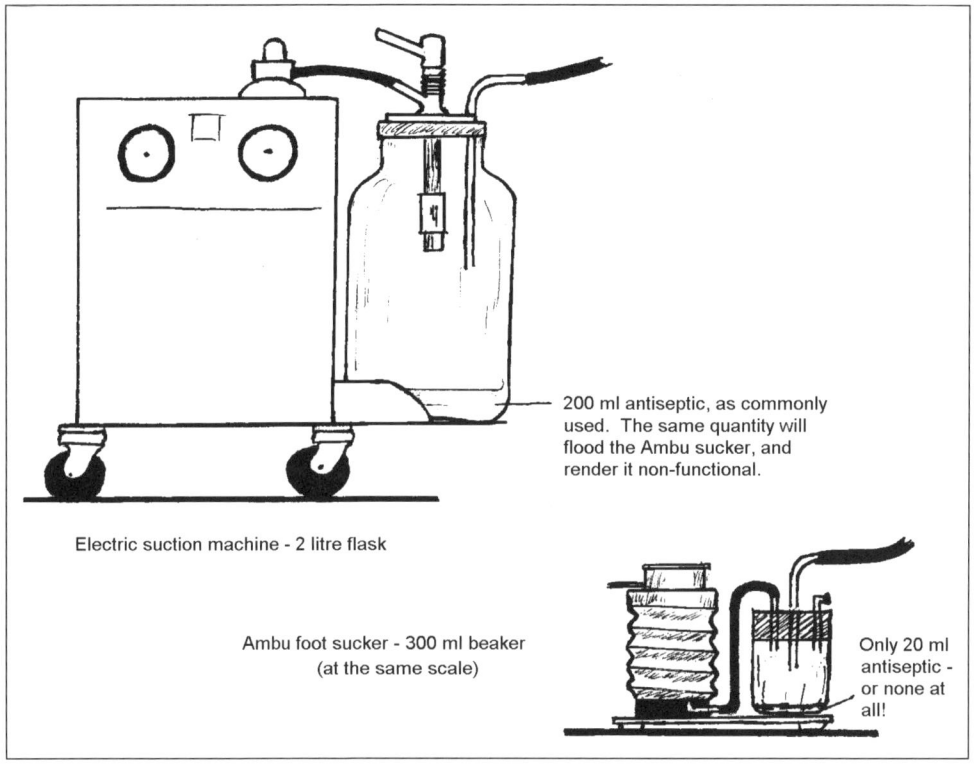

200 ml antiseptic, as commonly used. The same quantity will flood the Ambu sucker, and render it non-functional.

Electric suction machine - 2 litre flask

Ambu foot sucker - 300 ml beaker (at the same scale)

Only 20 ml antiseptic - or none at all!

The Ambu foot sucker is most valuable as a standby, particularly in paediatric wards or delivery rooms, should power not be available. It is very sturdy, and though its plastic suction jar is small, about 300 ml, it is sufficient for small volumes of mucus or meconium. However, if the nurse or aide who cleans the jar after use puts in the usual 200 ml of antiseptic, less than half the air space will be left, and it is highly likely that fluid will be drawn over into the bellows when the instrument is next used. Education of staff to put only 20 ml of fluid in, or none at all, is the only way to keep the sucker functioning.

Making splints and other equipment

There are many pieces of equipment which the carpenter and mechanic can make in the hospital workshop, sometimes with the help of a local blacksmith and welder. Wooden splints, Thomas' splints, gallows traction frames, walking irons, chart-boards, food trolleys and dispensing trolleys were all made at WGH Ilesha. Further ideas for making drip stands, wheel-chairs and aids for the disabled can be found in the Intermediate Technology publication, *Making Health-care Equipment* (42). (See also p.194).

Dr Awojobi at Eruwa in Nigeria has been making his own hospital equipment for years with the help of his local blacksmith, and reckons he can equip a small hospital for about £800. His ingenious designs include an operating table which pumps up to the required height using a hydraulic pump adapted from the type sold for use in repairing cars. A hospital water still (43), with the boiler adapted from a butane gas cylinder, and using other locally available materials, has worked for 10 years. With an industrial gas burner, the rate of production of distilled water is 6 litres per hour. The cost of making the still was only £50, as against £600 for an imported brand made of glass and operating on electricity (see Figure 6.13).

Figure 6.13: *Production of distilled water.*

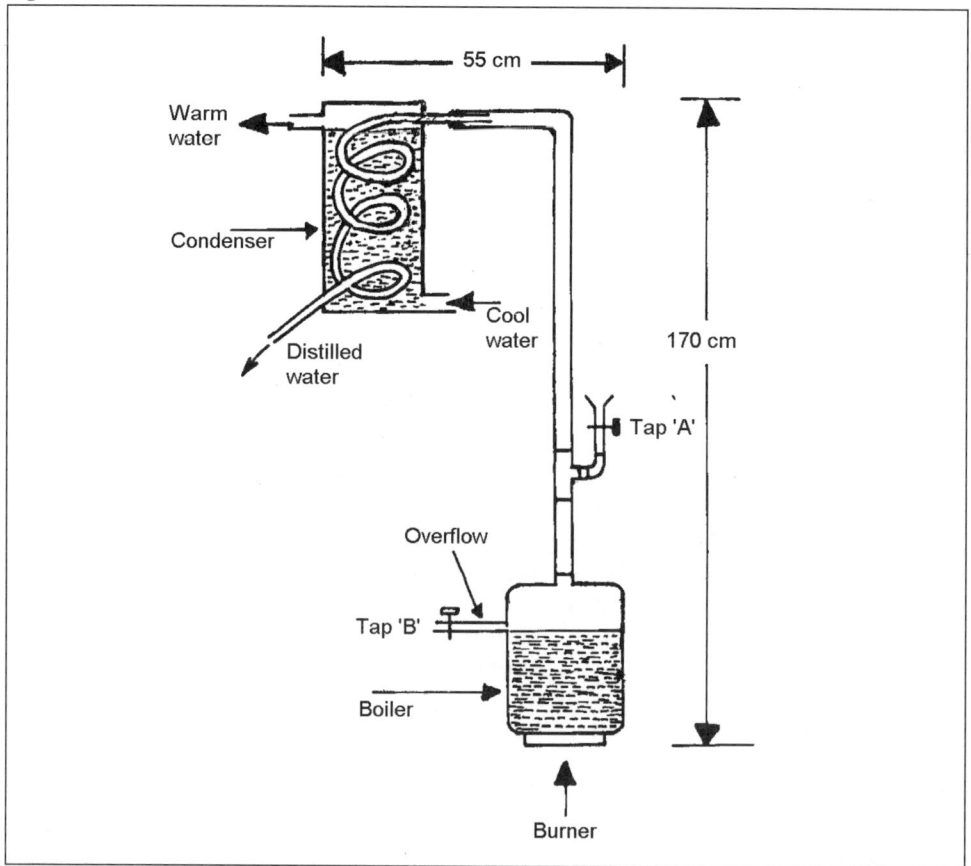

Care of buildings and furnishings
Cleaning of floors
Common domestic skills include dry sweeping of floors with a broom, or wet sweeping of concrete yards and swilling with buckets of water. Techniques of floor cleaning suitable for hospital use cannot be presumed. They have to be taught. This may include the use of scrubbing brush, soap and a little water, and then all excess water is picked up with a floor mop, or removed by rubber squeegee. This is the appropriate technique for hardened concrete or terrazzo floors.

Plastic vinyl tile floors need special care. How often one sees such a floor, which looked beautiful at first, and yet after 2 or 3 years it has been ruined. In places the tile edges are curling up, with corners knocked off, and in some patches many tiles have become loosened and lost. This is not just wear and tear. It is primarily due to wrong cleaning methods. The floor has been treated like a concrete yard with floods of water and a broom. Water in excess softens the adhesive between the tiles, and penetrates behind them. The tile edges curl up as the tiles dry. As people walk over them, and beds or trolleys are pulled around, the tiles are vulnerable to being scuffed, kicked or broken.

The rule for these floors is *minimum water*. Water must never be poured on. If scrubbed with soap and water, the water must be dried off at once with another large floor cloth. Black marks from rubber heels, or bed wheels, or due to some of the black adhesive oozing between the tiles, is best removed by a kind of 'dry cleaning' without water at all. Firm rubbing with a dry cloth and Vim (or similar) powder is much the most effective cleaning technique. Incidentally, never use kerosene. It is worse than water for penetrating behind the tiles.

Washing walls
Not only floors in a hospital, but walls as well need cleaning. This is so little appreciated by most ward orderlies that the hospital may find it best to employ one person full time on the job, and going round the entire hospital, under appropriate supervision. The job includes brushing cobwebs from ceilings and upper parts of walls and washing or scrubbing, say, from 5 feet (1.6 m) to floor level. Where gloss paint is applied to this area many scrubbings can be done before repainting is necessary. Many believe that walls that have been emulsion painted cannot be washed, as used to be the case with old fashioned non-washable distemper, or with whitewash. This is not true.

Emulsion painted surfaces are eminently washable, though not as long-lasting as gloss. White-tiled surfaces in sanitary annexes, or around wash-basins, need regular wiping, and well repay the work done. Washing the entire walls of operating theatres is, in some hospitals, a routine every Monday morning, because of the particular need for a near sterile environment. This is the work of theatre staff.

Broken white tiles should be replaced. It is at times found that tiles have been applied to a wall with large blobs of 'white cement' behind at each corner. A cavity is left behind the tiles. Such tiles are very vulnerable to damage when knocked by trolleys or other heavy equipment. In such cases the only permanent answer is re-tiling of the entire wall, with the tiles laid flat on the cement surface with no space behind. A 'tile adhesive' is used to secure fixation to the wall.

Painting

However well cleaned a hospital may be the painted surfaces do not stay smart indefinitely. The slowly increasing shabbiness of the buildings may not be noticed by the staff who use them every day, but they give a very negative impression to the patients and visitors. It looks as if 'nobody cares'. A new coat of paint in a ward can improve expectations, and heighten staff morale immeasurably.

There should be a regular repainting schedule of all buildings, related to the degree of wear and tear. Out-patient waiting halls, with large numbers in every day, will need doing every year. Wards may need doing every 3 to 5 years, and staff residences every 5 to 7 years – or when there is a change of occupant. For all this routine work, and for painting new structures when added, most hospitals should employ a full-time painter, with an apprentice or casual painter when needed. Those in charge of the hospital should have some knowledge of the painting materials needed and the standard of work to be expected.

1. For external walls, a cement-based paint such as Snowcem stands up well to all climates. The old-fashioned limewash (whitewash) is a cheap alternative, but needs frequent renewal. It is best kept for ceilings indoors. If there is an un-paved bare earth yard or parking place, or the open soil of a flower bed next to a white wall, the first metre of wall will become splashed and brown in the rainy season. Some paint that first metre red, or black, in expectation of the splash mark. The splash may however be prevented by having a concrete storm drain round the building, extending out to eaves level; or alternatively by having a grass lawn, regularly cut, up to the wall base (see p.149).

2. For internal walls there is a choice between emulsion paint and gloss paint. The latter is slightly more expensive, but is easier to keep clean. Good quality emulsion paint can also be used externally when special colour effects are required.

- *Emulsion paint* is miscible with water. It generally needs to be applied in two coats of full thickness. Some painters make the mistake of applying the first coat thinned down 3:1 with water. This practice should not be allowed. A few mls of water when the paint is near the bottom of the tin is all that is needed by way of dilution.

  Brushes should be washed in water immediately after use. Any paint splashes on the floor should also be cleaned off with water straight away. Once splashes have dried hard they become impervious to washing, and can only be scraped off with much effort. Emulsion paint can be applied to walls that have been relatively freshly plastered. The cement can continue to dry out through it.

- *Gloss* is an oil-based paint. It is not miscible with water, but with turpentine, or white spirit (turpentine substitute). Some painters use kerosene, but this is not advised. Patchy colour differences on a wall will show through a single coat of gloss paint if it is used directly. Gloss paint must be preceded by one or two coats of *undercoat* paint. These should be at full thickness, and applied very evenly, to provide a constant colour background. White gloss should have white undercoat; most colours need a grey undercoat. Application of undercoat in very dilute form, or with inadequate streaky cover, is a bad painting practice.

  Brushes should be cleaned with white spirit, or with a brush cleaning fluid like Polyclens, and finished off with soap and water. The same cleaning fluids should be used for removing splashes. If an oil-based paint is applied to a plastered wall which is not completely dry, it will become blistered and discoloured within a few weeks. At least three months should be allowed after plastering. If the room has to be used earlier a coat of emulsion may be used meanwhile.

- Plain wood surfaces on window sills or furniture are best protected with two or more coats of clear polyurethane varnish, well rubbed down with sandpaper between coats. This gives a hard smooth surface which is resistant to both water and heat. White spirit is the diluent, and this should be used for cleaning brushes.

Structural and general repairs

Broken window panes, leaks in the roof, damaged furniture, dripping taps, blocked drains, or blown fuses – these are the tasks which need the day-to-day attention of the maintenance team. All staff should take a pride in seeing that needed repairs are reported promptly, and effected as quickly as possible.

Items that cannot be repaired should not just be left in a pile on a side verandah to gather dust indefinitely. At regular intervals, perhaps once a quarter, the maintenance officer should bring them to the attention of the medical superintendent for a final decision as to what should be sold off or thrown away. In the public service, this is the responsibility of a board; hence the term 'boarding'.

One particular job, often neglected, is the care of castor wheels on instrument and ward trolleys, mobile drip stands, beds and wheelchairs. When new, these have a little oil on the axles. Before long, this oil dries up, and the wheels start to squeak when the trolley is pushed along. Castors which start to stick for lack of oil, or because of fragments of dressings picked up, eventually sieze up. The trolley, or bed, if it has to be moved, will just be dragged along, and the round wheel will soon have a square side. Regular maintenance with each piece of mobile furniture up-ended for inspection of the wheels, for oiling of the axles, and to remove bits of wool or gauze, can prove a great saving (see Figure 6.14).

Preventive maintenance of the buildings and hospital equipment should also be extended to the hospital vehicles, and to all the essential supporting services without which the hospital cannot function effectively.

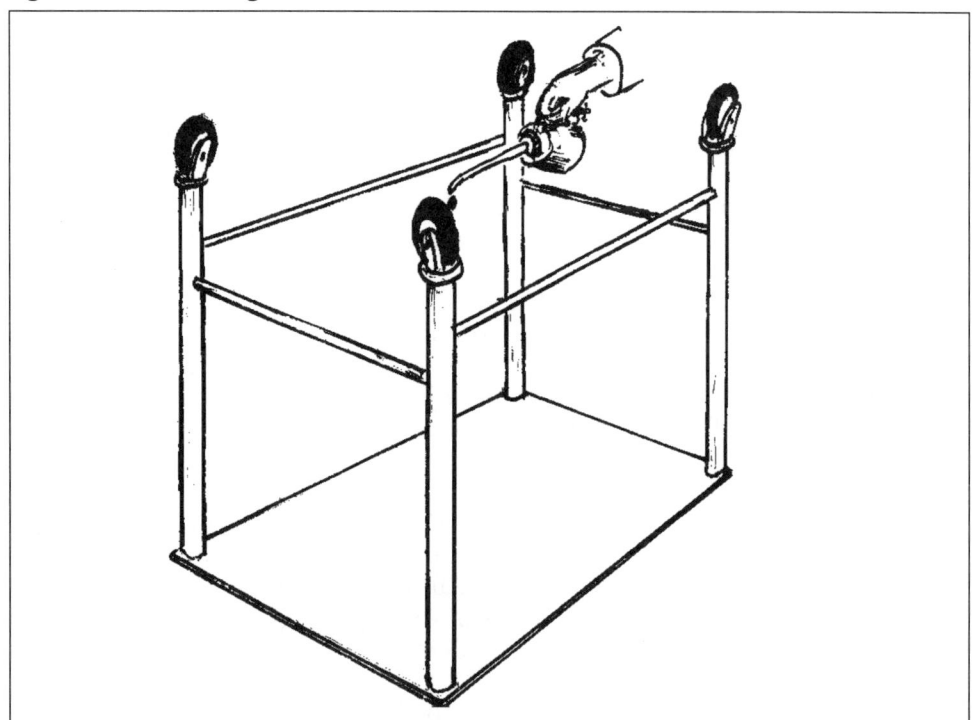

Figure 6.14: *Servicing castor wheels.*

CHAPTER 7

Supporting Services

The care of patients, whether in the wards, or in its outreach to the community is undoubtedly the hospital's main service. However, the medical administrator needs to be equally aware of the supporting services such as transport and communications, laundry and food preparation, waste-disposal and mortuary provision; and sanitation too. These are all of vital importance.

Transport and communications

The geographical terrain in developing countries may vary from riverine delta accessible only by canoe, to rugged highlands accessible only by mountain footpath or helicopter. However, in most countries, 95% of health facilities are likely to be dependent on road transport. A much smaller proportion of hospitals will have access to a telephone. It is this type of situation which we will look at in more detail.

Vehicles needed by a hospital

Road conditions, prices and availability of vehicles, and perception of need differ so much from one place to another, and it is not possible to generalise very far. Any vehicle that can be obtained will be useful. Where choices can be made the following considerations apply in situations where there are reasonable roads, whether tarred or not.

Those most useful
Light, general purpose vehicles are best (see Figure 7.1).

Figure 7.1: *Most useful vehicles.*

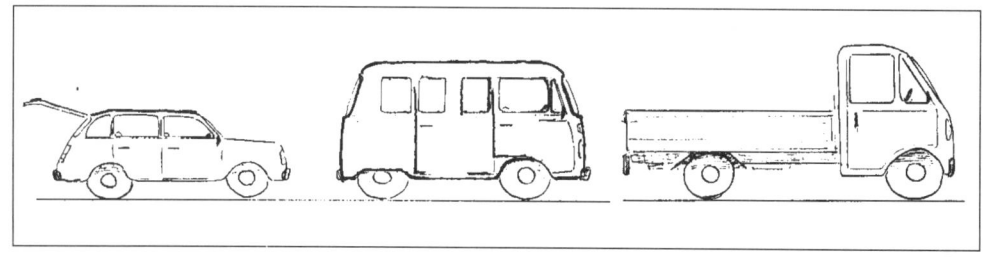

- Five-door estate car. This is not too expensive to run as a saloon for one or two people, but can carry five passengers when required. The back seat can be let down to enlarge the load carrying space, or to take a foam mattress and a recumbent patient. It can equally carry drugs and dressings, and health education equipment, for mobile primary health care outreach.

- The minibus, with seats for eleven, is also popular. Its engine is not usually very powerful, so when carrying a full load, much use must be made of the gears. However, with only the front seat occupied, it is still economical to run. Seats can be removed, and crates loaded on through the sliding side doors.

- A light lorry, of 2 to 5-tonne capacity, can be particularly useful for carrying heavier supplies, equipment or building materials.

Those less useful (see Figure 7.2)
- Land-Rovers, with four-wheel drive, are for very bad roads or open country. They are expensive on fuel and spare parts but they can generally get through when nothing else can. However, as soon as graded laterite or tarred roads are available, lighter vehicles are to be preferred. They are easier on the petrol – and easier on the driver too!

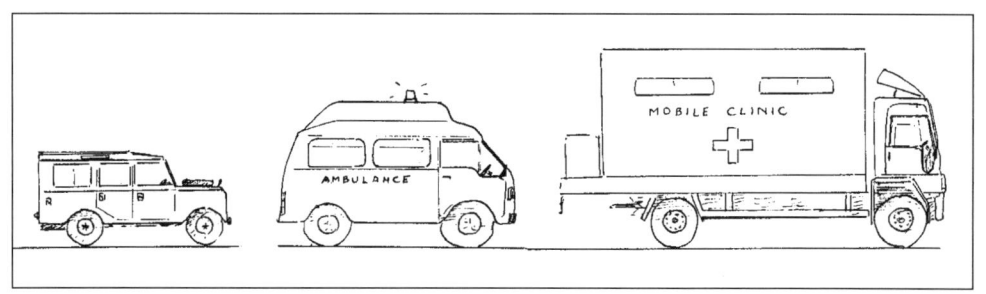

Figure 7.2: *Specialist vehicles – generally less useful.*

- The ambulance is often the first choice for a hospital vehicle by those without experience. It almost always turns out to be less useful than expected. It may occasionally be invaluable for transferring a patient from the hospital for specialist treatment elsewhere, but much less often for picking up a patient from home, or from the roadside, to bring him in. Only where there is excellent telephonic communication, and a primary care service through which the ambulance can be ordered, is that type of usage possible. More commonly the ambulance simply doubles up as another general purpose vehicle for carrying staff, or visiting outstations. Its expensive, specialist body work and interior fittings are rarely utilised, and its flashing light and wailing alarm (if fitted) may tempt the driver to speed even on non-emergency journeys.

- Purpose-built, fully fitted mobile clinics are also expensive to buy and expensive to run, and rarely fulfil the claims made for them. Some governments have spent huge sums on these, but the life of the vehicles has been very short. The money has been wasted. The even larger mobile consulting rooms, complete with air-conditioning and all mod cons, and a noisy 7kva generator on the back to run it all, are totally inappropriate for most rural situations. If the doctor or nurse have to travel to a primary health care clinic, or on a village survey, they will be more likely to see patients under a convenient tree than in the air-conditioned consulting room.

If possible, have more vehicles than you think you need

If the hospital is dependent on the road link for its supplies, or if it has a commitment to send staff to visit branch hospitals or a ring of primary health centres, then it is false economy to keep the number of vehicles down to the bare minimum. Vehicles do have to be withdrawn for servicing; they do break down; tyres do wear out when new tyres are often hard to obtain; vehicles do grow old and unreliable, and, unfortunately, accidents do happen. If the hospital has six vehicles it is likely to have only four on the road. The administration should endeavour to be generous in its provision of vehicles. Regular preventive maintenance servicing should be insisted on every 5000 miles (8000 km) or so.

Drivers
Who shall drive?

In the public service only officially employed drivers may drive government vehicles. This is a wise precaution, though a costly one in terms of manpower. In voluntary agency hospitals drivers are employed but certain senior staff are also allowed to drive. At WGH Ilesha they were probably responsible for more than half the mileage run by hospital vehicles on official business. Such a system is easy to operate, and saves the hospital a great deal of money.

> Staff who wished to drive at WGH Ilesha had to have official approval from the hospital administration. This was given when they had been some months with the hospital, and it was known they were familiar with the local road conditions and driving habits, and had demonstrated their driving ability with another authorised driver. When on the road they promised to take proper responsibility for the car, with due checks on tyre pressures, oil and water. When purchasing petrol they used their own money and obtained a receipt. The cash was refunded on their return.

Driver education

Even skilled drivers can get into bad habits, and become more prone to accidents. Excessive speed, dangerous cornering, poor road courtesy, failure to take a rest break when fatigued, and ignorance of the danger of even a little palm wine – all these can have tragic consequences. Vehicles are often poorly maintained. Tyres are allowed to wear till smooth. Few developing countries have yet passed laws requiring the use of seat-belts, and yet road research figures produced by Jacobs and Sayer in 1978 (11) showed that the 10 countries in the world with the worst accident rates (per licenced vehicle) were all in Africa; Nigerian rates were three times those of Kenya and 20 times those of Britain (see Figure 7.3).

Most countries have a printed highway code, and official drivers may be tested for their knowledge of this. Persistent reports of over-speeding, or driving under the influence of alcohol, should lead to disciplinary action. The hospital administration may wish to introduce a code of practice for

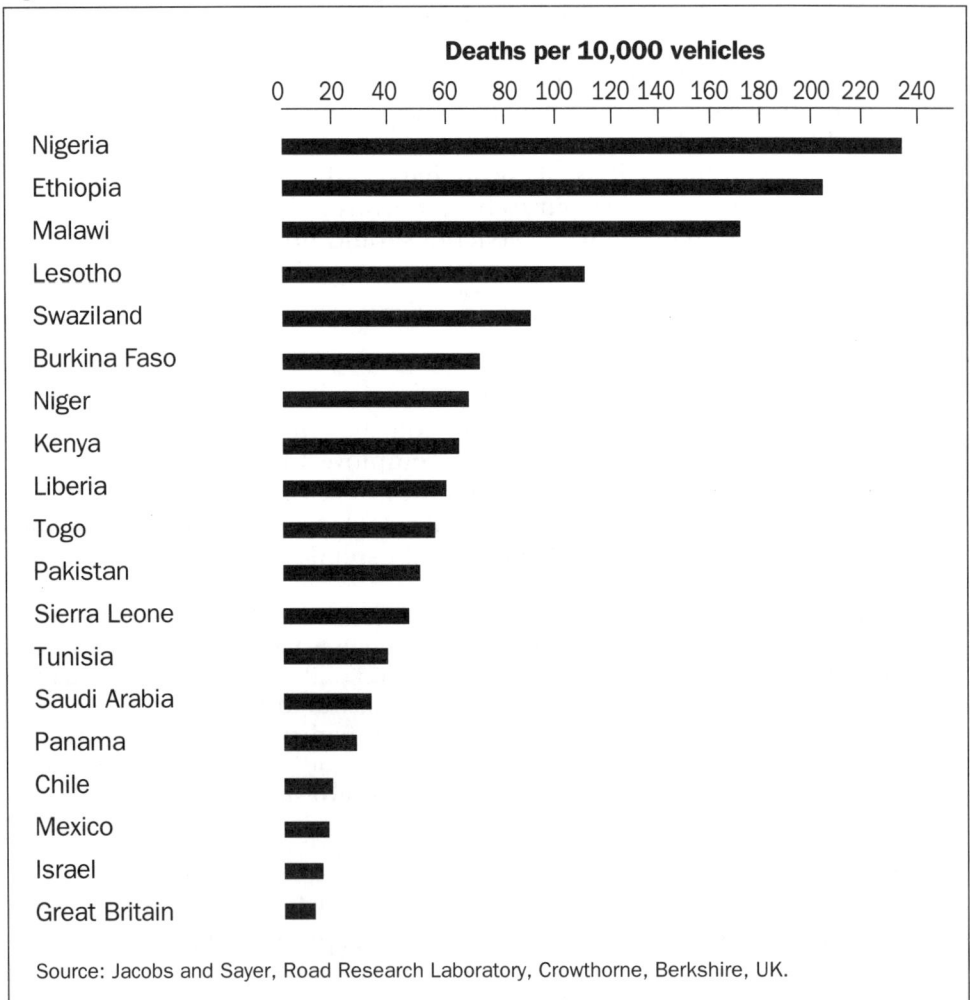

Figure 7.3: *Road accident fatality rates, 1978.*

Country	Deaths per 10,000 vehicles
Nigeria	240
Ethiopia	220
Malawi	160
Lesotho	100
Swaziland	90
Burkina Faso	75
Niger	75
Kenya	70
Liberia	60
Togo	55
Pakistan	45
Sierra Leone	40
Tunisia	30
Saudi Arabia	30
Panama	25
Chile	15
Mexico	15
Israel	12
Great Britain	10

Source: Jacobs and Sayer, Road Research Laboratory, Crowthorne, Berkshire, UK.

their drivers. The one produced for WGH Ilesha contained hints about local driving habits, road signs and likely hazards, and was addressed particularly to those new to driving in Nigeria.

Personal mileage
The hospital may choose to forbid personal mileage in official vehicles. This assumes that senior staff have their own cars, or that public transport is available. Alternatively the hospital may have a system whereby senior staff, who have been approved for driving hospital cars, can book a hospital vehicle for a personal trip, at a time when it is not required for official purposes. The car's log book must be strictly kept, and the staff can then be billed for payment at so much per kilometer – or per mile.

Communications
Enquiry office and signposts
The first line of communication is to help patients visiting the hospital to find their way to the department they want to go to. Staff often forget how confusing a maze of strange buildings can be. Not all patients or visitors will be able to read, so the first requirement is a well-placed enquiry desk, manned at all times throughout the 24 hours of the day. At night this should be well lit so that newcomers can find it without difficulty. The task of the receptionists at the enquiry desk is one of the most important in the hospital. They should be patient with strangers, sympathetic with those who are frightened or distressed, and slow to take offence when any show impatience or fail to understand.

Signposts to the various departments should be at all turnings, and some form of colour coding may be adopted, for example all signs to the maternity department in green, and all to the children's ward in yellow. Each ward and each department should be clearly labelled at its main entrance. Each door should have a label to indicate the use of that particular room. All signs should be reviewed from time to time to be sure they are up to date.

Postal and courier services
A hospital messenger, equipped with pedal bicycle, or light motor cycle, is a valuable member of staff. He can distribute urgent local messages, pick up mail from the post office, and collect letters from the various departments in the hospital for taking to the post. National or international courier services are relatively expensive, but the speed and certainty of delivery make their service worthwhile for very urgent and important matters.

Telephone
The reliability of telephone communication varies from country to country. When working well it is a boon. The system may involve just one line and one or two receivers, or be much more complex.

At WGH Ilesha a PBX sub-exchange was installed with 50 extensions, so that every ward, department and residence had a receiver. The sub-exchange was in the admission room, and manned 24 hours a day by clerks on duty there. They had other duties to perform, such as answering enquiries or preparing in-patient charts for new patients just arriving, so were occasionally a bit slow in responding to phone calls. However, they had a job with great variety and interest, and gave long service with increasing skill. Calls going outside the hospital were handled by them, and the destination and caller recorded in a book.

The internal intercom function of the PBX greatly increased the efficiency of the hospital. It was particularly useful at night for communication with the doctor on call-duty. Before the intercom service was available, a message would be sent by the staff-nurse or night sister on duty through a nightwatchman, or ward-aide. Once the doctor had been woken up there was no way the bringer of the message could answer questions to clarify what was needed. The doctor just had to get up and go and see. Once there was a telephone receiver by his bed, he could receive a call direct from the night sister, discuss the case with her, and sometimes authorise appropriate safe management until the morning. On the other hand, if the sister indicated a top-level emergency, he knew he must fly! Current technology brings such an intercom service within the reach of most hospitals.

Radiophone

Radiocommunication is usually subject to registration with a national body for use of an agreed wavelength. Transmitters on high frequency (HF), of the single side band type, can send messages for hundreds of miles, the radiowaves being reflected from the ozone layer in the stratosphere. Sets are economical and easy to maintain. There is usually considerable interference from 'static', but the spoken word is audible enough by those who have become accustomed to using it. A simple aerial wire, slung between two posts, about 10m (30 ft) from the ground, is sufficient to pick up HF waves.

Very high frequency (VHF) transmission has to be from a very high mast, up to 50m (150 ft), or from the top of a high building, and takes place direct from one point to the other, not via the stratosphere. Reception is therefore very clear, but is limited to distances of about 100 kilometers (63 miles) and is much more expensive to install and maintain (see Figure 7.4).

The radiophone is invaluable in situations where no telephone is available, or the telephone service is extremely poor. It is particularly useful between an outlying hospital and the city offices of suppliers of drugs or equipment, or the headquarters of the hospital management board. Fixed times must be arranged each day when the transmitter and receiver will be manned, whether or not there is a message to be sent.

The radiophone has been recommended for the link-up between hospital

1. High frequency transmission (HF)

2. Very high frequency transmission (VHF)

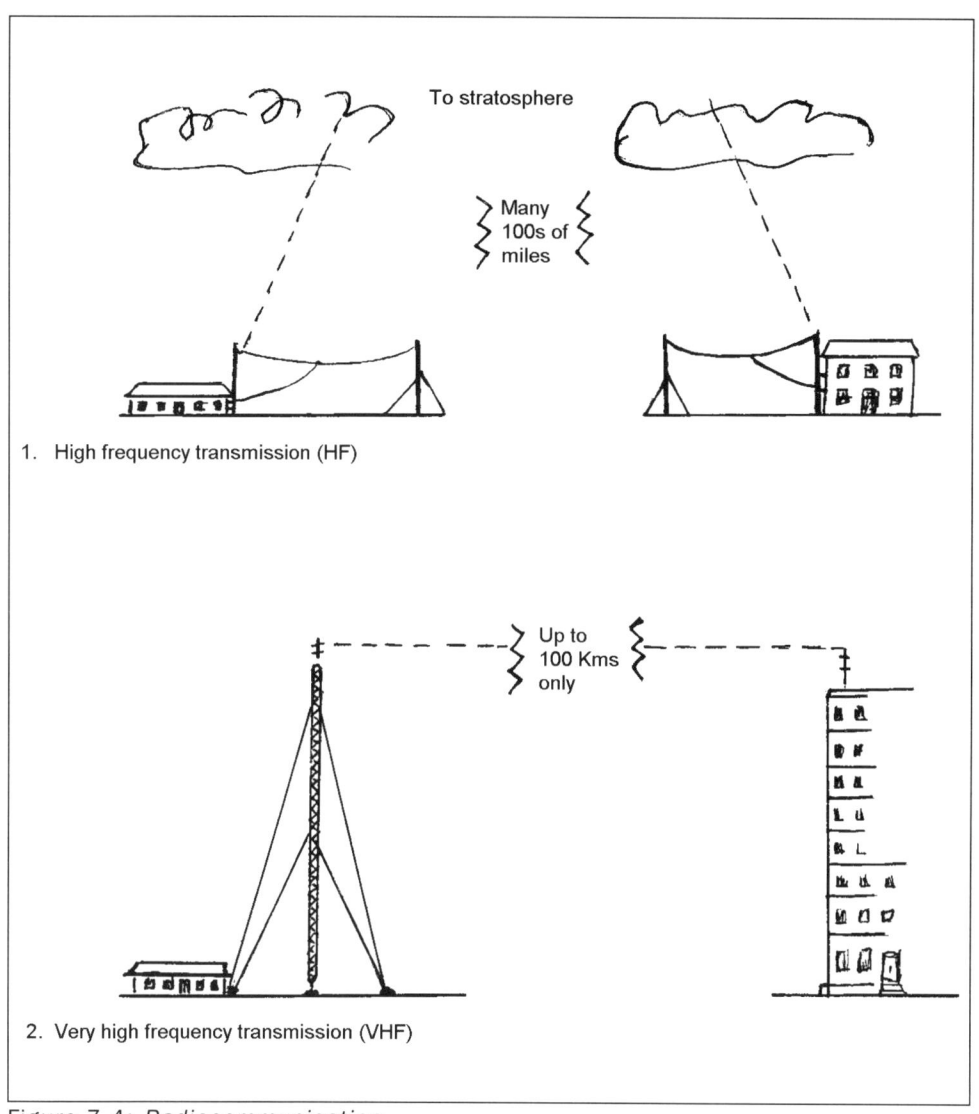

Figure 7.4: *Radiocommunication.*

and primary health centres under its supervision. That presupposes that there are well-educated staff in those centres who can use and benefit from advice or instructions given.

Laundry and kitchen

These two supporting services are often housed in adjacent blocks on the hospital site, so will be considered together.

The laundry
Collecting the linen
Hospitals in the tropics manage with much less linen than hospitals in temperate countries, but nevertheless the daily quantity of sheets, drawsheets, and pillow-cases can be very considerable. Blankets are needed, even in the tropics, when nights can be cold at certain seasons – for example during the harmattan winds of January–February in Nigeria, or at higher altitudes. Cellular blankets, of cotton or man-made fibre, are a great advance over the old woollen blankets which so quickly spoiled with washing. Linen from patients on barrier nursing for infectious disease may have to be soaked in disinfectant in the hospital sanitary annexe first. A bath or zinc tub on each ward should be provided for this.

Daily collection of soiled linen from every ward takes place by aides or orderlies under the supervision of the ward sister who prepares the inventory. Soaked items will have to be collected wet. The system *must* be daily wherever possible, because damp linen left around in tropical climates quickly becomes spottily discoloured with black mould. The operating theatre may have its own system for washing of caps, gowns, operating towels and laparotomy sheets, or share with the main hospital laundry.

Washing by hand or machine
Hand washing is labour intensive, but still the most practical in many situations. Adequate supplies of soap or detergent must be given out, generally under matron's supervision.

Hospital administrations often omit to provide sufficient space for hanging washing out to dry. Spreading linen on the ground, or over bushes, should be discouraged, and lines of galvanised fence wire at 2 metre (6 feet) height stretched between posts of 50 mm (2 inch) galvanised piping set in concrete, are ideal. If breezes blow, pegs will also be needed (see Figure 7.5).

Figure 7.5: *Laundry drying.*

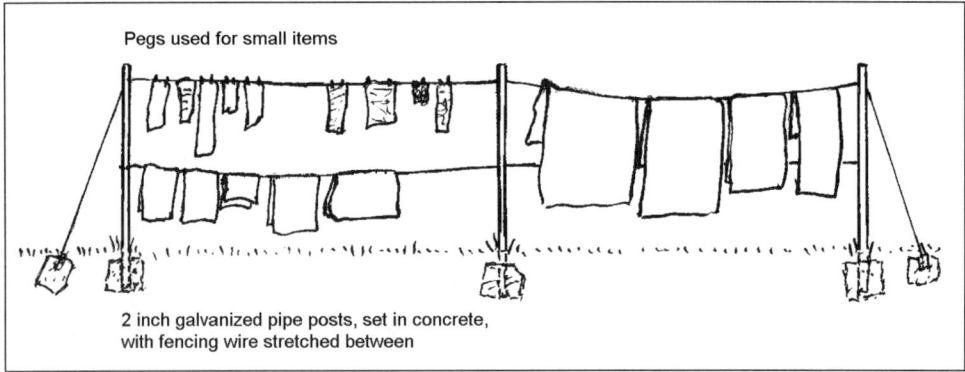

The sun does not shine every day, even in the tropics, and alternative space for drying under cover is necessary for the rainy season. Again, space for this is often forgotten, and one way of judging whether a hospital is well organised is to ask how the laundry is dried in the wet season.

Machine washing and drying is, of course, an excellent option, but not all hospitals can afford the capital outlay, or the running costs. This in turn can be considerably reduced by solar pre-heating (see p105) of all hot water used. The most useful machine of all is the spin-drier. One which reaches 1000 rpm leaves the washing slightly damp, but greatly speeds up the process of final drying when the washing is hung on the lines. If only one machine can be bought, then that is the one. It is economical to run, and ensures that all the day's washing can be completed in the day. A tumble-drier, which rotates and heats the linen till thoroughly dry, is valuable in the wet season, but not necessary in the dry. It is expensive to run, as also is a steam pressing machine. Most hospitals stick to hand ironing of the selected items for which it is deemed necessary.

Return of linen, repair and replacement
Clean linen is sorted for return, according to the inventory of each ward. Torn or worn linen is routed back via a linen room for repair or replacement. Hospitals can well employ a full, or part-time seamstress, with sewing machine, in a room adjacent to the linen store room.

The hospital kitchen
Not all hospitals supply food for their patients. WGH Ilesha was the first in Nigeria to do so. The hospital served a community which was 95% of one ethnic group, Yoruba, so food preparation according to local tastes was not difficult. Hospitals serving a very cosmopolitan population, with many cultural traditions, find it much more difficult.

If food is not provided then the hospital must expect each patient to have several relatives living in, or just outside the ward, to provide their patient with what he or she needs. A covered space for the relatives to camp, and cook, needs to be made available. To accept this situation puts a major limitation on the effectiveness of dietary treatment, so essential for some conditions.

Purchasing and storing ingredients
The matron, or a caterer under her supervision, may have to give some time every day to purchasing food supplies, rice, maize, tomatoes, onions, peppers, beans and meat, or whatever is eaten locally, from the local farmers and traders. A food store, close to the kitchen, will be necessary for items which can be obtained in bulk, and stored without risk of spoiling by rats, weevils or becoming over-ripe.

126 *Medical Administration for Front-line Doctors*

Figure 7.6: *The smoke-free wood-burning (HERL) stove.*

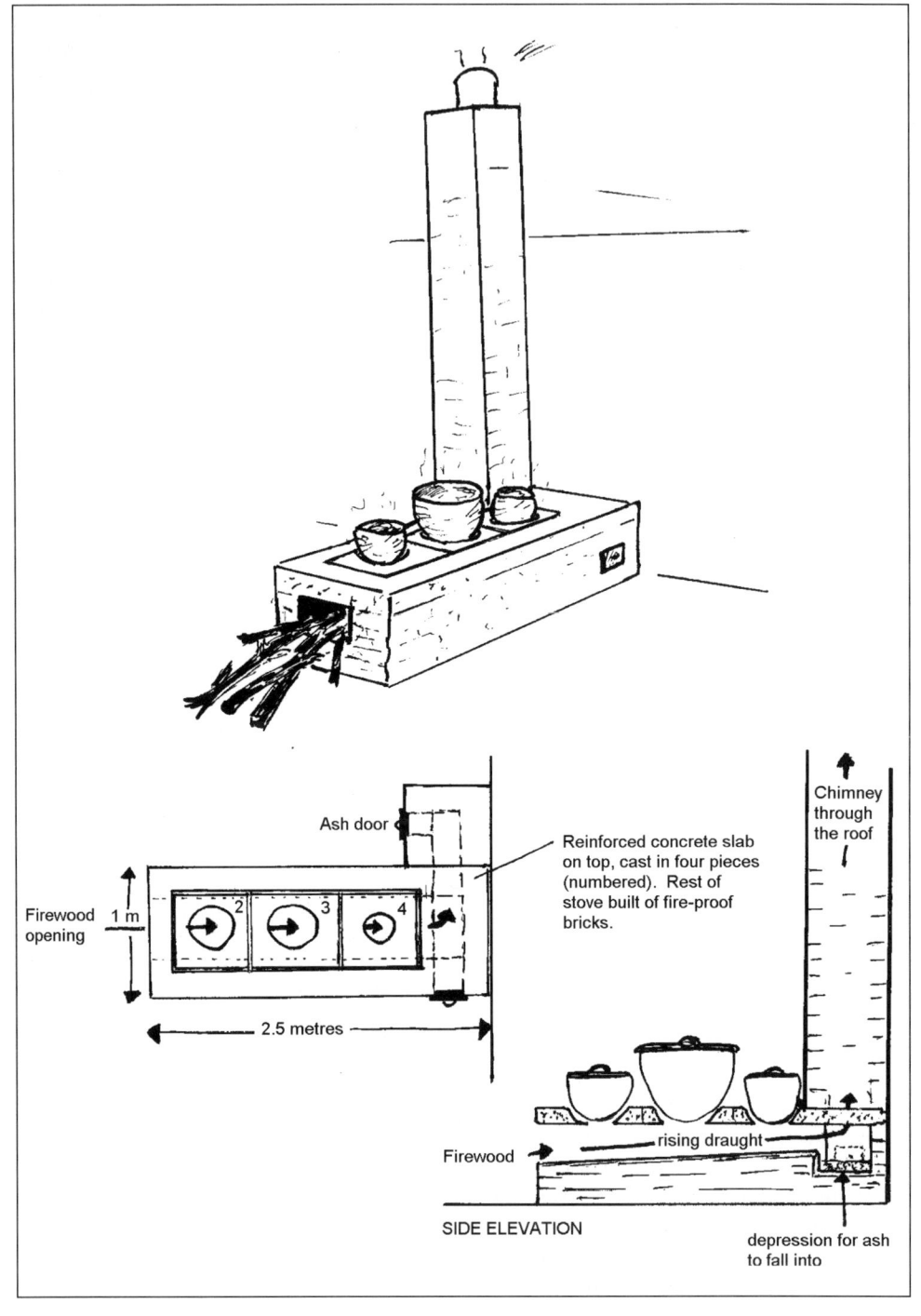

SIDE ELEVATION

Kitchen facilities

Consideration must be given to the type of stove to be used, at the minimum of expense and the optimum of convenience. As already indicated electricity is excessively expensive. Bottled gas is less so, but hospital requirements are heavy if gas is used for all cooking. An industrial size of storage cylinder and bulk delivery of gas would have to be arranged. Kerosene stoves are an alternative, but the life of such stoves tends to be short. Wood burning on open stoves causes much smoke, and soon blackens the kitchen walls and ceiling. Nevertheless, the use of wood for fuel is still common in developing countries. It can be adapted satisfactorily for hospital use, with minimisation of the smoke nuisance, if the stove is properly designed. The Herl stove at WGH Ilesha (see Figure 7.6) stood the test of time for over 30 years. A gas cooker was used for special diets only.

The principle of the stove is that all smoke is drawn up the chimney. Soot and ash from the chimney fall into the ash sump, and can be removed very easily each day, or as required. Cooks like it because it can be fed with long pieces of wood, which burn at the inside end, and are pushed inwards as combustion proceeds. The system is relatively fuel efficient.

Apart from the stove there must also be generous working tops for food preparation, and facilities for pounding yam, or grinding pepper, according to local custom.

Ward pantries

Each ward needs a mobile trolley for collecting the food and a ward pantry. Expensive, heated stainless steel trolleys, are not essential in the tropics where food is not normally eaten piping hot. Wooden trolleys, which can be made locally and fitted with 4 in (100 mm) castors, are quite adequate (see Figure 7.7). The ward orderly can collect the food from the hospital kitchen in large stainless steel, covered pans. Plates, bowls and cups are kept on the wards. Food can then be served in the ward pantry under the supervision of the staff nurse, taking note of any special dietary orders for each patient. All washing is then done by the orderly in the ward pantry, and the large containers returned to the hospital kitchen.

Milk kitchen

Feeding of children in a large children's ward has its own problems. For some, of course, breast feeding is all that is needed, and some older children can take adult diet. However, some of the smallest children need supplementary formula feeding, and others slightly older need special weaning foods of high calorific density, and relatively high protein. For these a 'milk kitchen' on the ward itself can allow stricter supervision of cleanliness, and refrigeration provided. In the one at WGH Ilesha nurses alone were allowed on the clean side (see Figure 7.8).

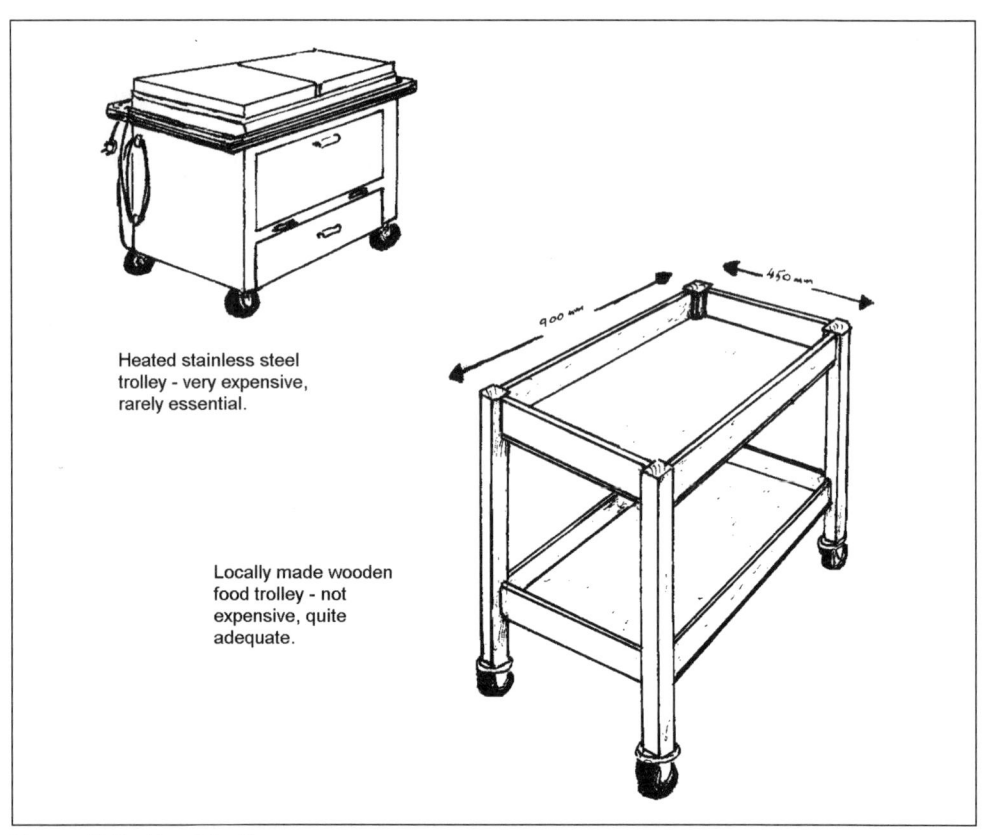

Figure 7.7: *Food trolleys.*

Heated stainless steel trolley - very expensive, rarely essential.

Locally made wooden food trolley - not expensive, quite adequate.

Figure 7.8: *Milk kitchen plan.*

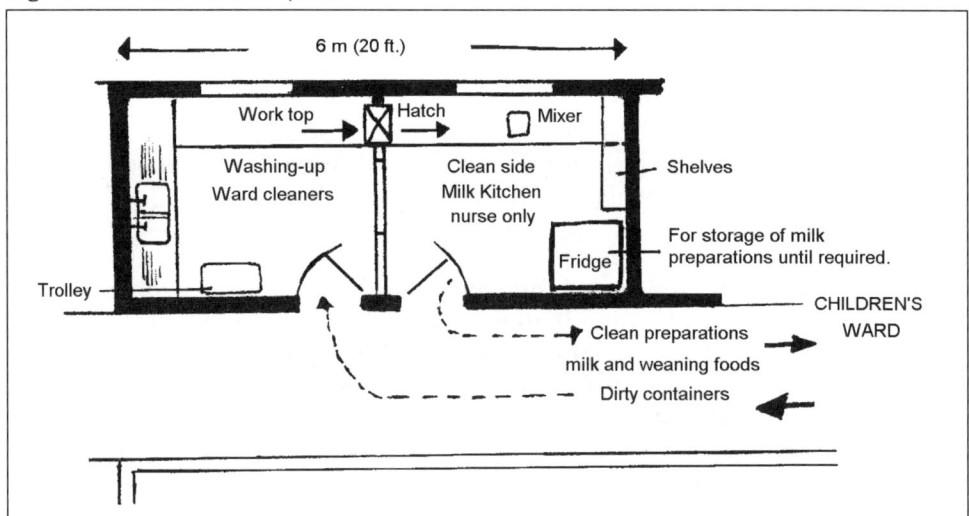

Mortuary care and waste disposal

The hospital mortuary
Siting and access
The mortuary needs careful siting at a point on the periphery of the hospital grounds, on the lee side for prevailing winds if unrefrigerated. Otherwise the smell of a body left too long will be apparent to the whole hospital. There should be good access for vehicles bringing bodies of casualties found dead outside the hospital, or taking bodies away for burial, and also convenient access for orderlies to bring the bodies of those who have died in the hospital. This access needs to be well lit for equally easy use by night as well as by day. If at a distance from the wards, a concrete path should be provided (see Figure 7.9).

Mortuary facilities
Refrigeration of bodies is highly desirable, but the installation and operation of this facility is expensive. Without it, bodies must be moved by relatives the same, or the following day, because of the smell of decomposition, which can become unpleasant for everyone within 3 or 4 days. Problems may arise with bodies of paupers brought in by the police, or accident cases far from the victims home, when no relative can be found.

For such cases the hospital itself has at times no choice but to use its own staff to take such bodies on a lorry to the 'strangers' cemetery', or wherever is acceptable, for burial. At Ilesha this unpleasant task was made a little more

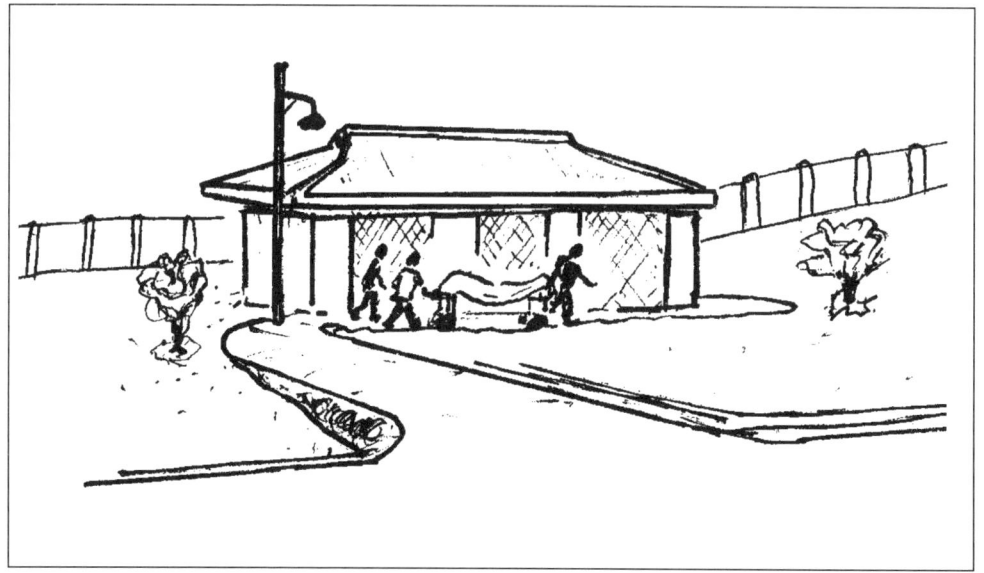

Figure 7.9: *Mortuary access.*

acceptable by the use of mortuary rubber gloves and aprons, and lots of a pungent phenol disinfectant such as Jeyes Fluid.

An autopsy table and instruments have to be provided, and encouragement given to the doctors to do post-mortem examinations on all who die in the hospital, particularly those cases where the cause of death is not obvious.

However, permission for autopsy is frequently refused, because of fear or misunderstanding, or simply because of the need to get the body back to the village of origin as quickly as possible. When little children die, the mother frequently prefers, after her initial distress is over, to put the child's body on her back, to carry it home as if sleeping. She knows that otherwise, the drivers of public vehicles will double the fares they charge her. If autopsy is insisted upon, the mother may simply run away, and leave the child's body in the hospital. The doctor often has no choice but to accept that a post-mortem cannot be done.

Once refrigeration has been installed, it may well be accepted as a social service (by those in the community sufficiently well-off to pay) for the bodies of senior relatives who have died to be kept for some days or weeks. When all arrangements have been completed, and the extended family gathered in from far and near, elaborate funeral celebrations can then take place.

Waste disposal

Keeping the hospital clean, neat and tidy is a very necessary service, both for the general appearance of the place, and for the prevention of spread of disease through house-flies, cockroaches or rodents. Ideally it is desirable to separate waste at the point of collection into material which can be:

- *placed in a compost pit*, to make fertiliser: includes all biodegradable items, such as food waste and garden waste

- *incinerated:* all paper, dressings and plastic which can be destroyed by burning

- *tipped in a pit* as the only means of disposal: all tins, and metal objects.

The separation is likely to be only achieved in part.

Refuse collection

Each ward, department and hospital residence needs a dustbin for general refuse. Galvanised bins with strong covers, reasonably dog and goat-proof, are best. Food waste from the hospital kitchen and the ward pantries may be collected in separate containers for putting on compost pits, or for feeding livestock such as pigs and poultry, if such are being kept. Food waste from staff residences can only be controlled by the householder.

The refuse collector should be provided with a wheel-barrow, or better still a 4-wheeled trolley and given a regular schedule for emptying the bins all round the hospital and grounds. Food waste should be disposed of as directed, and all general rubbish taken to the point of disposal. Some hospitals may be in urban centres with municipal vehicles coming to collect refuse, but the majority are likely to have to manage their own disposal.

Controlled tipping and incineration
A point in the grounds, low-lying and as little visible from the hospital as possible, should be chosen. If there is a natural pit to be filled, so much the better. Otherwise a pit should be dug and used until full, then another pit prepared. Waste engine oil from hospital vehicles or generator may be burned in the pit to fire the rest and reduce bulk.

Traditional incinerators do not always function well, owing to the variety of waste material. A well-planned incinerator should have two combustion chambers, one above the other. Easily combustible material, particularly paper, could be placed in the lower fire box. Damp dressings and mixed material, much of it non-combustible till dry, could be placed in the upper fire box, where eventually most of it would burn. An exit door for easy removal of all tins and other residue in the upper box should then be within easy reach of the tip.

Special problems
The disposal of placentae from the maternity department is a daily requirement. If there are no local customs or taboos these can be added to the general waste, or, better still, taken to a deep pit, with concrete cover, kept for the purpose. Blood clot, products of abortion, macerated or anencephalic foetuses, and amputated tissues from the theatre, may be treated in the same way. Mothers of stillborn infants should be allowed to see the child, and take it home for burial if they wish. Otherwise it is the hospital's responsibility to see to disposal.

Sanitation

Water-borne sanitation has become accepted as the standard practice in countries and towns where a regular and generous water supply is available. In many rural situations this is not the case, and alternative methods of sanitation have to be used entirely or in part. In many Asian countries, such as China, human faeces is considered far too valuable to be flushed away down pipes to some distant sewage farm. All is carefully collected in farm sewage tanks, stored for a week or two, then returned to the land. The fertility of Chinese soil, which produces three crops a year, year after year without fail, is a tribute to the value of this recycling technique. They have had the system for 3000 years, and feed nearly a quarter of the world's population on only 1/7th of the world's cultivatable land surface.

African culture would not tolerate this use of human faeces for direct fertilisation of land. In small village communities, defaecation is usually on an area of waste-land or rock at a short distance from the village. Dessication by sun, washing away by rain, and natural processes of degradation, soon cause it to become part of the soil. If people are taught to shovel some earth on the fresh faeces after it has been passed, then fly breeding is also reduced to a minimum.

In villages of less than 100 houses this system may not be so unhygienic, even if inconvenient. However, when the village grows to become a town, the village ecology is no longer tenable. Areas of waste land are diminished or non-existent, or too far for regular use by those at the town centre. Alternatives have to be found through the building of toilets of some kind. In the design of these, care may have to be taken to allow the squatting position for defaecation to continue to be used.

Sanitary systems where water supply is limited
The bucket latrine

The old-fashioned bucket latrine is mentioned here though not recommended. The toilet seat is set in a frame over a galvanised bucket, and a trap-door in the wall behind the frame allows the bucket to be removed daily from outside the toilet for emptying. A sanitary worker has to be employed to do this emptying, often in the early morning before the working day begins. He fills a larger container, and that in turn is emptied into a septic tank or pit. In countries of Asia where faeces is valued as a fertiliser, this work is not looked down upon so much. In Africa such work is considered very lowly, and the system is demeaning.

The chemical closet is a modification of the bucket latrine, but a cup or two of chemical liquid, such as Elsan, is placed in the pan after emptying, and this both counteracts the smell, and acts as a digestant and disinfectant. Emptying once a week may be sufficient. The contents should be placed in a refuse pit, not into a septic tank, as the biodegrading bacteria in the faeces have been destroyed. The system is still used in mobile caravans and buses which have a toilet on board, and it may be of temporary value in a hospital. No construction work is required, so the cost of installation is not high, but the cost of the fluid to be added soon adds up.

Pit latrines

Where hospitals draw in many villagers who have never seen or used a modern toilet before, then the pit latrine is still the best option, at least for those just attending out-patients. Those admitted may be given instruction on the use of water closets if provided.

Methods for construction of the standard pit latrine are widely known. Excellent detail is given in Werner's *Where There is No Doctor* (29) and other manuals. The concrete platform to place over the top of the pit can be cast in a mould near the point of use, then placed in position, and the 'little house' built over it. In theory, the hole in the platform for defaecation should always be kept covered with a wooden lid between use to prevent flies entering to breed. In practice the edges of the hole soon become fouled, so faeces mess up the lid as well. Before long it ceases to be used. The latrine odour is free to come out, and the flies to enter and multiply as they please. No wonder people do not like ordinary pit latrines, and tend only to use them by compulsion.

The Ventilated Improved Pit (VIP) latrine is a marked advance. By one or two ingenious design modifications, at minimum extra cost, the standard pit latrine is rendered almost free of odour and of flies. The design has come from work done in Zimbabwe, and has been popularised throughout the developing world. One, two or more may be built together (see Figure 7.10). A full description can be found in *Rural Water Supplies and Sanitation* by Peter Morgan (13).

The essential features of the VIP latrine are as follows.

- The pit is no different from a standard latrine.

- The concrete platform is cast with two holes in it, not one. There is the usual hole for defaecation, and a second hole of 110 to 230 mm (4–9 in) diameter for the ventilation pipe.

- The platform is placed over the pit, and the shelter built on top with the entrance preferably facing north (if north of the equator), never east or west. This minimises morning or evening sunlight entering the structure.

- The ventilation pipe should be placed over the second hole, just outside the shelter, and projecting 1 m (3 feet) above it. It may be made of PVC of 200-225 mm (8 to 9 in) diameter, if such piping is available, or it may be built of bricks or 100 mm (4 in) blocks, to an external size of 450mm (18 in) square; 225 mm (9 in) square internally.

Zimbabwe: encouraging families to build latrines

The government in Zimbabwe is encouraging families to participate in constructing and maintaining ventilated pit (VIP) latrines, to improve sanitation in rural areas. The Blair ventilated latrine is very popular because:

- it does not smell
- it does not attract flies
- it is safe to use
- it is very private
- it costs little to build
- it can be used as a private bathing place
- it is easy to maintain and lasts for many years.

Ministry of Health
Box 8204
Causeway
Harare
Zimbabwe

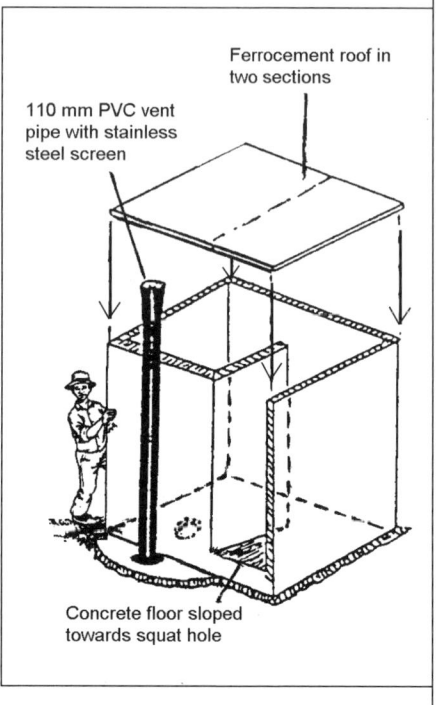

Figure 7.10: *Ventilated improved pit latrines as advocated in Zimbabwe.*

- The ventilation pipe should be painted black to increase heat absorption. The interior and ceiling of the shelter may also be painted black to minimise light reflection from outside.

- A mosquito gauze screen should be placed over the top of the vent pipe. Aluminium wire screening will have a longer life than cheaper forms of gauze.

- No lid is required to cover the latrine opening. In fact it must be left open.

- The door should open inwards, and be provided with a spring so that it is always kept closed, whether or not there is anyone inside. This is to prevent light entering. In some designs a screen wall light trap is provided, as in the entry to an X-ray dark room, and no door at all. Users knock outside before entering to be sure the latrine is vacant.

Supporting Services 135

The latrine works on the following principles (see Figure 7.11).

1. The black painted ventilation pipe absorbs heat, and promotes a rising current of air. Air is therefore drawn in through the latrine hole, which must always be kept open. Latrine odours are carried up through the pipe to a higher level, and the air in the shelter remains fresh and odour-free.

Figure 7.11: *Working principle of the VIP latrine.*

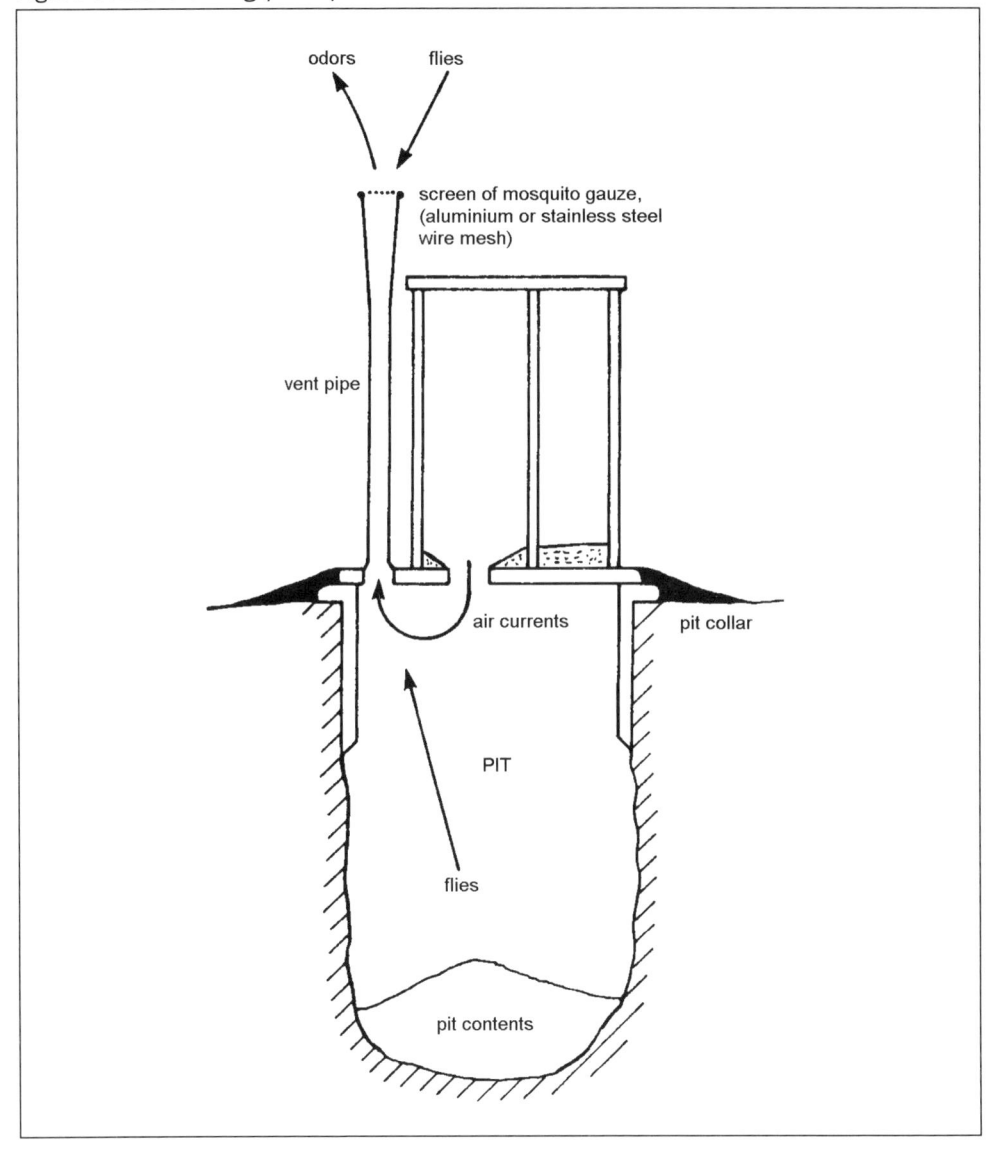

2. The inside of the shelter is kept relatively dark, so that more light enters the pit through the ventilation pipe than through the latrine hole. The flies that can enter through the latrine hole are more likely to exit through the ventilation hole, being attracted by the light. Any flies that breed will also go the same way. However, the mosquito gauze will trap them at the top of the pipe, and they will eventually die and fall back into the pit. Hence the VIP latrine is kept fly-free as well.

The aqua privy, and pour-flush systems
These require some water, but relatively little compared with full waterborne sanitation. The aqua privy is in fact a septic tank with the latrines built directly on top of it. The tank does initially have to be filled with water up to the effluent outlet level. The concrete slabs on top of the septic tank have 100 mm (4 inch) holes in them as latrine openings. From the lower surface a 4 inch (100 mm) pipe descends about 600 mm (2 feet) to just below the water level. This therefore provides a water seal against odour and flies. Water from a bucket does have to be used, at least once a day, to wash down any faeces which has soiled the edge of the opening. A latrine attendant is therefore essential (see Figure 7.12).

An open, screened area may be provided over one end of the tank, to which mothers can take their children. A tap should be provided, and an opening into the tank. Mothers can let their children perform there on a potty or piece of paper or leaf, then put the results in the tank by hand, and wash their children. This is better than allowing the children to defaecate in the open, and leaving scavenging dogs to clear up the mess.

Faeces in the septic tank digests, and the washing water tops up the water level. The effluent that comes from the outflow end is virtually odour-free. It may be collected in a bucket, and used for watering flowers, or it may be led into a soakage trench to be absorbed into the soil. After many years the sludge in the tank will have to be emptied.

Other forms of 'pour-flush' toilet, simply use a toilet pan, placed at a short distance from a septic tank. A bucket of water poured down the pan after use carries the faeces to the tank. Proper water closets are really not much better when mains water supply becomes so depleted that cisterns will not fill, and flushing has to be done by hand with waste water from buckets. That situation is unfortunately all too common.

Sanitary arrangements where water supply is good
Water-borne sanitation has all the advantages of freedom from smell and flies, good hygiene and convenience. It is the only way of coping with sanitation in the modern house or hospital, and in the urban situation. However, as noted under water supply, the amount of water required per

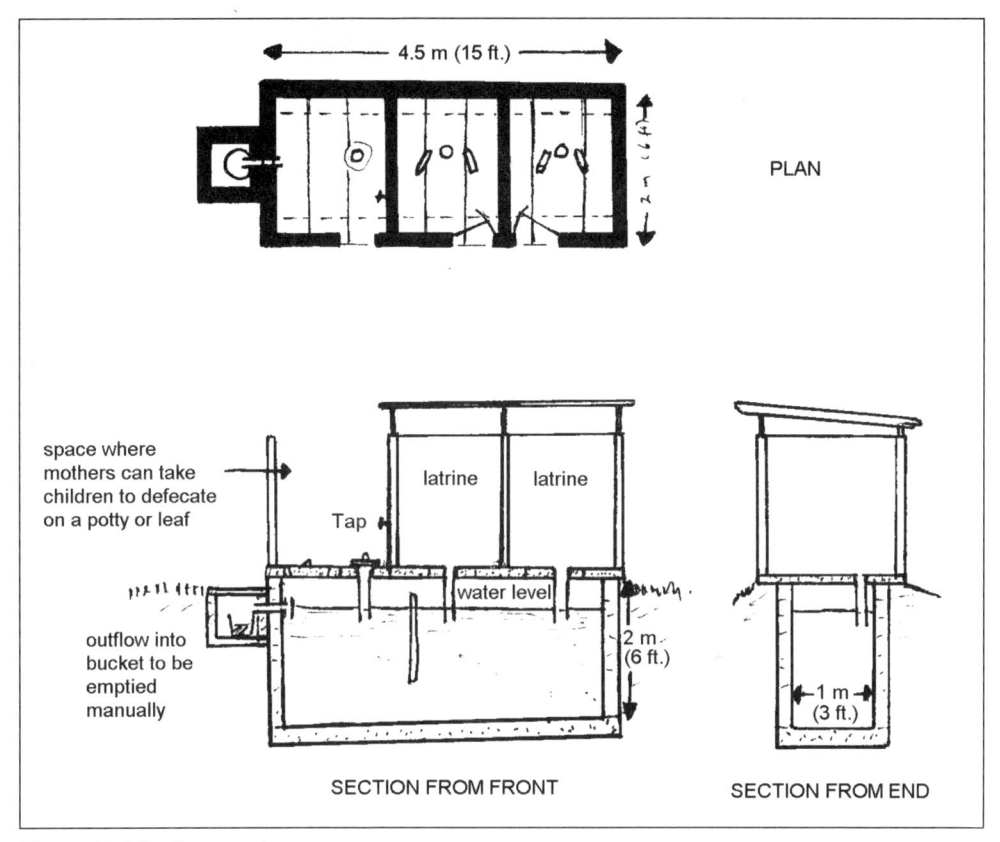

Figure 7.12: *Aqua privy*.

user per day is in the region of 10 gallons (45 litres). Without water-borne sanitation the amount required is only about 3 gallons (13.5 litres).

Water closets (WCs)

A decision may have to be made as to whether to install only pedestal type toilets, or whether to have some squatting type toilets for those used to that position for defaecation. If no concession is made to those who for their whole life have squatted, then they will try to squat on the pedestals. Plastic toilet seats break very quickly under this treatment, and even the ceramic toilet bowls may have a relatively short life. Strong wooden toilet seats, when obtainable, have their advantage in this situation.

If squatting toilets are provided the following points should be noted. The concrete floor around the pan should slope gently towards it from all sides, to allow for easy cleaning each day. The foot rests should be correctly placed, on each side of the pan. A water tap should be provided close to the toilet, so that those who clean their anus by hand can wash themselves straight away.

It is wise to provide toilet paper to all using water closets, preferably a roll to each patient admitted. If this is not done they may use newspaper, banana leaves, tow or other materials which take too long to digest in the septic tank, or may block the soil pipes on the way. The nuisance created by a blockage, and the expense of repair, is likely to be greater than the cost of supplying toilet paper.

Staff who clean the toilets must be told not to put any kind of antiseptic into the pan, as they may have been taught to do for cleaning the floor in the sanitary annexe. Antiseptic in the pan will be flushed into the septic tank, and the septic digestive process in the tank will cease, so that the tank soon fills to the top, and has to be manually emptied. This should only be necessary every 5 to 8 years, not every few months.

Care must also be taken not to allow malfunctioning cisterns or broken taps over a squat toilet to run water continually into the pan. This may soon flood the septic tank, and the overflow will then flood the soakaway with incompletely digested effluent. This is a calamity. The only answer is laboriously to dig out the stones from the old soakaway pit, or construct a new one.

Strict supervision of staff caring for sanitary annexes pays dividends. At one hospital in Ibadan, Nigeria, the matron herself includes a visit of inspection to every ward toilet on her daily rounds.

Water-borne – to where?
Centralised disposal in sewage farms for a whole town or village is the ideal, but not yet common in developing countries. If such a service is available, hospitals will obviously make use of it. The 'waste stabilisation pond' system is excellent in some circumstances (12). More commonly there has to be dependence on septic tanks for each house or ward or compound. Tanks have to be placed where they can easily be connected, and where there is room also for the soakage pit, or trench to absorb the effluent.

Pipework connections
Sewage is a mixture of solids and liquids. To ensure that the solids are carried along and not deposited, the mixture in the pipes must be carried along quite quickly, with the minimum of interference on the way. In particular the sewage must pass smoothly and quickly round bends. Inspection chambers at bends, which impede quick flow, are likely to be the cause of blockage by slowing transit, and allowing solid faeces to deposit. Some inspection chambers are necessary, but these should always be placed on a straight section of pipe where the sewage can still flow quickly despite the opening (see Figure 7.13).

Figure 7.13: Inspection chambers.

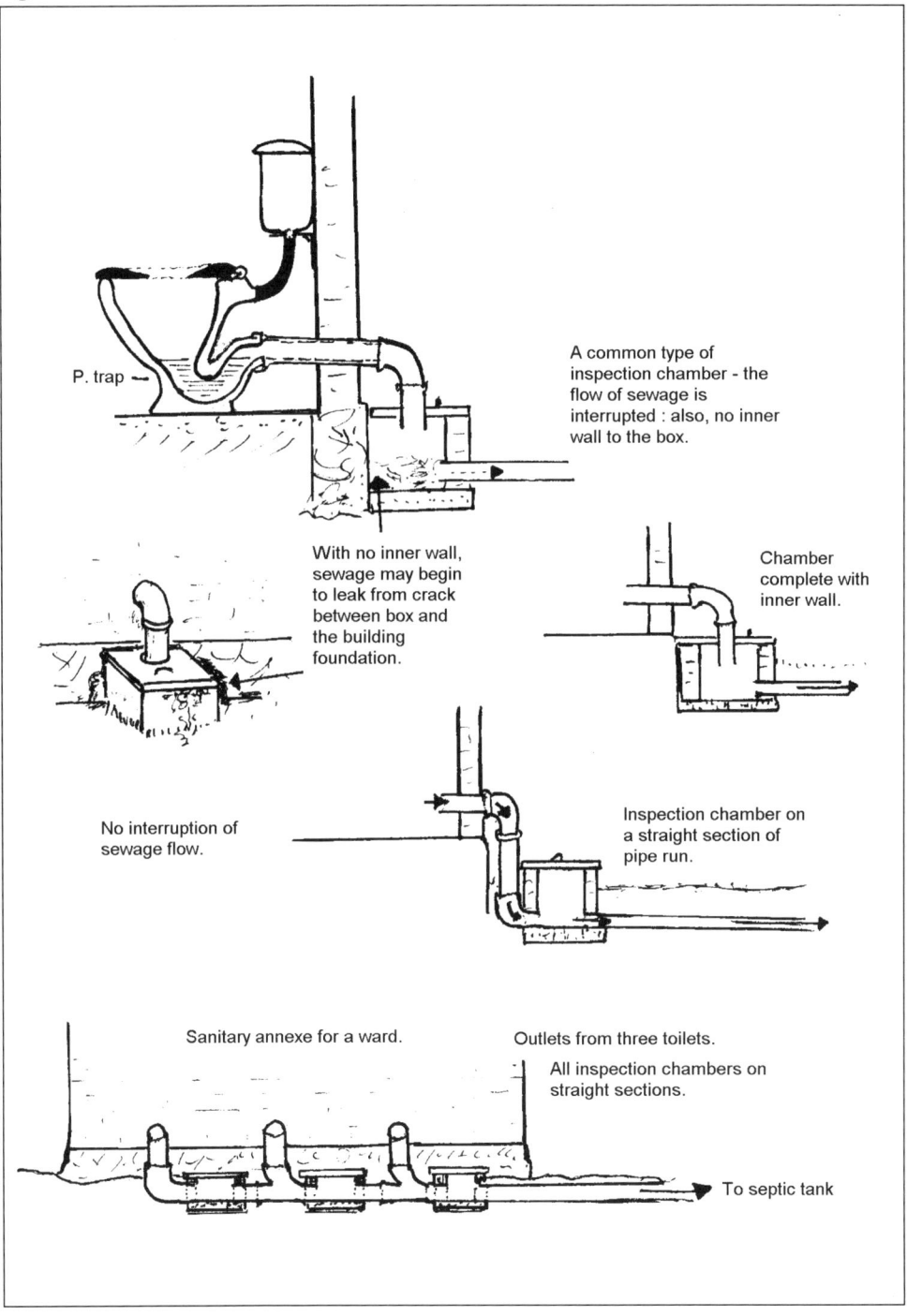

140   *Medical Administration for Front-line Doctors*

Design of septic tanks
Long experience has shown the design of tank that works best, and the desired size per estimated number of users (see Figure 7.14).

Sewage enters through the entry inspection chamber, and falls into the tank through a T-junction. Digestion takes place in the first compartment. This is an anaerobic process, and there is no need for a ventilation grille on the top of the tank. The gas produced can exit with the effluent. Non-digestible material gradually sinks as 'sludge' to the bottom. The digested portion becomes entirely liquid, and largely odour-free. It passes under the baffle

Figure 7.14: *Standard septic tank and soakaway.*

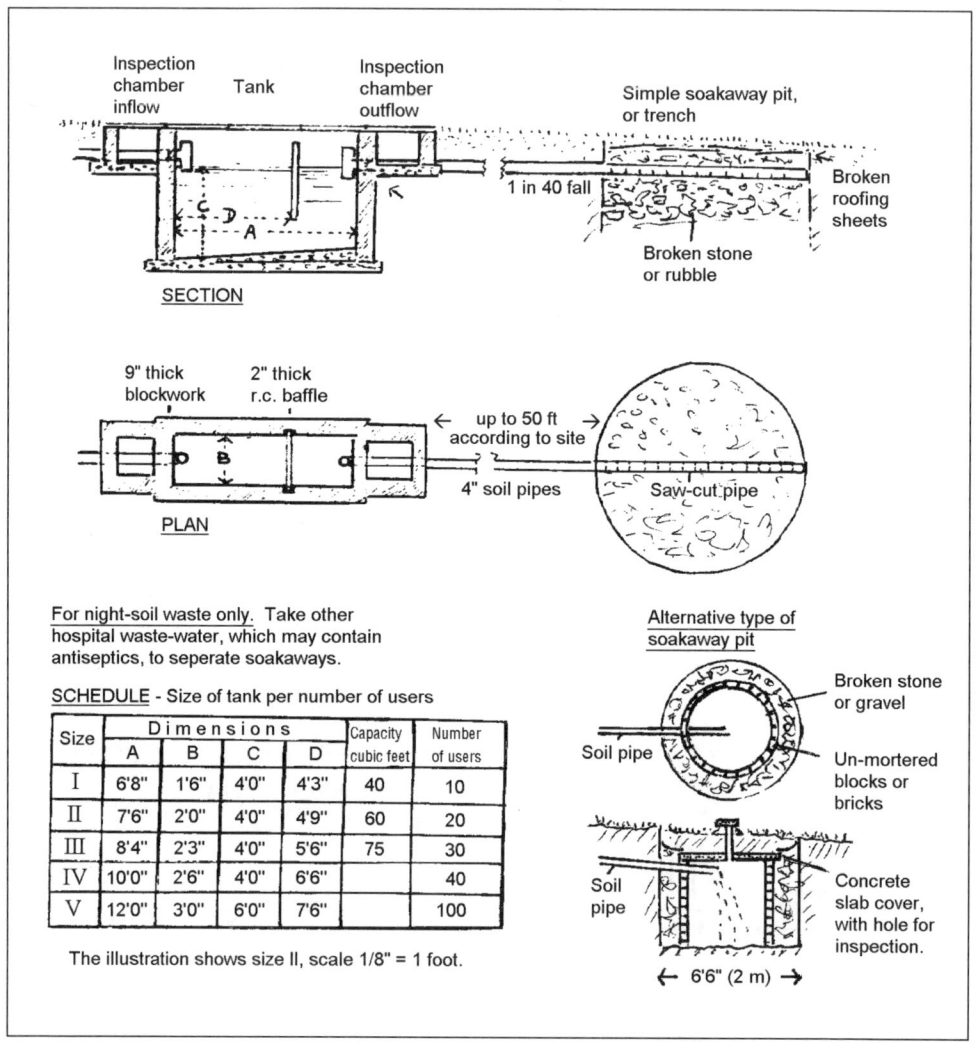

For night-soil waste only. Take other hospital waste-water, which may contain antiseptics, to seperate soakaways.

SCHEDULE - Size of tank per number of users

Size	Dimensions				Capacity cubic feet	Number of users
	A	B	C	D		
I	6'8"	1'6"	4'0"	4'3"	40	10
II	7'6"	2'0"	4'0"	4'9"	60	20
III	8'4"	2'3"	4'0"	5'6"	75	30
IV	10'0"	2'6"	4'0"	6'6"		40
V	12'0"	3'0"	6'0"	7'6"		100

The illustration shows size II, scale 1/8" = 1 foot.

into the second compartment with any excess water. This is the 'effluent' which gradually overflows through the exit pipe. This is placed 100 mm (4 in) lower than the entrance to the tank, so there is always a gradient of flow to-wards the exit. Effluent can be inspected in the outflow inspection chamber.

Soil pipes carry the effluent to a soakaway pit, or long soakaway trench. The latter is excellent if there is plenty of space, preferably on land sloping away from the hospital buildings. The trench of to 1 m (2 to 3 feet) depth, and 20 m (60 feet) long, filled with gravel, covered with soil, allows the effluent to be absorbed into the top-soil. If space is more limited the pit system has to be used. This should be simply dug out to a depth of about 3 metres (10 feet). It should not be lined with concrete, as absorption into the top-soil has to take place throughout its circumference. It may be filled with large stones to above the level of the effluent pipe, roofing sheets laid loosely on top, then soil to surface level, and allowed to grass over. An effective alternative is to dig the pit as before, 2 metres wide, then build a circular open brickwork tank in the centre, 1.5 metres wide, to within 0.5 metres of the surface. Fill the space between pit-wall and tank with stones or gravel. Run the effluent pipe into the tank. Place a pre-cast concrete cover over the tank, with a hole in the centre and inspection pipe from it to above ground level. Place plastic sheeting over the gravel, then back-fill the whole and grass over, leaving just the inspection pipe, which will need a cover.

Emptying of septic tanks
The inspection chambers should be checked from time to time. As long as the sewage flows across the channel of the entrance chamber freely, without back flow from the tank, and effluent in the outflow chamber is clear, then all is well. If the tank is full, then all use of the toilets draining into it should be discontinued. The tank should be opened, all liquid material pumped out, or lifted out in buckets, and carried away in 44-gallon drums to be dumped. Urban sanitary departments have special tankers with strong suction pumps for doing this work.

The solid material (sludge) at the bottom then has to be dug out and removed to a site distant from buildings. Later, when its odour has gone, this material can make excellent fertiliser for the fields. Sanitary workers often do no more than remove the liquid material, leaving the sludge behind. This restores the septic tank to normal operation for a time, but, as its capacity is much less, it may need re-emptying again in a year instead of five or more.

Developing efficient supporting services in a hospital, and good modern sanitation, comes only with steady effort. There is always room for improvement – and demands for further extensions too.

CHAPTER 8

Improving and Extending Hospital Buildings

Hospitals grow. Buildings have to be modified. Some of the modifications relate to the way buildings function in the tropical environment – the effects of sun and storm. Additions are required to make good omissions from the original design, and to meet the needs of expanding demand, or a new area of service.

Architects, building engineers and planners should be consulted and used whenever possible. In many places they are just not available. The medical administrator may have to make do with advice from a general builder or draughtsman. In time, he will acquire quite an experience of building design and construction through having to be unofficial 'clerk of works' and supervisor. His knowledge of how the building will be used – its functional flow – is always of the greatest importance.

Protection from the elements

All climates vary. A tropical climate can be warm and pleasant (or at least hot and tolerable) for much of the year, and health work at the primary health care level can even be done out of doors in the shade of a convenient tree. However, hospitals have to continue to function whatever the weather, and allowance must be made for seasonal changes bringing excessive heat, cold nights, driving rain, and storms with terrifying wind and lightning. These are equally part of the tropical environment.

Some buildings prove functional even in the most extreme conditions. Others must be modified, for the sake of patients and staff: the ventilation is too poor, the sun shines direct on working areas, or the rain soaks the patients' beds or waiting benches every time there is a storm. If a good architect has been employed he should be able to anticipate these design faults, but so many buildings go up without such help. To turn to air-conditioning as the remedy in every case of poor ventilation, for example, is an excessively expensive option, both to the hospital, and to the nation which has to supply the energy.

The sun
Orientation of buildings

Where there is space to choose, tropical buildings should mainly run east to west. On the side facing the equator (south face in the northern hemisphere, as in Nigeria) there should be a roof overhang of at least 2 m (6 feet), which allows for a verandah of 1.6 m (5 feet). While the sun is hottest at mid-day walls and windows on that side are shaded. Early morning and late afternoon sun will enter any windows facing east or west, and these should be avoided if possible. The sun's angle will be lower, and the rays not quite so intense, but still hot enough to be uncomfortable (see Figure 8.1).

Figure 8.1: *Orientation of buildings (from* A model health centre (6) *– modified).*

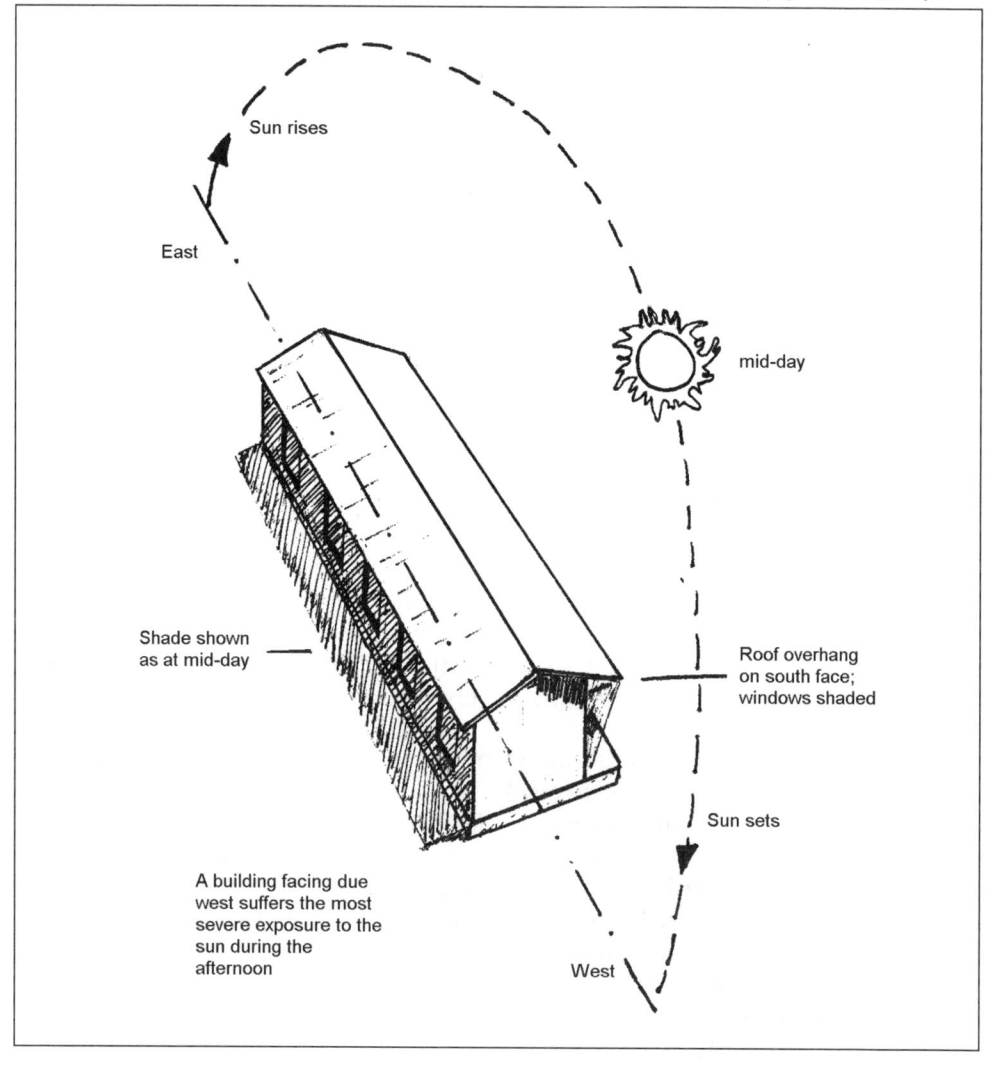

Curtains

Where the site requires buildings to run north to south, west facing windows may need shading with curtains or plastic louvre (Venetian) blinds to protect those in the room from the afternoon sun. Curtains which are just tied up with a piece of string look untidy, and can generally only be knotted up to get them out of the way, when the sun's heat is less, and more light is needed. The use of modern curtain runners requires the upper hem of the curtain to be fitted with 'rufflette tape' into which curtain hooks can be attached at about 150 mm (6 inch) intervals. These can then be hooked into the metal or plastic runners on the rail. Smooth movement of the curtain is then made easy (see Figure 8.2).

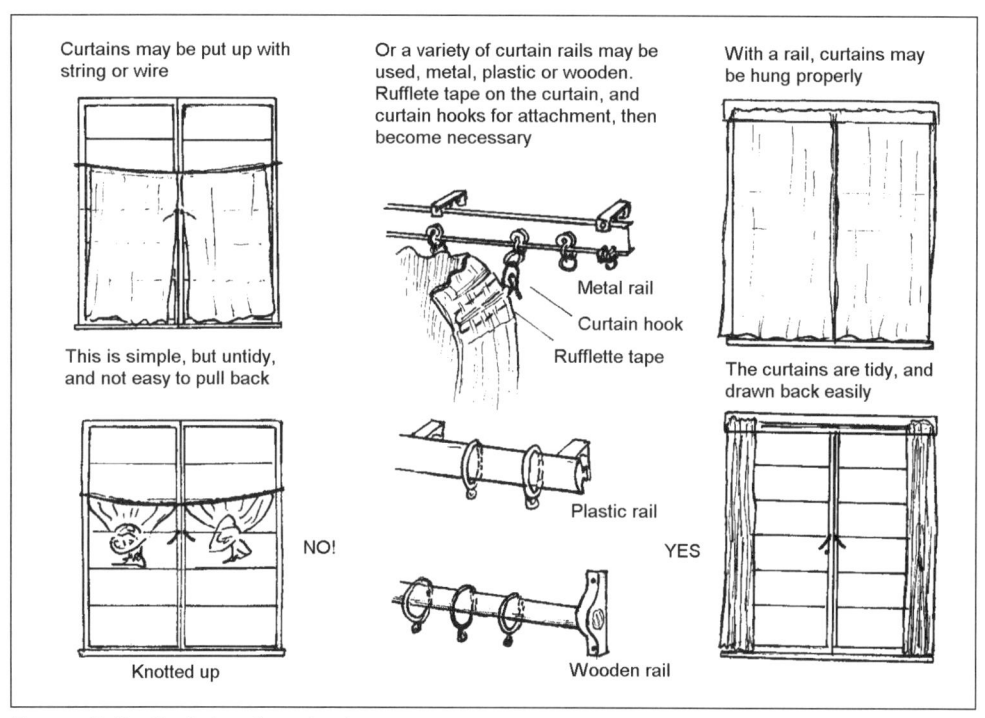

Figure 8.2: *Curtains for shade.*

Heat resistant roofs and ceilings

Corrugated iron roofs are still widely used, as being so much longer lasting than thatch, and the roofing sheets are generally available. They absorb heat and, to counteract this, movement of air through the roof-space should be allowed for, cool air being drawn in from the eaves, and the heated air given a vent to the exterior from gable ends (see Figure 8.3). If the rooms below are protected with a ceiling of flat asbestos-cement ceiling sheets, working conditions are reasonable. In wards and residences where people sleep, the openings into and out of the roof-space should be screened to prevent the

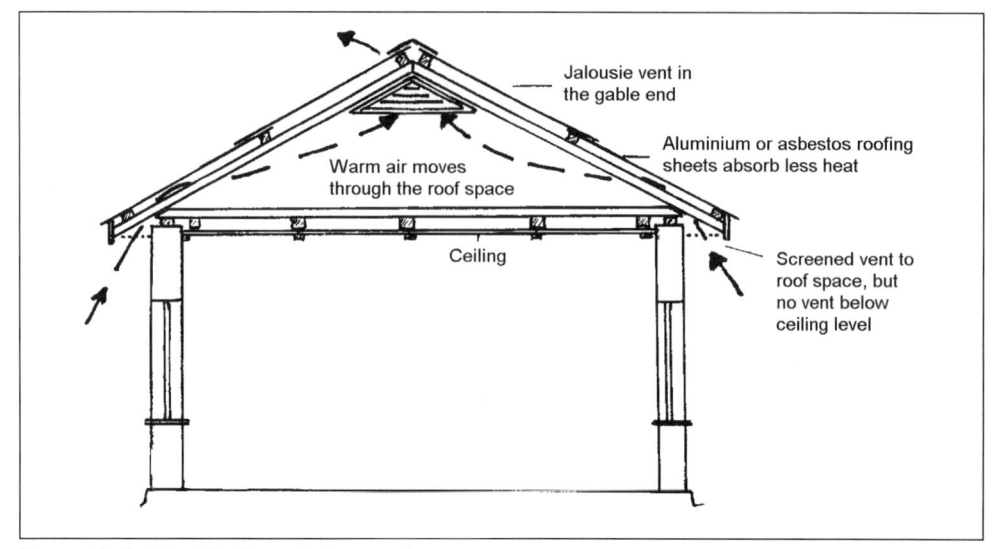

Figure 8.3: *Ventilation of the roof-space.*

space being populated with lizards and rodents which can cause so much noise as they scamper around at nights.

Aluminium roofing sheets reflect more of the heat, and have the advantage that they do not rust, but in other respects behave like corrugated iron. Corrugated asbestos cement roofs provide the best heat protection, though being heavier, roof timbers need to be stronger. Unfortunately the smart white appearance of an asbestos roof tends to blacken after a few wet seasons through the growth of algae. The matt black surface absorbs more heat, and counteracts to some extent the heat resistant properties of the asbestos cement. Apart from applying a white cement paint to the roof, there is no way to avoid this. Algicides cannot be used for fear of contaminating the run-off water, and the ground around.

In some countries asbestos is being phased out for occupational health reasons, and alternative fibres are being combined with the cement to provide roofing sheets which are as good (such as Unicem). A cottage industry is growing up in Uzuakoli, Nigeria, and elsewhere in forest areas, using palm fibre as the reinforcement for cement roof tiles.

Room ventilation
The two important factors are that air can traverse the room from one side to the other, and that hot air can escape from below the ceiling.

1. *Through ventilation.* Buildings should, where possible, be constructed lengthwise, one room deep, with windows on either side and ventilation

across the room. This gives the most comfortable working environment. Residences built four square, with windows in two adjacent sides, give reasonable ventilation, but rooms with a window on one side only can be very stuffy to work or sleep in. Where rooms are built on either side of a central corridor, some cross ventilation can be obtained with a louvred vent above the door, or even a window on to the corridor with opaque glass louvres and curtains. These allow air movement, but decrease security and privacy, and also admit corridor noise and dust, and at night the unwanted illumination from corridor lights left on, if there is mains power.

Figure 8.4: *Air vents at ceiling level.*

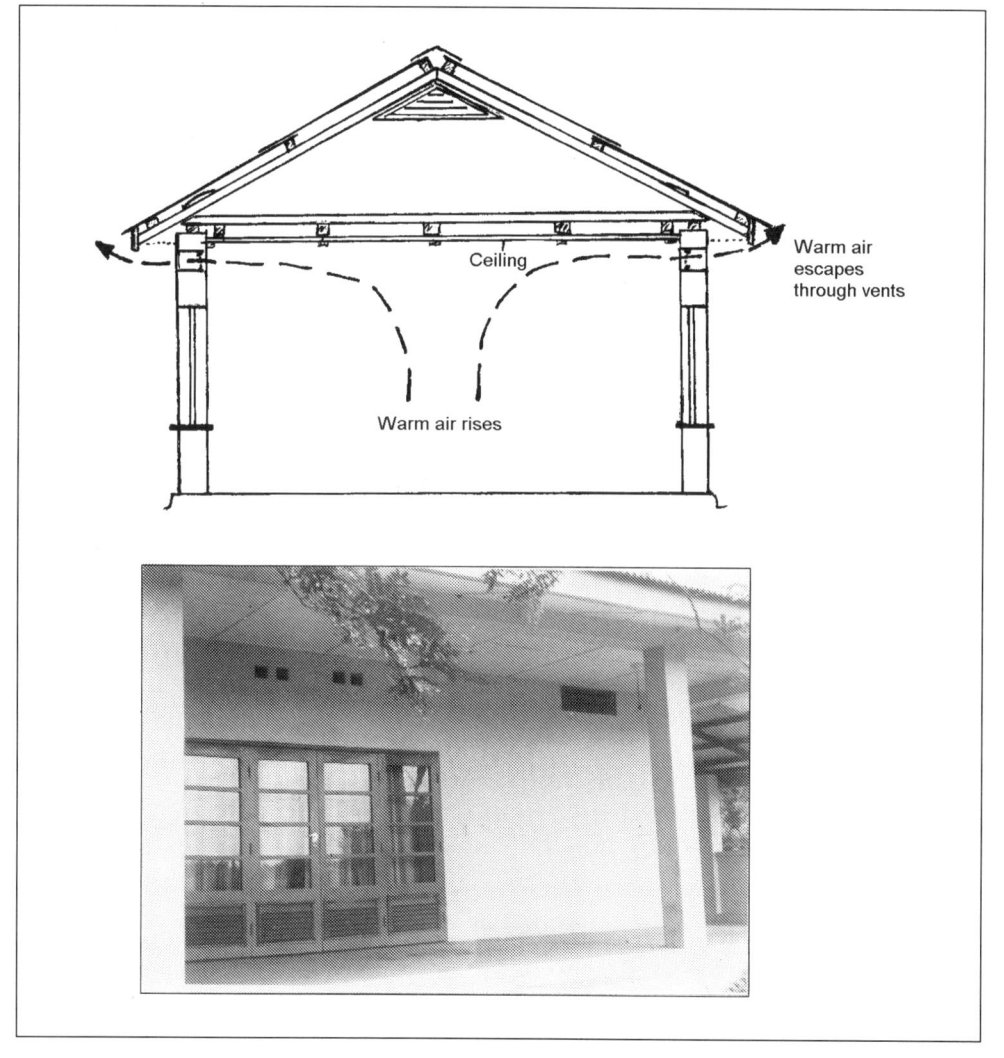

Where the windows of a building are screened against mosquitos, one has to weigh the advantages of reduced insect nuisance against the partial obstruction to air movement by the gauze screens. Many feel that the degree of ventilation loss is still acceptable.

2. *Air vents at ceiling level.* A simple design feature, so often forgotten, is the inclusion of air vents at just below ceiling level, one or more in every room (see Figure 8.4).

Hot air rises, and hot air must be allowed to escape. If the room ceiling is at 3 m (9 feet 9 inches), and doors and windows 2 m (6 feet 6 inches) or 2.3 m (7 feet 6 inches) high, there remains a dead space below the ceiling of nearly 1 m depth where stagnant hot air gathers. A common solution is to install a ceiling fan to stir up the hot air and force some of it out through the windows. It is much simpler to incorporate air vents on each outside wall. These should be of adequate size, say 225 x 450 mm (9 x 18 inches), and are generally placed above doors or windows. Two hollow cement blocks on their side may be sufficient, but it is better to leave a space in the blockwork and put in a small wooden frame to which mosquito gauze can be fitted if the building is to be screened.

Rain and wind

Tropical rainstorms can be very heavy. The noise of rain drumming on the corrugated iron roof of a lecture room or health education shelter can drown out the voice of the speaker. This is another good reason for using asbestos cement roofs on such buildings since they are relatively quiet in a rainstorm. But rain does not only fall vertically; it may also be blown almost horizontally, and a few storms soon show up a building's weaknesses, particularly on the side of the prevailing wind.

Problems of open blockwork

Architects and builders often like to use this around waiting spaces or external staircases. Open blockwork walls provide shade. They provide good ventilation, but they may also let the rain in disastrously. In a waiting space they can be a real problem. Patients sitting close to the ventilated wall have to retreat to safety in a storm. Staircases or covered ways can be unpleasant to negotiate when the rain is blowing through; but at least one is only passing, and an open block wall is better than nothing. Such walls are really only suitable for car ports, or screen walls where the entry of rain does not matter.

Secure windows

As soon as rain blows up it is essential to be able to close windows quickly and easily. Glass louvre windows have an advantage in light vertically falling rain, since no drops can enter, but if the rain is blowing hard they may still allow some water through even when tightly closed.

Side-hinged casement windows, if left open, may allow even light rain to enter unless protected by very wide eaves. Latches and window bolts should be checked from time to time for effective functioning. Severe storms can blow rickety wooden windows right off their hinges if not secured in time. Metal-framed windows at least are not in danger of that. Neither do they shrink or warp as wooden ones do.

Storm water drainage

Roof edges do not have rain gutters in tropical countries, except when the water is being collected for storage. As rain pours off the roofs on to the ground around a building it can cause trouble in various ways:

- splash discoloration on the walls, if falling on to bare earth,

- erosion of the footings,

- rising damp in the walls, if the ground slopes towards the building.

Figure 8.5: *Ice-plant hedges beside covered way.*

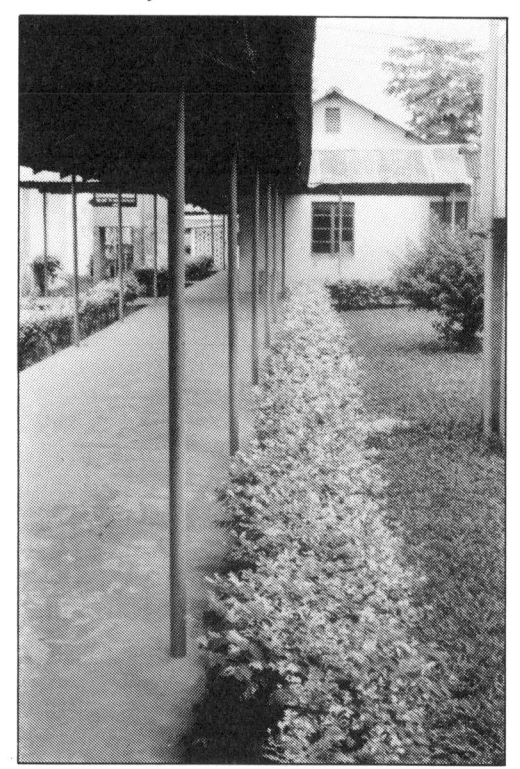

Having grass lawn up to the walls of buildings can prevent splash and erosion. The grass must be regularly cut. A low hedge of ice-plant (see Figure 8.5) can be planted around a building, or beside covered ways, along the line where the roof water falls. It is slow-growing and strong enough to withstand the rain and prevent erosion.

Concrete storm drains around buildings are favoured in many compounds, and are essential on the side of a building where the ground slopes towards it. The gutter must be placed correctly under the eaves along the line where the rain reaches the ground. This is not necessarily vertically under the roof edge. Rain falling from corrugated iron and asbestos roofs behaves differently, due to differing surface tensions (see Figure 8.6). Rain from corrugated iron falls out and down, so the drain should not be too close to

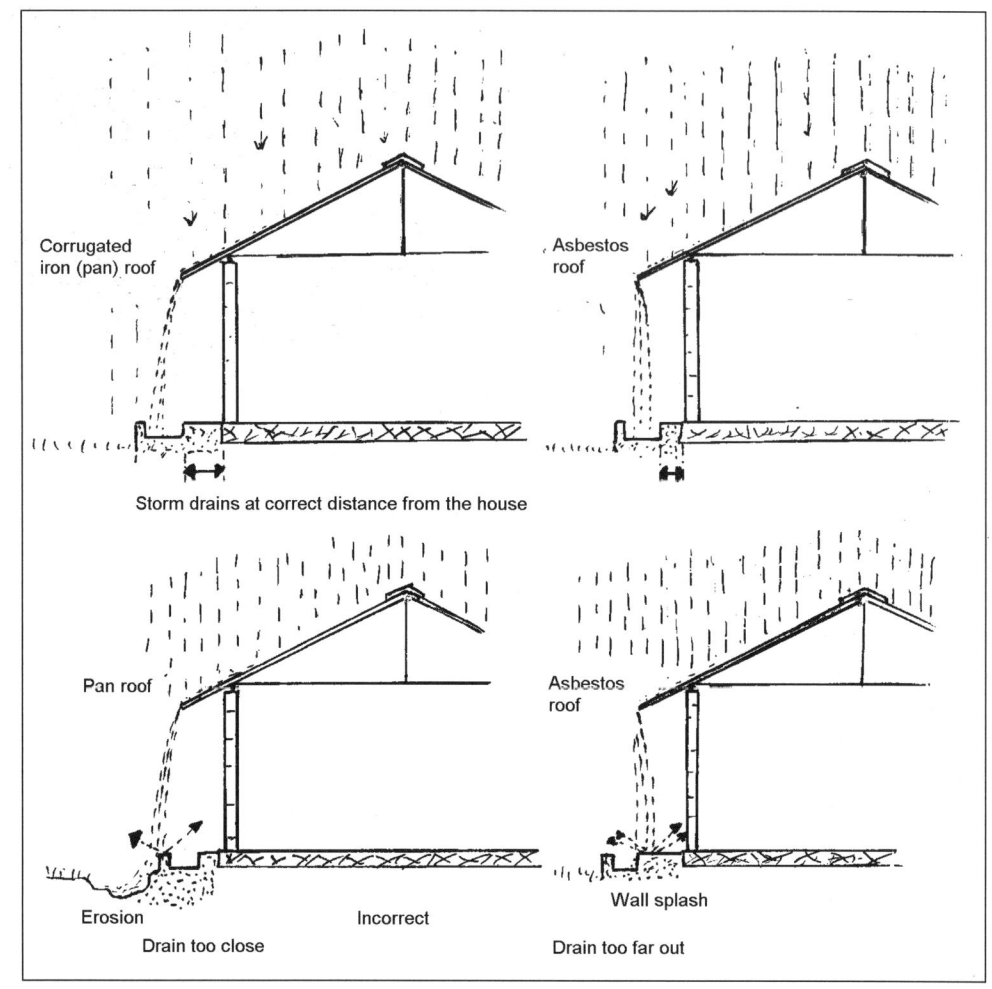

Figure 8.6: Rain falling from different types of roof to a drainage ditch.

the building. Rain from asbestos roofs tends to angle back towards the building, then down, so the drainage gutter should be closer. Incorrectly placed gutters allow the rain to fall on the concrete apron causing splash, or beyond it causing erosion.

Trenches to carry storm rain away from buildings down slopes to unused ground should be built. These should be of adequate size and depth to cope with the heaviest storms, for example 1m (3 ft) wide, and nearly as deep, and concreted where erosion can be expected. If not concreted they should be shaped in a V-section, and allowed to grass over to prevent erosion (see Figure 8.7). The grass on a sloping edge can be easily cut with a cutlass by a labourer keeping the grounds tidy. A square cut drain is less easily cared for.

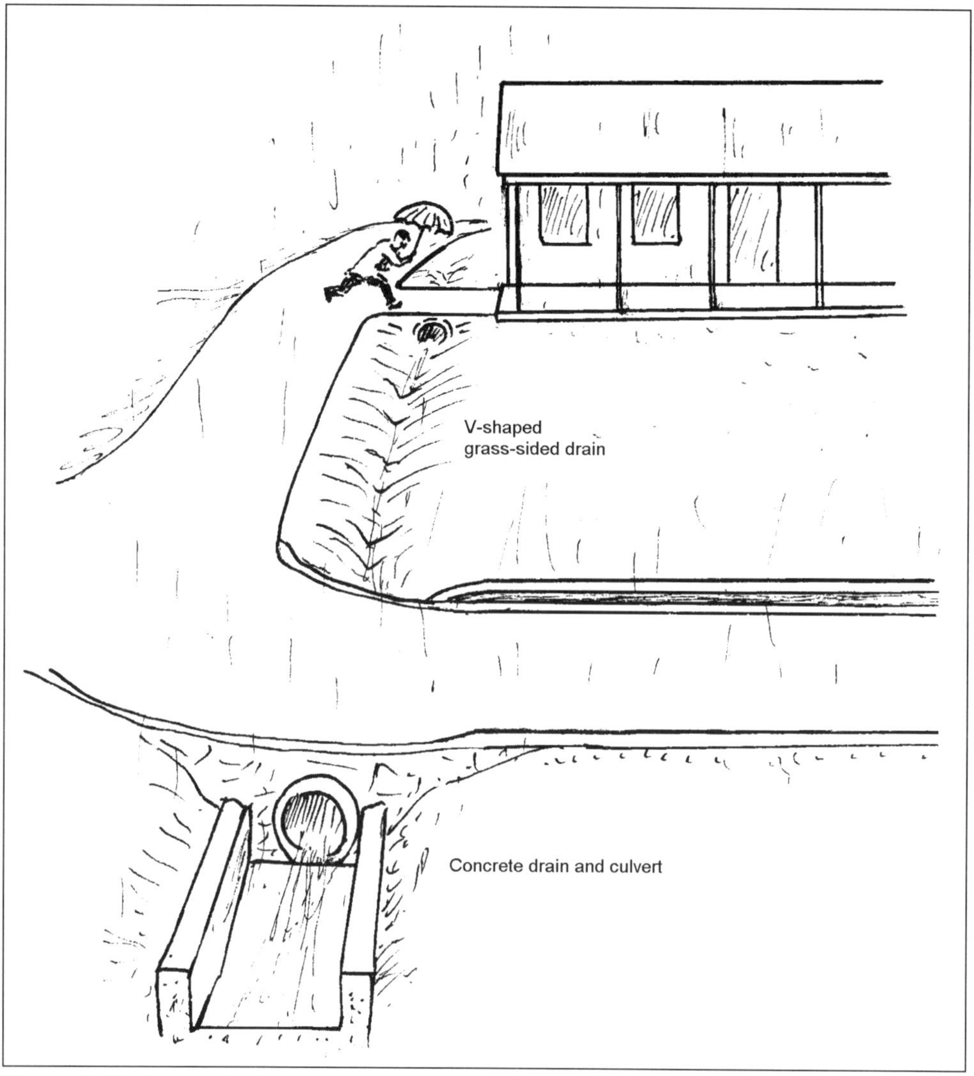

Figure 8.7: *Storm drains.*

Culverts are essential to carry storm drains under roads and footpaths at all low points where water otherwise accumulates. Large soil pipes or pre-cast concrete culvert rings should be used.

Wind damage

Concrete block or brick built buildings are largely immune to wind damage, apart from damage to roofs. Rising, twisting winds may get under the roof eaves, rip off a corner, or even lift the entire roof. It is worthwhile for hospitals to have an insurance against such an eventuality. Building contractors should also be watched when roofs are being put on. If the roof is insecurely fixed to the wall with nothing more than strips of metal banding taken over the wall-plate and sunk into the blocks at each side, then disaster may follow.

The durability of a roof lies in its fixing to the wall-plate and the wall-plates bonding to the wall (see Figure 8.8). The wall-plate is the piece of 100mm x 75mm (4 x 3 inches) timber laid all round the top of a concrete block wall. It should be specified in the contract that this should be fixed by means of coach or rag bolts set in the concrete which tops the wall. When the nuts are screwed down on the wall plate a firm and safe anchorage is provided for all the roof timbers which are nailed or bolted to it.

Figure 8.8: *Wall plates.*

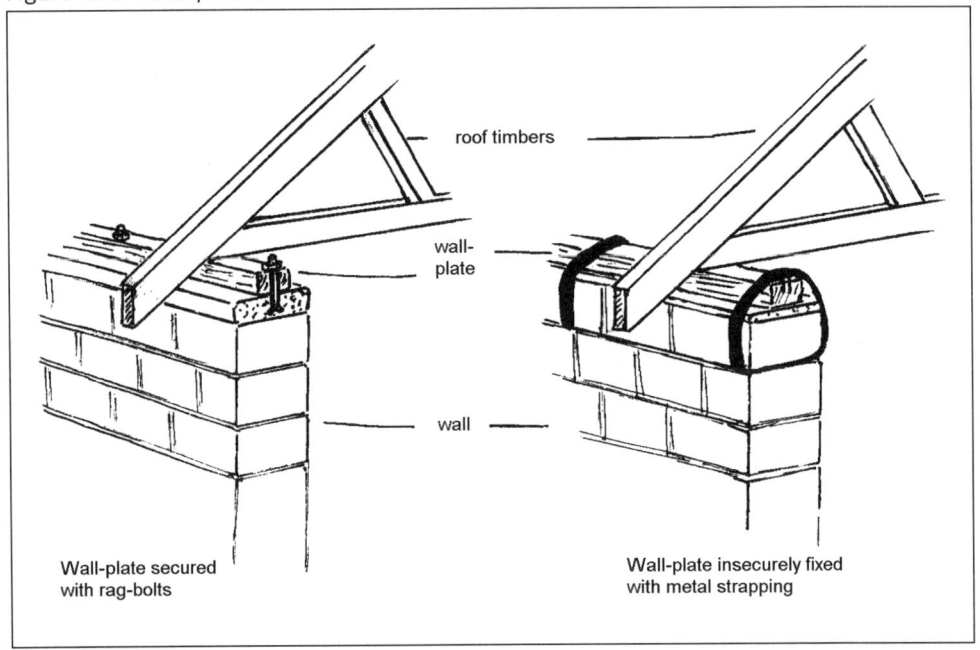

Lightning and fire
Lightning can strike anywhere, anytime, and in tropical storms it can be frightening. Normally we think little about it, but buildings should be adequately protected. Precautions against lightning strike, and against fire from whatever cause, should always be taken in public buildings.

> When WGH Ilesha was rebuilt in 1953 copper lightning conductors were fixed to the two highest points, the overhead water tank and the bell-tower of the hospital chapel. Despite these, during 1962–63 the hospital buildings were struck by lightning three times. On the first occasion it earthed in the

water pipes of a house and wrenched a shower-rose and connecting pipe out of the wall, leaving a large hole. Fortunately no one was under it at the time. The second strike burnt a hole in the meter board of the hospital gatehouse, and the third terminated in the refrigerator of a doctor's house, giving three people shocks, and temporarily paralysing the doctor in his right arm. Action to protect the whole hospital against lightning was then taken, with the help of a visiting consultant engineer. He also reviewed the entire electrical installation to eliminate possible causes of fire. It was an object lesson in the measures which should be taken to protect tropical buildings.

Good earthing

Laterite soils in the tropics tend to have a high resistance, so the earth rods for the electrical system should be more than just a piece of 20 mm (3/4-inch) water pipe sunk 600 mm (2 feet) in the ground. Steel-cored copper rod should be used. This usually comes in metre lengths, which can be joined together. The first should be hammered in, then a second attached and hammered in too, plus a third if possible, providing an excellent earth to a depth of 2 to 3 metres. Each ward, department or residence should have its own earth, and this should be linked by a heavy copper earth wire to the ring main supplying all the sockets in the building.

The use of earth linkage circuit breakers (ELCBs)

The customary large 30 amp fused main-switch for each building may now be supplemented, or replaced, by an *earth linkage circuit breaker*. The mains supply goes through this to the distribution fuse box, and it is linked direct to earth. It automatically disconnects if there is an overload or a leak to earth due to faulty equipment, or if there is a sudden surge on the mains supply or a lightning strike. The switch goes up and power is cut off. The red button does the same thing and can be used for testing. Power can be restored by simply putting the switch down (see Figure 8.9). It is much easier than mending a fuse.

Figure 8.9:
Earth linkage circuit breaker.

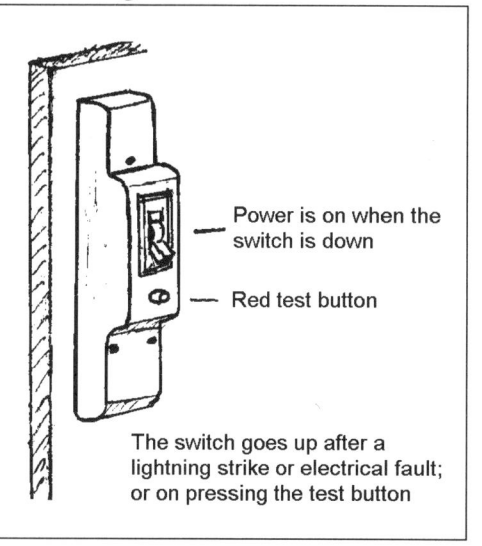

Power is on when the switch is down

Red test button

The switch goes up after a lightning strike or electrical fault; or on pressing the test button

However, if there is still an earth leak or overload due to faulty equipment, it will immediately trip again. Electric irons, kettles, refrigerators, bed-side switches and other equipment should all be examined for bad connections, and the distribution box checked for blown fuses.

Lightning arresters

The overhead distribution lines around a hospital compound can themselves 'attract' lightning, that is they may provide a natural source for earthing, in the same way as a high building or tall forest tree. It is therefore wise to fit lightning arresters to the overhead poles at the ends of main distribution lines, or a point where the direction changes (see Figure 8.10).

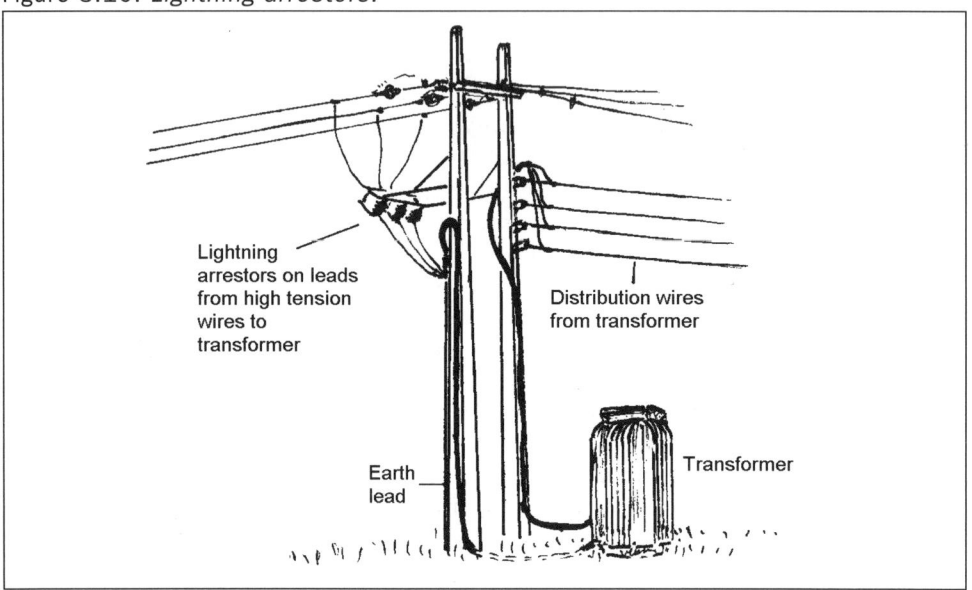

Figure 8.10: *Lightning arrestors.*

Arresters look like large porcelain connectors, with a lead from each wire on the pole. They are linked to earth, and filled with a substance, silicon carbide, which at normal voltage is a non-conductor. However, in the presence of a sudden surge of 10,000 times normal, its resistance drops dramatically. Lightning is thus safely earthed. In the presence of a super strike the arrestor may be shattered, and need replacement. After installation of arresters on the distribution lines at WGH Ilesha there were no further reports of damage from lightning strikes in 20 years.

Fire prevention

Fires are not common, but when they do occur are generally traced to faulty electrical connections, or careless disposal of cigarette ends. The electrical system should be examined from time to time in a programme of preventive maintenance.

Fused, square-pin plugs should have the correct strength of fuse, 3 amp or 5 amp for lighting equipment, and 13 amp only for heating elements, or heavy users of power like a deep freeze. A 3-amp fuse may be deliberately used on delicate equipment like record players or electronic items to protect them from mains power surges.

The fuses in distribution boxes should be checked to be sure they have the recommended strength of fuse-wire in them (see Figure 8.11). If any have been repaired incorrectly with copper wire that will not melt with overload, this should be put right, and those responsible warned about the danger of such a practice.

Figure 8.11: *Fuse wire card.*

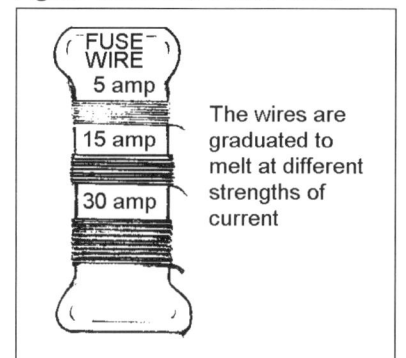

The wires are graduated to melt at different strengths of current

Excessive use of three-way or multiple adaptors on a single socket should be discouraged (see Figure 8.12). It is safer to provide more sockets. The connection of electric irons or toasters to lighting outlets which have no earth should be forbidden. Additional spurs from a ring main should only be taken via a standard junction box on the wall, or in the roof space.

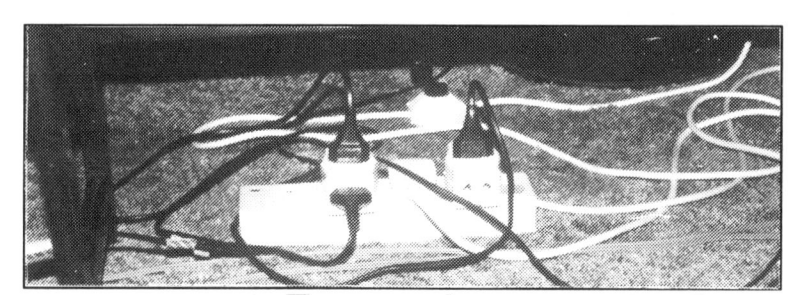

Figure 8.12: *Excessive use of adaptors on one wall socket.*

Wiring does deteriorate with time in tropical temperatures. Insulation exposed to sunlight, movement and kinking, or excessive heat, as in the mains service leads or in the wires at the entry to light sockets, leads to irons or hanging switches above beds, are particularly vulnerable. Insects such as mud-wasps and spiders may also make their home in ceiling roses, sockets and switches where the slot for the cable entry gives them room to enter. All these wiring faults can be potentially dangerous and a fire hazard.

Fire-fighting precautions

Every institution should have some kind of *fire alarm*, either electrical or hand-operated, and this should be test operated from time to time, with due notice to the staff, so that they know what it sounds like, and what the sound means. Where staff should go in case of fire should also be rehearsed, so that panic might be minimised in the event of an actual fire.

Fire-fighting equipment, such as foam extinguishers, should be at strategic places in each ward or department. These need regular servicing from a local agent, or fire-brigade if there is one. If there is a chief fire prevention officer he would also advise about the siting of water hydrant openings to which their hosepipes could be attached in an emergency.

Planning for growth

As said at the beginning, hospitals grow. It is a mistake to imagine that the initial set of buildings will be sufficient for long. The reasons are not far to seek.

1. The population of most developing countries is growing at 2% to 3% per year, and urban centres even faster.

2. A well run hospital tends to attract patients from a widening radius as its name becomes known.

3. Extension or improvement of the roads in the area brings more people within easy travelling distance.

4. Health expectations rise when the hospital proves it can help in conditions previously accepted as incurable.

5. Promotive and preventive health activities in the community may bring primary care workers into contact with people formerly outside the range of the hospital. Such workers cannot ignore the need for curative care among people they see, or the credibility of their health education will be lost. So more patients are brought to hospital.

Small primary care clinics may best be allowed to *grow in numbers*, by building more clinics on new sites to bring health care even nearer to where the people live. On the other hand many health facilities will exand on their initial site as they grow in the range of service offered. A first aid post may develop into a primary health centre, and that into a maternity home, and finally into a full comprehensive health centre or hospital.

A centre built as a district hospital, providing secondary care, should always be planned with growth in mind.

The site as a whole

- *Hospital sites should be large enough to allow for growth.*

- *Hospital buildings should be compact enough to allow for easy supervision.*

The appropriate balance between these two requirements is not always achieved. Consider two possibilities.

1. *A compact design on a small site – little chance for growth*

   A hospital designed like this (see Figure 8.13) may look attractive, and work very well in its early years. It is compact, and easy for a small staff to supervise. However, to make additions to it for more out-patient consulting room space, or for a children's ward, for example, is difficult, if one is to do it without spoiling the overall appearance, and making the place look cluttered and untidy. The site is small. The building is not designed to have natural 'growing points' from which extensions can take place.

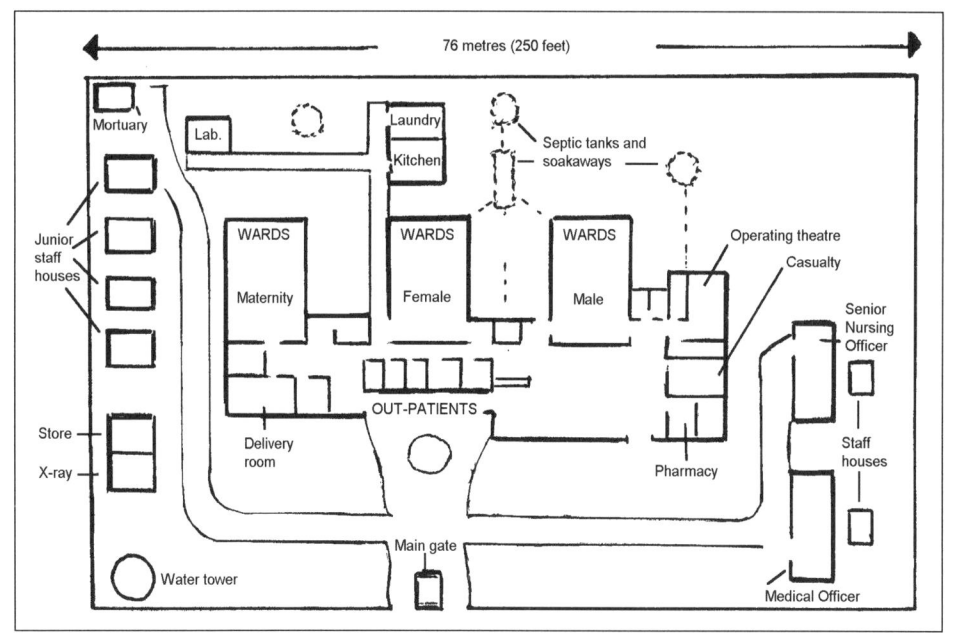

Figure 8.13: *Small site, only 250 feet long compact plan, but little space for extensions.*

2. *A diffuse selection of buildings on a large site – room for growth, but hard to supervise (see Figure 8.14)*

   It is correct to have a site large enough for growth, but it is a mistake to spread the initial buildings too far apart, making intercommunication between departments difficult, and supervision virtually impossible.

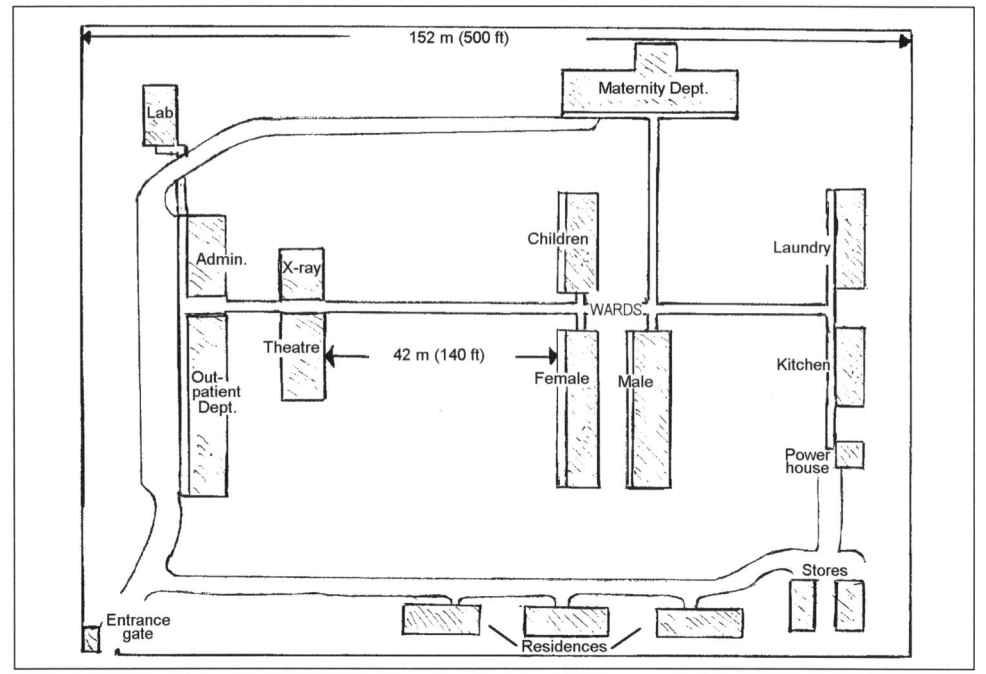

Figure 8.14: *Hospital layout, site 500 feet long and four times the size of that in Figure 8.13; good but rather diffuse for easy supervision.*

Phased growth

It is obvious that a balance has to be kept between allowing for growth and achieving sufficient compactness for easy supervision. This may be done by having a compact initial group of buildings as 'Phase I', and leaving space on the site for Phase 2 and Phase 3, with the expectation that the use to which Phase 1 and 2 buildings are put at first will alter in the larger institution. (See Figures 8.15, 8.16, 8.17.)

The federal government of Nigeria had plans for such phased growth in the buildings sketched out for its primary health care 1980–85 development plan. In it the small initial clinic could grow to a primary health centre, and ultimately to a comprehensive health centre with 30 beds, a theatre, laboratory and X-ray.

All hospital functions grow together

If a hospital is increased in size with, say, the addition of a 30-bed ward, it is necessary to consider what other facilities will also need to be added. More nurses will be required, and if nurses are housed on site, then additional accommodation for them will be needed; likewise, if another doctor is employed, another out-patient consulting room may be required, and possibly extension to technical facilities, such as the laboratory or X-ray. A balanced development should be aimed at.

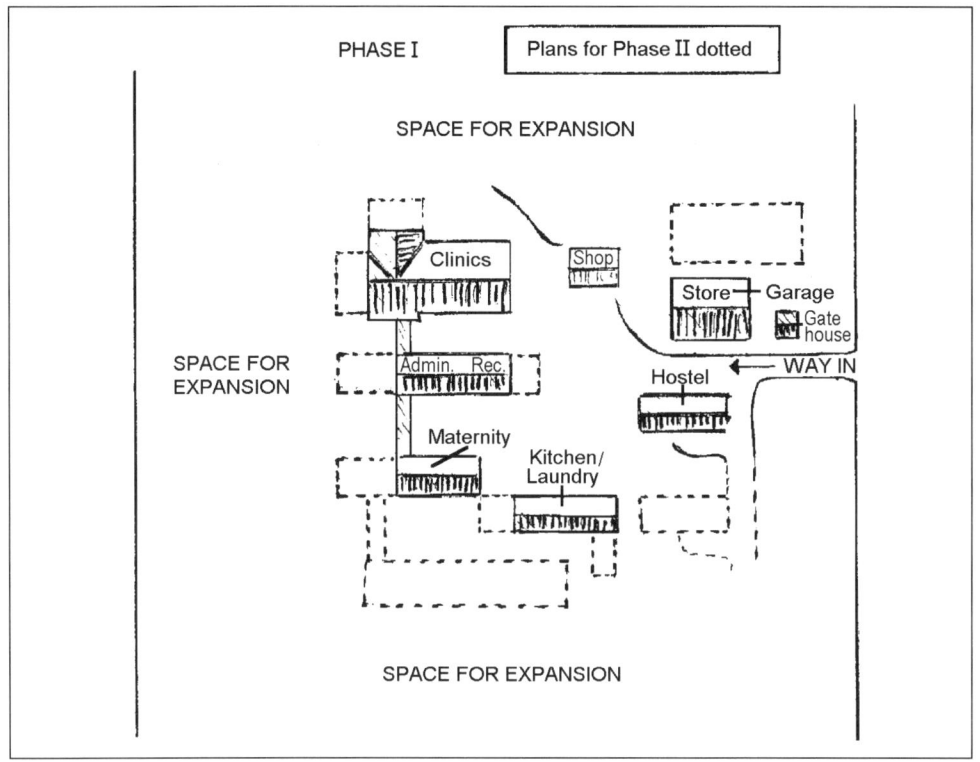

Figure 8.15: *Phase 1.(Plans for Phase 2, dotted).*

When WGH Ilesha was rebuilt with 120 beds in the 1950s, it found itself faced with the need for planning further extensions in the 1960s. Fortunately a qualified town planner offered his services. He resurveyed the entire site to be sure the existing buildings were correctly placed on the drawings, then used the 'growing points' which had been provided, and the surrounding vacant areas, to show where different buildings could be added in a 10-year development plan. This allowed for a balanced increase in number of beds, nurses' accommodation and enlarged training school, senior staff residences, X-ray department, administrative offices, out-patient consulting rooms, medical records, theatre, pharmacy, laboratory and laundry. The plan was duly followed to completion during the next 12 years, though not exactly as originally envisaged (see Figures 8.18 and 8.19).

Private hospitals
Private hospitals, which use one or two adjacent large residences adapted for the care of patients, inevitably suffer from the effects of a cramped site as growth takes place, and every square metre gets taken up with essential extensions, for improved toilet facilities, hospital stores, a larger laboratory or whatever.

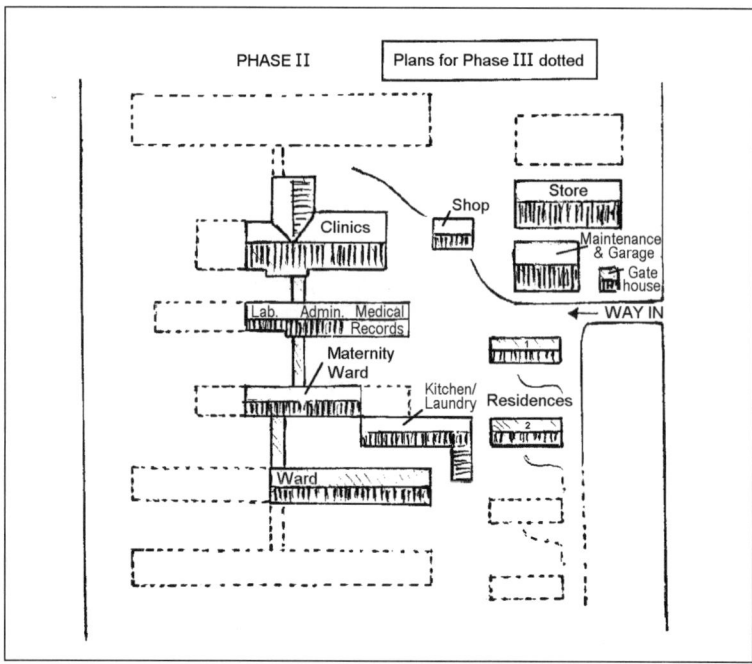

Figure 8.16: *Phase 2. Plans for Phase 3 dotted.*

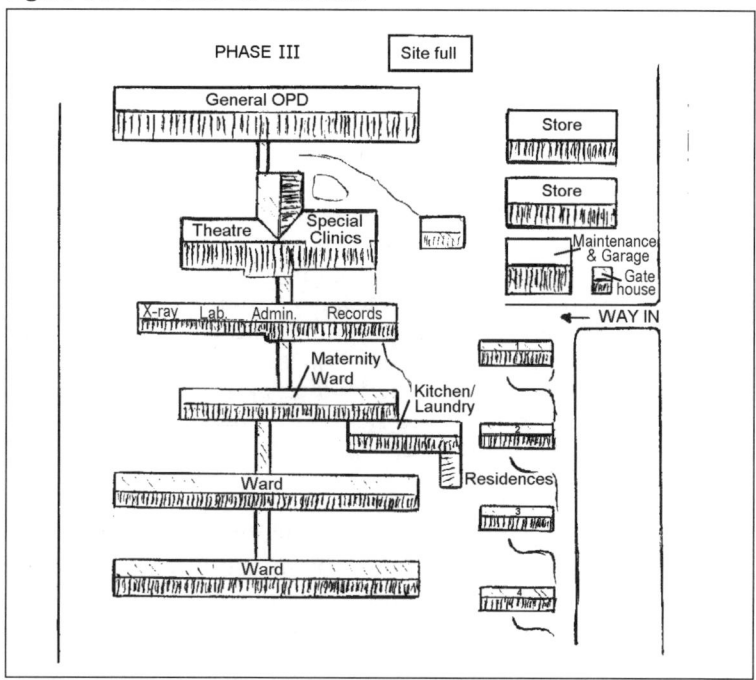

Figure 8.17: *Phase 3. Site full.*

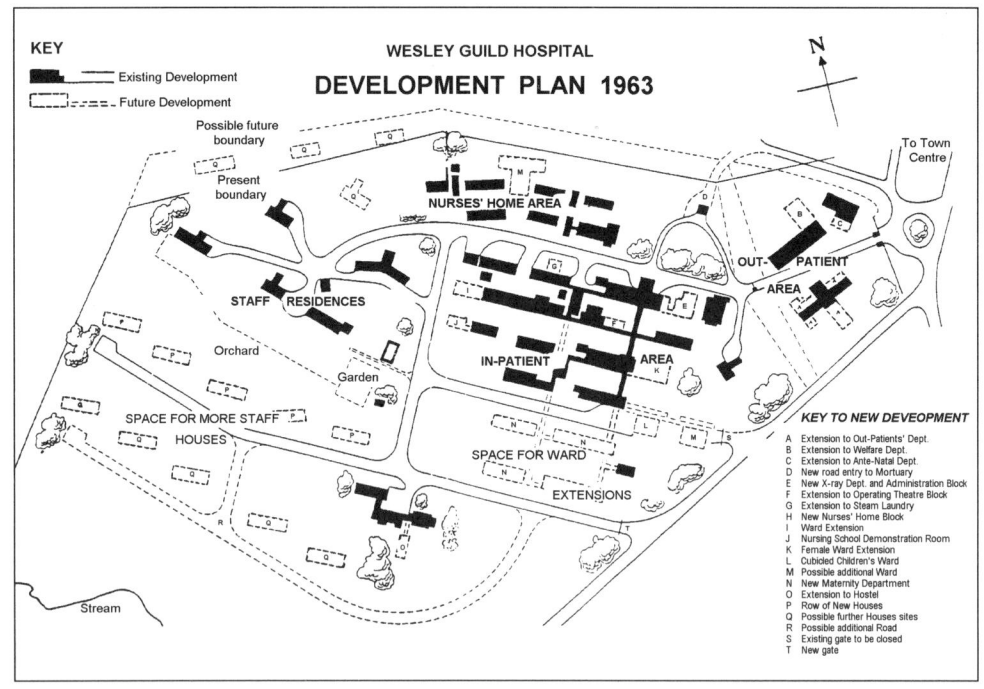

Improving and Extending Hospital Buildings 161

Figure 8.18.

Figure 8.19.

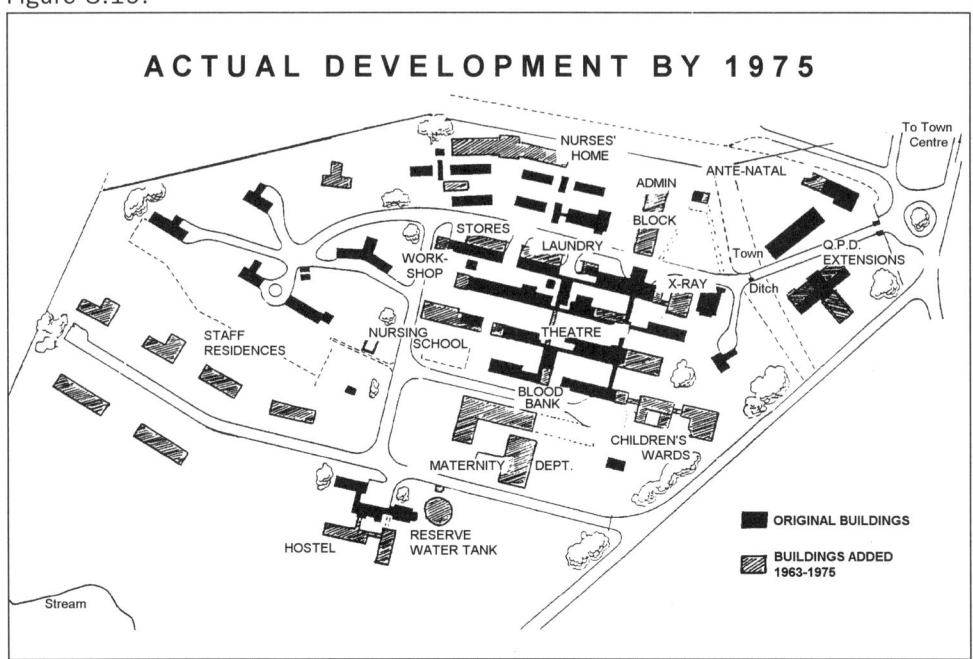

When purpose-built hospitals can be put up on a new site, the above principles of phased growth and balanced development can be followed. Urban sites may have to consider vertical development, with a lift system between floors, and ramped walkways for the occasions when power fails.

On more spacious sites there will be no need to go beyond single or two storey buildings, which do have advantages for hospital purposes, for example in wheeling patients from one department to another.

A perimeter fence or wall

In the urban situation the site is likely to be fairly circumscribed, and the need for a boundary wall a first priority. In a rural area, however, on a large site, a fence or wall round the entire site can be extremely expensive. In some countries this has to be constructed as soon as the site is obtained in order to establish and retain the right of occupancy. In other situations the land border may be marked with stone pillars at each of the corners and points along it. The building of a definitive fence or wall may be deferred till seen to be inescapable.

When that time comes it is worth considering what kind of protection the fence is to provide. Is it to prevent human intruders and improve general security? Or is it to prevent cows entering and causing havoc? Or is it to enable the hospital to do some landscaping of the compound with the planting of flowers, trees and hedges? For that the fence needs at least to be strong enough to keep out stray goats and sheep.

> At WGH Ilesha an economical fence was built along the most vulnerable border of the site, which served three purposes.
>
> 1. The low wall at the bottom prevented vegetation creeping up all over the fence, and gave support to the concrete posts.

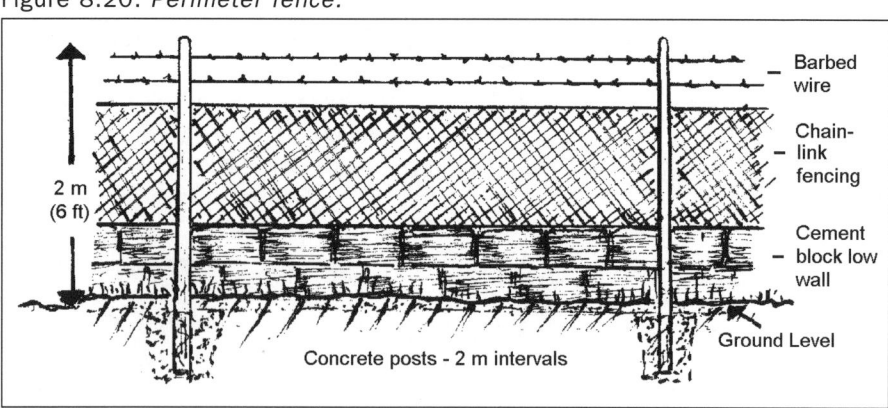

Figure 8.20: *Perimeter fence.*

2. The chain-link fencing wire effectively kept out goats and sheep. A 2 m (6 foot) roll was cut to 1 m width to make it go further and reduce cost.

3. The two strands of barbed wire discouraged human intruders (see Figure 8.20).

Building contracts

Before starting any new building or building extension, plans have to be drawn and these should contain as much interior detail as possible, e.g. sanitary fittings, drains and soakage pits, electrical sockets and lights, fixed cupboards or working surfaces, types of windows or doors (not forgetting ceiling-level vents, see p147), and whether a floor should have a terrazzo finish, vinyl tiles or plain smooth cement.

The more that can be included in the initial specification, the less will have to be added later – generally at increased cost as a 'supplementary item'! There should be an agreed Form of Contract which can then be attached to the Plans and Specifications, and Estimates of cost sought from local builders. When one Estimate has been accepted, the builder can be called, and the Contract completed and signed and witnessed by both sides.

The *Form of Contract* may be a standard one as used by the government or the proprietor, or one specific to the hospital. From hard experience one learns that this is essential. However friendly, trustworthy or well-known the builder, a word of mouth agreement can lead only too easily to misunderstandings and bitter arguments! The contract form is mutually beneficial because it contains items which protect both the builder and the employer. At the very least it should include:

- Agreement that the contract is based strictly on the plans and specifications which are attached.

- The contract price, and the time to be allowed for completion.

- The points at which payments will be made as building proceeds, and the proportion to be given, e.g. 30% on completion of foundations, 30% on reaching the wall-plate. No 'mobilisation fee' should be paid in advance, but by giving a fairly substantial part of the cost in the early stages, the builder without great capital resources should be able to manage. Some contracts include 'penalty clauses' for taking longer than specified, but these may only cause initial estimates to be inflated.

- When the builder considers the work complete, there should be an inspection, any deficiencies seen made good, and then an Interim Certificate of Completion given by the employer. Up to 90% of the contract price should then be paid.

- As long as the contract has stated it in advance, the final 10% can be kept as a *Retention Fee* for an agreed period, say three months, or one wet season. This will ensure that the builder makes up any further defects or deficiencies that come to light during that period. A Final Certificate of Completion is given at the end and the builder paid off and absolved of further responsibility.

Departmental plans

Care should be taken in each department to allow for maximum convenience of patients and staff in moving from one area of service to another. There should be a natural 'flow' from one point of service to the next.

This principle will now be considered in relation to certain departments where it is particularly important.

Out patient departments

The counters for patient registration should be opposite the main entrance, and beyond them there should be *adequate waiting space*, with comfortable chairs, or benches with back-rests, sufficient for the average daily attendance. This can often be in a hall which can also be used for health education talks or demonstrations. Smaller secondary waiting spaces outside consulting rooms, laboratory or pharmacy, should also be provided. It is a mistake to expect patients to wait in a dark corridor, or narrow verandah, crowding around, and often obstructing, the entry door to a consulting room for example, yet this deplorable practice is so often seen.

Some hospitals also have arrangements for screening, or a preliminary consultation given to all patients by experienced nurses, and arrangements for this should be incorporated in the natural flow. Some patients will be sent for simple treatments straight away without seeing a doctor, others for laboratory tests before referral, or for repeat dressings. Others may be sent to see a doctor for emergency care even before the normal doctor's clinic begins. The flow should allow for all these movements (see Figure 8.21).

Even where hospitals do not route patients through a preliminary nurse consultation, there is need to ensure the maximum of convenience in *cooperation between doctors and nurses in the care of patients*. The Kwun Tong United Christian Hospital in Hong Kong has a well-planned out-patient department on the ground floor of its nine storeys. Here there are covered waiting halls outside doctors' consulting rooms on either side of the central nursing area. Patients are called from the waiting areas into the consulting rooms, and from the central area nurses can be quietly called by the doctors to help with emergencies, assist in procedures, or simply act as chaperones. After the consultation patients can be conveniently referred through to the nurses for an injection, dressing or other nursing care. The patients then

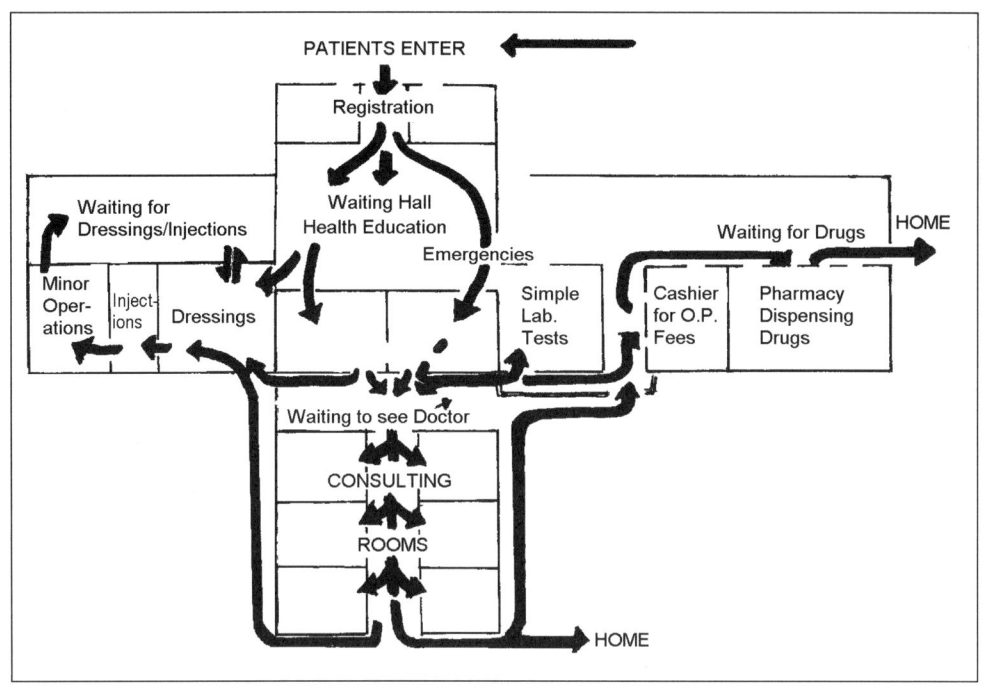

Improving and Extending Hospital Buildings 165

Figure 8.21: *Out-patient department plan and flow diagram.*

move on directly to collect medicine, book their next appointment or return home (see Figure 8.22).

The flow pattern for an under-fives clinic has been considered elsewhere by its originator, Professor David Morley (14). The clinic requires a very simple building which allows a convenient flow from the entrance:

1. to registration, with weighing and charting of the weight
2. to a waiting hall for health education
3. then nurse consultation, receipt of medication, and referral for immunisation, special nutritional care or oral rehydration
4. return home, or see the doctor if very ill or in need of admission (see Figure 8.23).

No health centre or hospital in a developing country should be without such provision for paediatric out-patients.

Ante-natal clinics also require similar care in ensuring smooth patient flow for the various services required: registration, urine examination, weighing,

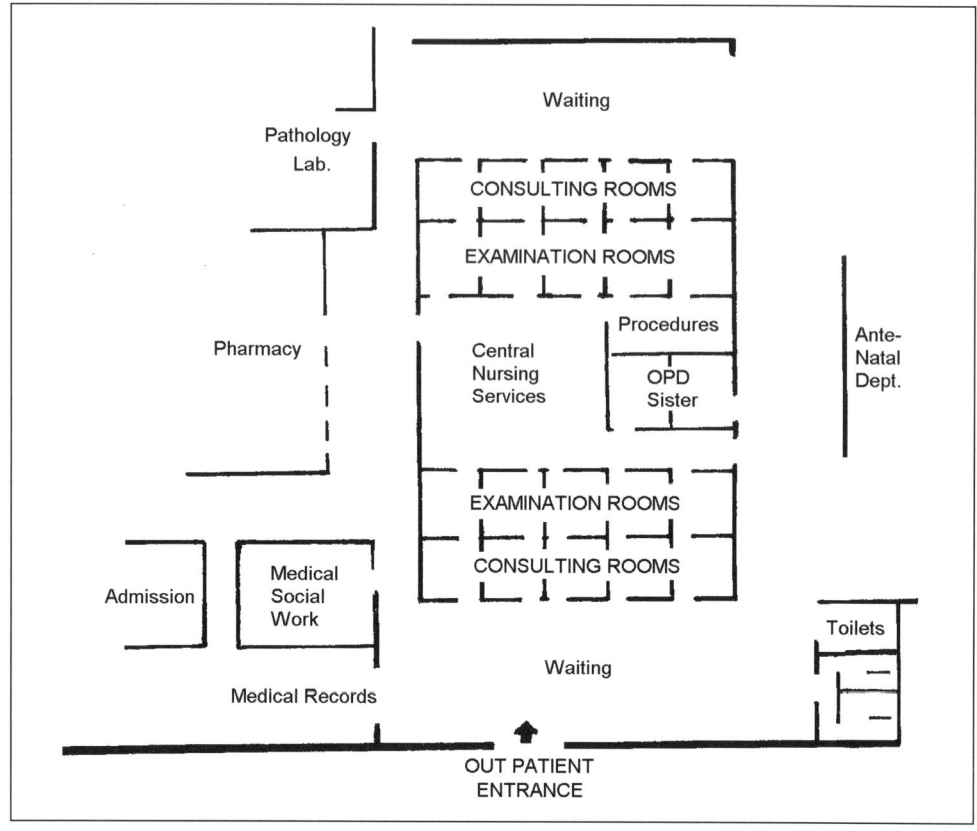

Figure 8.22: *Out-patient Department plan, Kwun Tong UCH, Hong Kong.*

Figure 8.23: *Under-fives clinic plan and patient flow.*

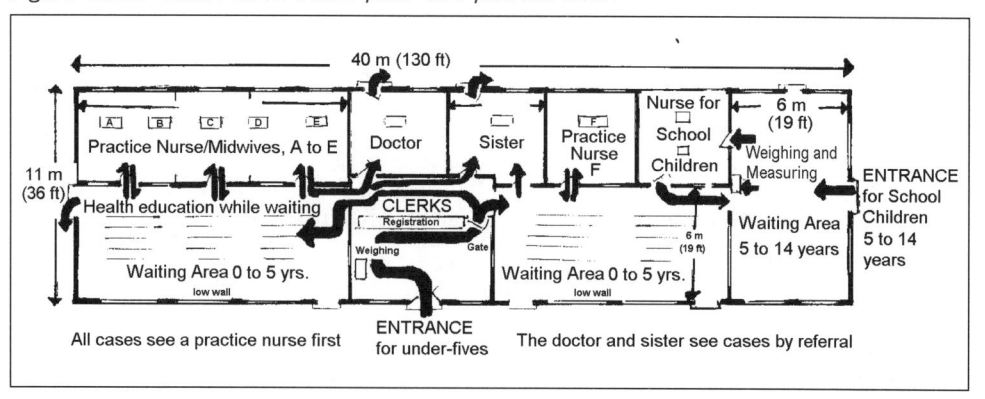

interview, blood pressure testing, abdominal examination, referral to doctor where necessary, and exit to collect any necessary medication (see Figure 8.24).

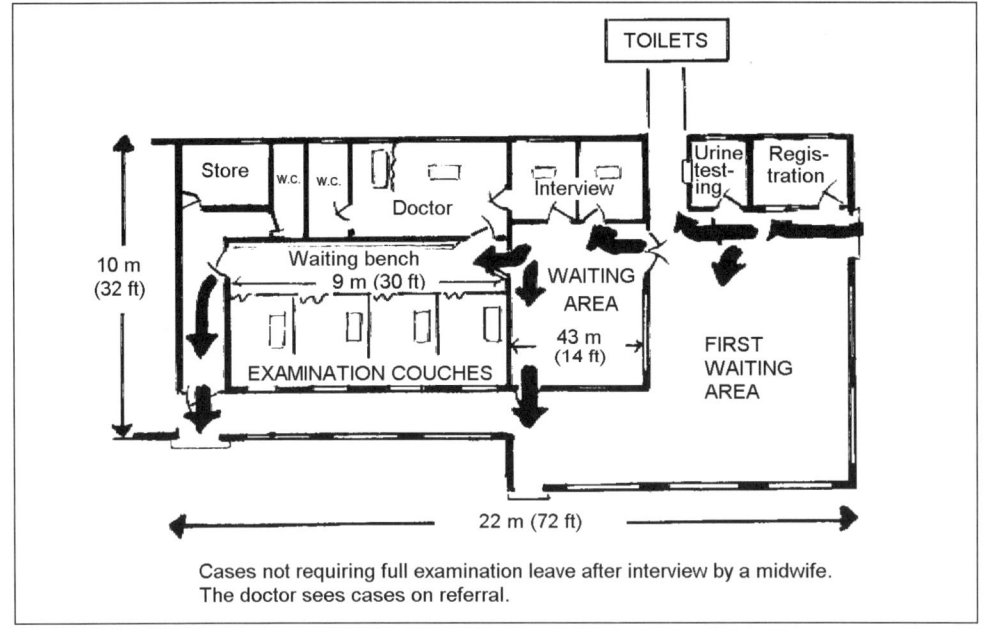

Figure 8.24: *Ante-natal clinic plan and patient flow.*

Theatres and maternity units

Operating theatres have specialist requirements in terms of flow which are well understood. The operating area is deemed 'clean', and there is generally a line near the entrance at which staff change from outside shoes to theatre boots and don theatre gowns, and patients are moved from ward trolley to theatre trolley. Staff in the clean area do not move out while on duty. Patients being returned from the theatre should be taken by a different exit, or via a recovery room, rather than being wheeled past patients who may be waiting to go in.

Separate small theatres should be provided for incision of abscesses and treatment of septic or trauma cases not requiring sterility, and for the application of plaster of paris for fractures.

The delivery unit in a maternity department presents similar problems in trying to provide a clean environment.

> The maternity department opened at WGH Ilesha in 1972 proved to be superb in terms of flow and convenience. Patients entered through a receiving room, complete with its own shower room and sluice, and thence to the first stage ward. When second stage started they could then be wheeled through to a delivery room, or to the obstetric theatre, if operative intervention was required. All dirty linen and used instruments from theatre and delivery

rooms could be dealt with in one sluice room, then taken through to a sterilising room adjacent. From there clean materials could be taken back to the theatre, or to delivery rooms (see Figure 8.25).

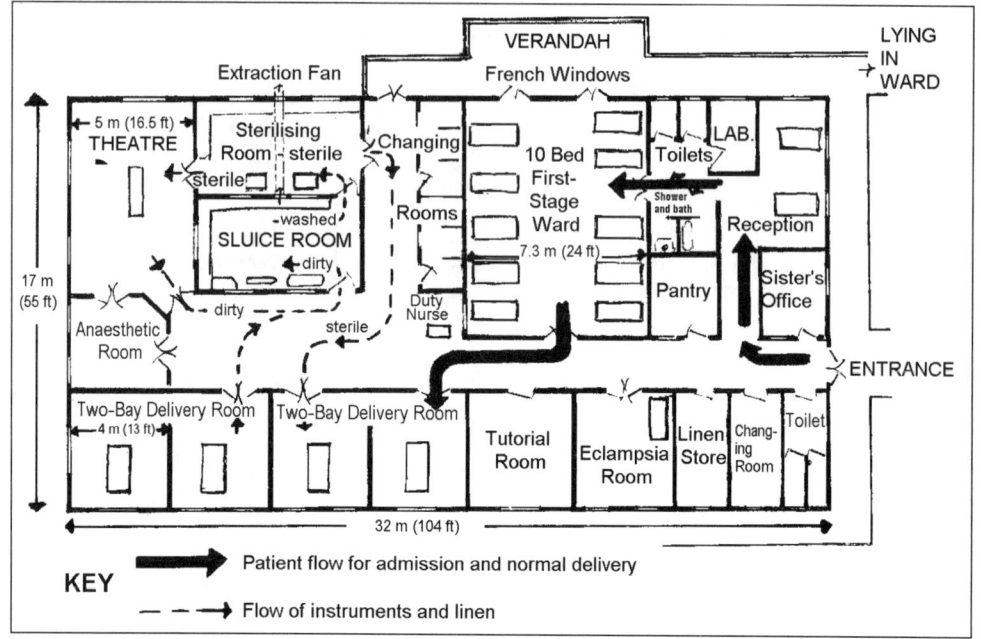

Figure 8.25: *Delivery unit.*

Children's wards

Many hospitals do not have special wards for children, a serious omission since half the population in many countries is under the age of 14. In fact, the majority of the paediatric patients are likely to be under five years old, and the paediatric wards may reserve their space for that age group. The six to 13 year-olds would then have to be nursed in a side ward near the adults.

For the under-fives it is essential that the mother, or other relation, be allowed to remain with the child to prevent it suffering from the 'maternal deprivation syndrome', which can be so emotionally traumatic. If cots are provided for the children the mothers may be advised to bring a sleeping mat on which they can sleep beside their child at night. Other hospitals provide adult beds for the children, so the mother can sleep together with the child at night. Whichever is to be the practice, a decision has to be made. What is no longer acceptable practice is for the mother to be excluded from the ward at night, and forced to go home, or sleep outside.

A Mothers' Shelter should be provided not too far from the ward where mothers can do their own laundry, shower, and rest during the day, when their own children are asleep. A kitchen area where they can prepare their own food is also necessary.

Most children's wards are still built on the conventional open plan, but they do carry more danger of cross-infection. As so many of the children have infectious diseases, there is an advantage in having *a cubicled ward*, with four cots or so per cubicle (see Figure 8.26). Children with measles, pertussis or typhoid, for instance, can then be given some degree of barrier nursing. Children with burns can also be kept in a separate cubicle with a cleaner environment. Nursing supervision is facilitated by direct vision through glass partitions from the nursing station to the cubicles. At WGH Ilesha two sluice rooms were provided, one for the nurses to use, and another for the mothers to use when emptying their children's potties.

Figure 8.26: *Cubicled children's ward plan.*

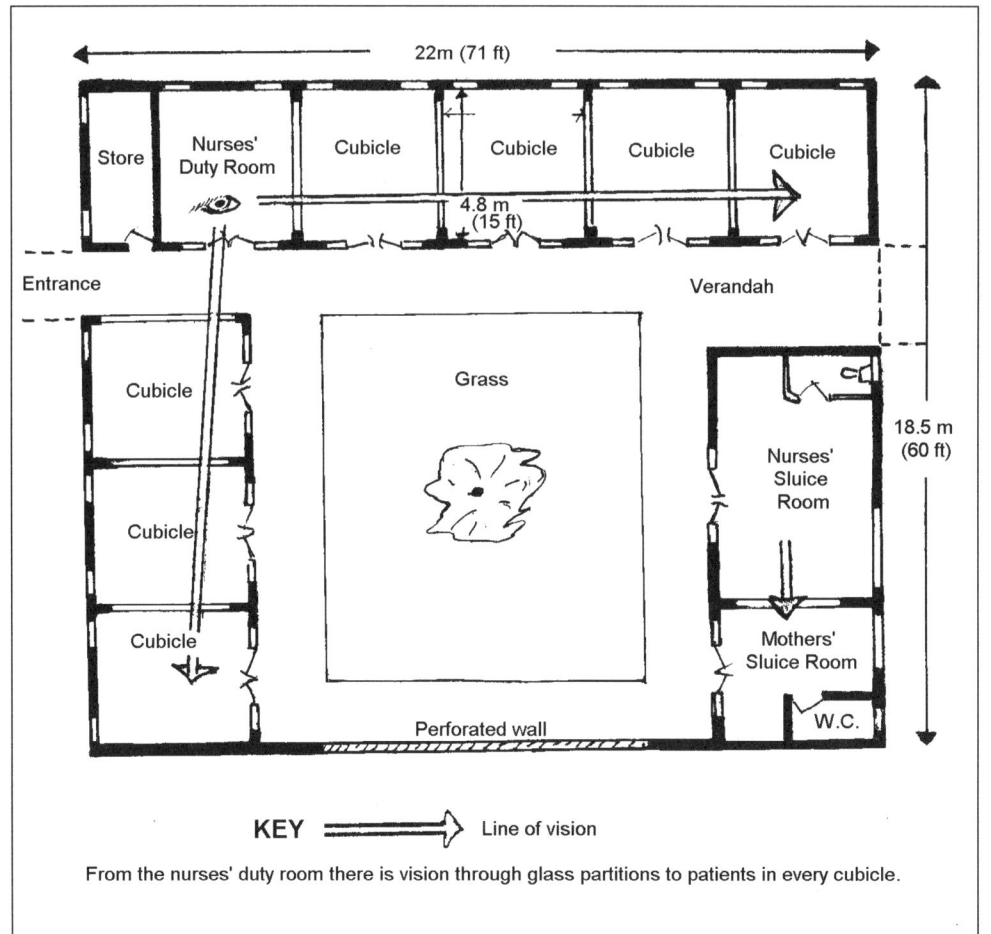

Provision of a *premature baby/neonatal unit* requires a compromise between the needs of the babies for a very clean, if not sterile environment, and their need for maternal contact and care, and for the mother's expressed breast milk till able to breast-feed directly. Survival on purely artificial feeding is hazardous for any infant in the tropical environment, and this is even more so for the premature or low birth weight child. It is generally deemed better to risk relatively early contact with the mother.

The experimental ward which was built at WGH Ilesha combined some of the features of the western type premature baby unit run entirely by nurses, with little input from the mothers, and the cubicled ward where the mothers were present all the time, and did most of the nursing. It proved admirably effective in practice (see Figure 8.27). The central nursing area was treated as clean, with the minimum of entry to it, except by the nurses on duty and the paediatrician. On either side were glass-walled cubicles, each big enough for two infants in small cots warmed with electric light bulbs, or in electric

Figure 8.27: *Neonatal and premature baby unit.*

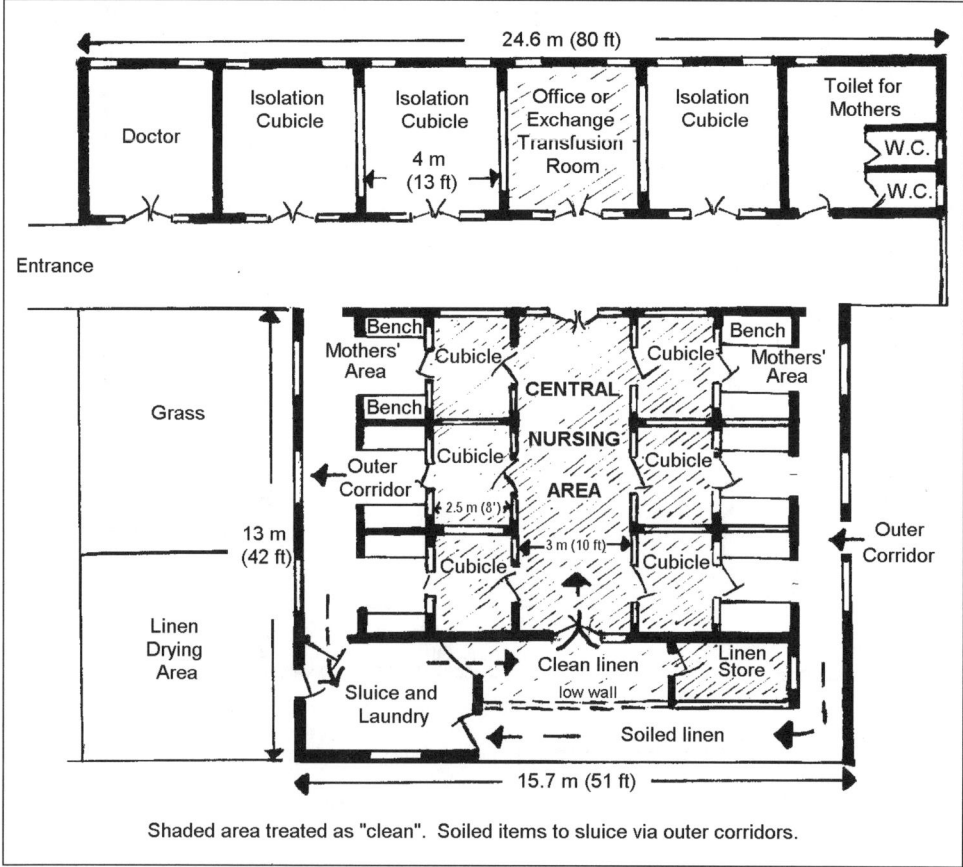

incubators, when these were available – and working. The outer wall of the cubicles had a second door onto a mothers' area, with partitioned benches where each child's mother could rest opposite her baby's cot. The nurses undertook all initial care of the infants, and the mothers produced EBM in a side room. However, as soon as the mother was needed she could be called in to her own baby's cubicle to share in the care. This was generally sooner rather than later (see Figure 8.28).

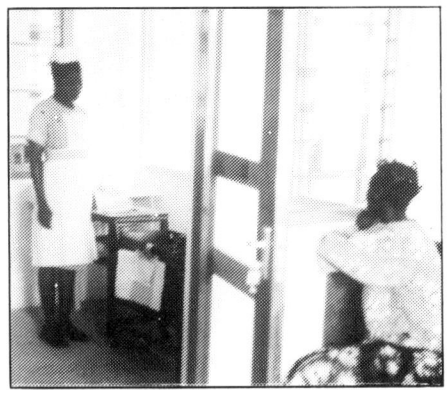

Figure 8.28: *The nurse cares for a premature baby; mother waits to be called.*

All soiled linen and utensils were removed through the outer doors of the cubicles, and taken via the verandahs to the sluice room. Here the linen was washed, dried, and returned to the clean linen store. From there it was collected by the nurses for distribution from the central nursing area to the cubicles as required. Siderooms, across the main corridor, were kept for neonates with tetanus, or suspected infectious disease.

To have good buildings which allow for functional flow is a great advantage, but the hospital can only work effectively if given adequate supplies and good diagnostic facilities.

CHAPTER 9

Hospital Supplies and Technical Services

When a doctor starts up a new hospital on his own in the private sector, or for a voluntary agency, he is likely to discover for the first time what a variety of supplies are needed for the medical, nursing and technical services of a hospital. He will have no choice but to get down to deciding what is needed, making the orders, collecting in the materials, arranging for storage, and working out means of issuing, and ensuring honest, economical and effective use of all the items so far as he can. The same is true of the government medical officer appointed to a district hospital, though here he will have help from the state authorities.

The problems in obtaining supplies vary greatly from country to country, and indeed in any one country from year to year as the economic situation changes. In some places the recession has become so serious that public service hospitals have had to use nearly their whole budget on salaries. Patients are sent out to buy drugs, dressings and other supplies for themselves from local pharmacies, before the prescribed treatment can be received. They pay heavily, and have no guarantee of quality. Such a situation should never be considered acceptable in the long term. Hope must be retained that the tide will turn. Hospitals *should* keep in stock all the essential drugs and supplies to effect the treatments ordered by the medical staff. It is on this assumption that we look now at the basic principles involved.

Supplies may be classed as *expendable or non-expendable*. Expendable items are used up. Non-expendable are not.

Into the latter category come all the major capital items of equipment, such as a vehicle, or a blood bank refrigerator or generator, which last for many years. They are, of course, expensive items which have to be specially budgeted for, and will normally be bought by the medical superintendent, subject to the approval of the hospital board, or by the government in a public service institution. The budget for purchase should also include sufficient for maintenance, and the balance sheet should allow for depreciation.

Initially the doctor in charge will find he has a heavy load in securing expendable supplies too. To have a good nursing superintendent/matron with whom to share this is the greatest relief. Other senior staff, such as hospital secretary/manager, pharmacist, laboratory superintendent, radiographer and caterer, can also be expected in due course, but only as the hospital grows and trained people become available.

The variety of supplies can be quite daunting. The development of responsibility sharing may be along the following lines.

Supply category	Responsibility Early on	Later
Drugs, vaccines, IV fluids	Med. Supt	Pharmacist
Anaesthetics, oxygen	Med. Supt	Pharmacist
Surgical and medical sundries	Med. Supt	Pharmacist
Instruments	Med. Supt	Pharmacist
X-ray film, chemicals	Med. Supt	Radiographer
Lab reagents, glassware	Med. Supt	Lab Supt.
Stationery	Med. Supt	Manager
Maintenance spares, building materials	Med. Supt	Manager
Diesel, petrol, gas, kerosene, firewood	Med. Supt	Manager
Cleaning materials	Matron	Manager
Dressings, nursing supplies	Matron	Deputy Matron
Linen, uniforms	Matron	Deputy Matron
Food for patients and nurses	Matron	Caterer

The pharmacy

Whose responsibility?
This is a sensitive area. Drugs are important. Drugs are expensive. They have to be bought, stored, issued and accounted for. A high degree of trust has to be built up between all those responsible.

The doctor's role
In some hospitals the medical superintendent, or his deputy, still keeps direct control of the pharmacy. The drugs in store are the physician's tools, and he wants to be sure they are always to hand in the quantity, strength and formulation that he needs. Drugs can be a source of temptation, and they can go astray. His concern is therefore understandable, and justified. However, his time is limited, and in other hospitals a nursing sister with a knowledge of drugs, or the matron herself, is given the responsibility under the medical superintendent's general supervision. When a pharmacist is employed a new situation arises.

The relationship between pharmacist and doctor

The pharmacist is a professional in his or her own right, and a colleague who should be ready, both to receive advice from the doctor as to the drugs needed for the conditions being treated, and to give specialist advice in return, for example as to the quality of drugs available, storage problems or ways of making economies. Honest dealing and absolute trust between doctor in charge and pharmacist are essential. As in the handling of money, where we have seen a system of cross-checking with two signatures is necessary, so in the handling of drugs the stock-ledger should normally have two signatures at times of stock-taking to confirm the quantities are correct.

> At WGH Ilesha it was accepted that the medical superintendent should hold a key to the main pharmacy store, so that he could obtain emergency supplies at night, or at a week-end when the pharmacist was not available. Should the medical superintendent have to be away, his deputy held the key. Any item taken, be it a drug from the shelves, or a cylinder of oxygen, was written down in an emergency issue book, and signed for, so that the pharmacist could know what had been taken, and adjust the stock book accordingly.

Some pharmacists are reluctant to give doctors emergency access to the stores in case they take drugs for private use; but if there is no other way to obtain an urgently needed item, to deny access may be to jeopardise a patient's life, and doctors should not allow such a situation to develop. The absolute trust must be mutual. Doctors must be strictly scrupulous in recording what they take. Only then can the pharmacist take proper charge of the drug store, and the senior doctor retain his right of entry.

What should be ordered?

Consideration has to be given as to the range of drugs that is to be made available in the hospital.

Rational prescribing

Prescribing a drug is not the only form of medical treatment. A listening ear, counselling, nutritional advice or a change of life-style may be more important. Every effort should be made to see that such drugs as are to be made available are used economically and rationally. Prescriptions should be limited in number, and in quantity. It is an abuse of drugs to give six preparations to one patient – something for each symptom – when the patient cannot really afford them, and anyway can only remember how to use two or three of them at a time. The simpler the regime the better.

A hospital formulary

Agreement should be reached between the doctors, in consultation with the pharmacist, and any others concerned with prescribing, such as the delivery room sister, as to the drugs which should be kept in stock, and the most convenient formulations. So far as possible preparations should be chosen which keep well under local conditions. For example, sugar-coated tablets deteriorate in the tropics once the original pack has been opened. Some mixtures, once they have been made up, cannot be stored for more than a few days. The final list should then be made into a hospital formulary which all prescribers in the hospital would be required to make use of.

The 1972 formulary for WGH Ilesha contained 400 items, 150 of them as tablets, 120 as injections (including 10 vaccines, and 10 intra-venous fluids), 40 as mixtures or suspensions, and approximately 30 each as ointments/drops for ENT & eye, ointments/pastes/powders for the skin, and lotions/solutions/liniments for skin or as antiseptics. No special effort was made to restrict drug use, except for a limit on expensive antibiotics and the like. Modifications were made from time to time as new treatments became available, and within economic reach of the patients, or as doctors expressed their preferences for particular treatments. Hospitals making a formulary now would probably have fewer mixtures, solutions and ointments, and more tablets and injections, since prescribing habits have changed.

Three policy decisions to consider

While preparing a hospital formulary the opportunity should be taken to:

1. *Agree on a hospital policy for the use of antibiotics*, for example limiting streptomycin and rifampicin to the treatment of tuberculosis; or limiting the use of certain expensive drugs to in-patients, or those on whom sensitivity tests have been performed.

2. *Agree on a hospital policy for the use of antiseptics and disinfectants.* Moist heat with an autoclave (or dry heat with a hot air oven) is necessary for surgical sterilisation, but there is an important place for disinfectants too. Chemical disinfectants are many and various, and which one is to be used for any particular purpose tends to be dictated by custom rather than by a reasoned policy. Expert advice (15), and a little thought, can reduce the number of items to be ordered as in the following example.

Chlorhexidine (Hibitane) can cover nearly all requirements, and is the nearest to an ideal antiseptic. It can be purchased as Hibitane concentrate (5 per cent), and made up for use as 1:2,000 or 1:5,000 in water for use in body cavities, or as 1:200 (0.5 per cent) in 70 per cent spirit for pre-operative skin sterilisation. For convenience it may also be purchased as the 4 per cent Hibiscrub for pre-operative hand cleaning, and as 1 per cent cream for obstetric use. *Savlon* (Hibitane with cetrimide) is favoured by some for cleaning contaminated wounds. Cetrimide has detergent properties.

Tincture of iodine is cheaper, and is the most rapidly effective skin antiseptic, but at times it can cause reactions.

Hypochlorites, like *Milton,* can be used safely on infant feeding utensils. *Phenolics,* like *Izal,* are cheap, though pungent, and useful for some instruments, and for environmental cleaning. Soap and water are, of course, the cheapest of all. For a policy on cleaning and decontamination of equipment or environment, see Appendix 2.

3. *Exclude from the list drugs of limited or no value,* except as placebo, or drugs which have been shown to be positively harmful in a significant proportion of cases, for example pyrazolone (Novalgin) or the hydroxyquinilones (Mexaform, Enteroviform). *MIMS (Africa)* may still list some of these drugs, but caution should be exercised, and advice obtained from non-commercial sources as to genuine indications and side effects. Some use the British National Formulary (BNF) which is renewed twice yearly. A back copy, obtained from a medical contact, can be very helpful.

WHO Model List of Essential Drugs

The whole process of preparing a Hospital Formulary has been made much easier since 1977 when the World Health Organisation took up the idea of an *'essential drug list' (EDL).* This included the drugs necessary to meet the needs of the majority of the population at reasonable cost, and where two or more drugs fulfilled the same purpose, one was chosen on the basis of 'efficacy, safety, quality, price and availability. In cost comparisons between drugs, the cost of total treatment, and not only the unit cost of the drug' was considered. Drugs which research had shown to be harmful, or of limited value, were excluded.

The idea of an EDL arose out of the concern that many developing countries were being persuaded by the international pharmaceutical companies to buy vast amounts of drugs which the countries could ill afford. It was found in Bangladesh, for example, that out of 4,500 registered brand products available in the country about one-third were useless, unnecessary and at times harmful. The original WHO expert committee on the use of essential drugs found that only about 200 drugs were really necessary. Review and updating has continued ever since.

In the 1992 Seventh Model List the number has risen to 290 drugs and vaccines, with 34 complementary drugs necessary for rare disorders. The final total is still only 324 drugs. To show the style of the drug list the opening pages are given in Appendix 3. It is expected that application of the EDL will vary country by country, according to the diseases prevalent and the economic situation. It will also vary at different levels in the health care system, a shorter list being applicable in primary care.

In 1982 Bangladesh set up its own expert committee to promote the selection and use of essential drugs, and to promote local drug production. The committee selected 150 drugs, following WHO recommendations, with local modifications, and reckoned it would save the country US$32.4 million a year. Since most drugs could formerly be bought from any medicine seller, and control throughout the country was not practicable, the only solution seemed to be to control drugs at the point of importation.

In the UK too, despite its wealth, a restriction was placed in 1985 upon the drugs which could be prescribed under the National Health Service. This was done by the government for reasons of economy. The restrictions were limited to certain groups of drugs such as tranquillisers, analgesics, antacids and cough medicines. Professional approval for this has been gained. Medicaments not on the restricted list can still be bought from retail pharmacies by those prepared to pay.

A similar initiative was taken by Nigeria in 1987 with the introduction of the National Drug Formulary and Essential Drugs List. The EDL contained only 205 different drugs listed by generic name, and only these were to be ordered for use in all health facilities under government jurisdiction. Many other countries are doing the same, and medical administrators should be aware of these developments.

Hospitals, therefore, now have an excellent basis on which to prepare their own Formulary. The latest WHO Model List should be obtained from the national WHO headquarters, and any government list in operation put beside it for comparison. A hospital list, agreed between the senior staff responsible can then be finalised and distributed to all prescribers.

How should the ordering be done?
Once the formulary has been drawn up, the task of deciding what to order and keep in stock is made much easier. Generic names should be used wherever possible, though the pharmacist should beware of sub-standard or fake preparations from dubious sources of supply. He should patronise only reputable companies.

Piece-meal or on-demand ordering; spot buying
Most hospitals order from local drug companies, or travelling salesmen, as and when the opportunity occurs. In times of economic recession, or rapid inflation, there is no other way. One takes what one can, when one can. Occasionally one can snap up a bargain, as when a company has a closing down sale. Such spot buying can have economic advantages. Should there be doubt about the quality of a cheap offer one can request a 'certificate of analysis'. Beware of frauds.

Large packs of drugs are generally much more economic, but may be less convenient when it comes to making issues. A balance has to be kept. For example, if the OPD only dispenses about 50 40mg tablets of frusemide per week, a pack of 5,000 tablets is going to last two years. A smaller pack would be advisable, even at higher unit cost. Alternatively smaller empty bottles can be collected, and large packs broken down into these in the pharmacy before issue. This takes time, and if time is at a premium, the convenience of smaller packs may be preferred.

Annual tendering

In times of relatively stable economy there is great advantage in presenting drug firms with a list of the entire annual drug requirements of the hospital, and asking them to submit competitive tenders for those items in which they are interested. Low prices can be given in return for bulk orders, and in particular when a large package of items can be ordered from one supplier.

> When a pharmacist was appointed to WGH Ilesha and annual tendering introduced in 1963–64, the drug bill for the year was cut by 27%, despite a 16% increase in out-patient attendances, and a 22% increase in in-patients. Ten years later the pharmacist reported (16):
>
> 'This rather lengthy process entails making estimates of turnover for the following financial year of about 200 separate items. Tenders are invited from about 30 or 40 indigenous companies, and these are processed to determine the most reliable and the most economical quotations. Awards are made in January each year to between 20 and 25 companies, the whole process having taken four months of intensive work from start to finish. Apart from savings to the drug budget, which are often between 30 and 50% of current wholesale prices, the system also provides much valuable information about alternative suppliers, and even alternative treatments.'

Fears that there will not be the space to store a year's supply at a time are unfounded. Arrangements can be made that drugs for which quantities are large will be delivered on a quarterly basis, or as convenient, until the year's tender has been completed. Satisfactory prices, and satisfactory performance in delivery, will of course be taken into consideration in the next year's round of orders. This gives good local companies the chance to prove their reputability.

National supply sources

Governments are in the best position of all to obtain drugs cheaply for their institutions by obtaining tenders at national, and even international level. Central purchasing of such great quantities should lead to the very lowest prices. That this does not always happen is unfortunately true. Commercial suppliers expect the government to pay well, and all the tenders may be inflated by such expectations.

In many countries the voluntary agency hospitals have coordinated their buying of essential drugs, and this has led to supply of basic pharmaceuticals at wholesale prices to the members of their national associations. The Church Health Association of Ghana (CHAG), and the Christian Health Association of Nigeria(CHAN) and others, have organised pharmacy supply bodies. CHAG Drug Committee supplies 34 drugs to mission hospitals and health centres, and CHANPHARM about 50 drugs. These are supplied cheaply, on the condition that the mark-up for service will be kept as low as possible, for the benefit of poor patients, and in keeping with the hospitals' non-profit orientated basis. Such hospitals can also make use of supplies from Equipment to Charity Hospitals Overseas (ECHO) in UK, which stocks about 120 drug items, as well as equipment, at far below commercial prices. The prices are low because they only have to cover costs, and not make a profit for investors, and are, of course, also the result of prudent bulk buying. However, such overseas sources can only be useful to institutions with access to sterling or other hard currencies.

Emergency orders
Within the best of systems emergency shortages arise, and it is important that the hospital has the means for meeting such needs. In private or voluntary agency hospitals this presents no problems. The medical superintendent or the pharmacist are simply given the authority, and the cash if necessary, to go out and buy. An emergency shortage is a crisis affecting the care of patients, and the solution to it is accorded top priority. Under the government system, where all supplies come from a central stores far away in the capital, emergency requirements can only be met if there is money in a local bank account, under hospital control, and an authority to incur expenditure to purchase approved drugs in an emergency (see p.13).

Storing and issuing
The store building
Pharmacy stores are generally given insufficient space. This was soon apparent at WGH Ilesha, as the hospital grew. The original stores, with the hospital at 120 beds, and the expanded building to cope with a hospital of 200 beds, are shown (see Figure 9.1).

> The larger building allowed for an unloading bay, a sliding steel door for the goods entrance, a transit room for unpacking, a room for storage of bulk liquids, sacks and gas cylinders, and a main store with shelves from floor to ceiling, and doors kept locked, with access only to authorised persons. There was an extra secure cupboard for narcotics covered by the Dangerous Drugs Act (DDA), and a refrigerator for vaccines and antisera. The stores clerk had an office beside a service door and hatch from which issues were made to the wards and other departments. The pharmacist's office was elsewhere, but most of the central stores were placed under the pharmacist's control, with the assistance of the stores clerk.

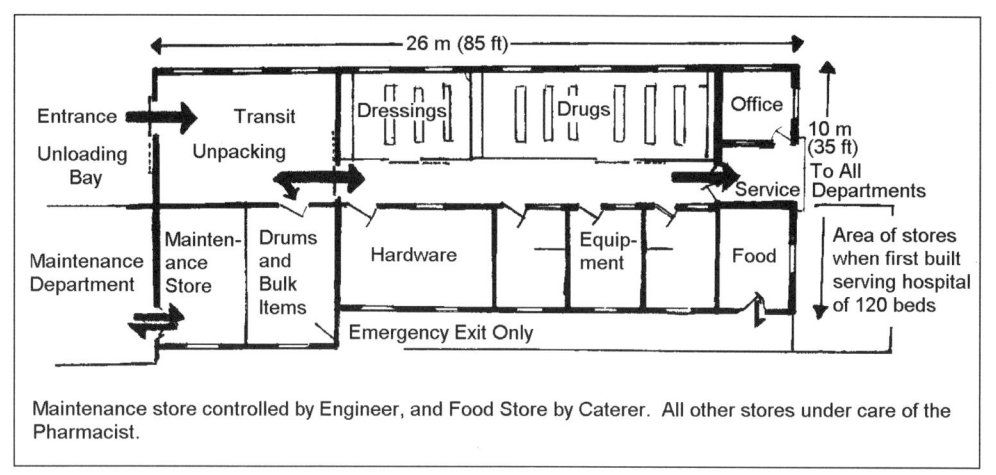

Figure 9.1: *Central stores plan.*

In such stores all doors should, of course, be given strong locks and bars, and all windows should have a strong security mesh cover, the mesh being fine enough to prevent hands passing items through.

Arrangement in the store

Any arrangement will do so long as it is systematic and clear, so that all who have to find items can do so easily, and without delay.

> Drugs at WGH Ilesha were arranged on the shelving in the main stores in roughly alphabetical order, with tablets at one level, injections at another, and liquids or bulk items at the top. It was found convenient to keep the small tubes and dropper bottles for ENT and ophthalmic use in a separate case of narrow shelves.
>
> The main drug shelves were 600mm (2 feet) deep, so it was possible to keep the stock in use at the front, and the reserve stock behind. As soon as the reserve stock was started, then it was known that the re-order level (ROL) had been reached. Some hospitals have a system of dual shelving, with the stock in use above, and the reserve stock below. The effect is the same, an automatic visual reminder that the time has come to re-order.

All stores must keep some kind of card index system with a stock card for each item. Stores that have sufficient staff may also keep a 'bin-card' attached to the shelf for each item of stock stored. This card should be removed from the shelf for action when the ROL is reached.

If the drug is one that is coming by quarterly delivery from a bulk order on annual tender, then the reserve stock has to be sufficient to last till the expected date of arrival. If it is an item that is just ordered as required, the reserve stock should be enough to cover the time taken to make and post the order to the company supplying it, and for them to prepare, pack and dispatch it to the hospital.

All receipts of items for the stores must be recorded on the stock cards by the stores clerk, and all issues as items go out. Until computerisation becomes generally available there is no alternative to these rather time-consuming methods.

Issuing

Issues should be made from the main stores at an agreed time each day when the pharmacist and stores clerk, and any other staff needed, can be present.

From the main stores drugs will be issued to the out-patient department dispensing area from which all OP prescriptions are dispensed on presentation of OP card and receipt. Drugs are also issued to each of the wards, and to the maternity department, theatre and emergency room, in accordance with requisitions made by the departmental nursing sisters. These wards and departments each have their drug cupboard (and DDA cupboard) which are, in effect, *sub-stores*. Supplies to these stores should be dated by the pharmacy to indicate the 'shelf-life', and the pharmacist should inspect ward supplies at intervals to ensure there is no overstocking, and to remove any items out of date. From the ward sub-stores the sisters will replenish the drug trolleys from which in-patients are served. The emergency room, or casualty, and the maternity department, will need larger sub-stores in order to cope with anticipated needs after working hours, and over week-ends. Other wards may be instructed to call on these for certain items in an emergency.

Central enveloping of ward prescriptions by the pharmacy for each individual in-patient has been adopted by a few hospitals as a means of reducing losses on the wards through misappropriation, or through ward sub-stores going out of date. This can be very time-consuming for the pharmacy staff. The method can, however, be made to work efficiently, if combined with the use of modified ward drug trolleys. These can be brought to the pharmacy each day and stocked according to the day's needs.

> At Tansen Hospital, in rural Nepal, ward drug trolleys, made locally from wood, have a compartment for each patient identified by bed number. The pharmacist collects the trolleys after the morning ward round, together with lists of what each patient needs for the day. She clarifies with the ward nursing staff anything which is not clear. Back in the pharmacy the compartments are filled with enough of each medicine as prescribed for the one day. PRN drugs are estimated. For example 'Aspirin PRN' receives 6 tablets. The trolleys for the 3 wards (120 beds) are all back by 11.00 am when it may be time to give patients their medicines again. The night nursing supervisor and doctor have a key to a 'night cupboard' for the supply of emergency needs. Drugs from here are labelled red, so the bottles can easily be picked out by

the pharmacist next morning, re-filled and put back in the night cupboard. Thus with two hours work each day the in-patient needs are cared for, and drug losses are eliminated (17).

Hospital manufacturing and pre-packaging

When a hospital is large enough to employ a pharmacist much can be done to save the hospital money. The preparation of stock mixtures will of course be routine, and many are still very acceptable for simple treatments. Mist magnesium trisilicate, Mist potassium citrate, Mist potassium iodide, Mist ammonium carbonate are all old favourites, and the cost minimal.

More extensive manufacturing may be done when local conditions and the pharmacist's expertise permit. Space will be required for this, and some simple apparatus or machinery. The expense involved will soon be repaid. The most cost-effective area will be in the manufacture of liquid preparations for oral or intravenous use, with great savings through not having to pay for the transport of water, or glass containers. However, an effective system for quality assurance should be implemented. This includes a check on documentation, and the regular controls in use. Some products may need to be subjected to simple tests for the consistency of the production process.

1. *Suspensions and syrups.* Chloroquine syrup, promethazine elixir, and simple cough linctus are all used extensively.

    A mixer of adequate size for hospital use is the main item of equipment needed, and 50ml bottles with caps for putting the fluid into.

2. *Intravenous fluids.* Commercially available fluids now come in plastic bag containers, thus eliminating the weight of glass in transport costs, but they are still expensive when compared to the cost of making one's own. One hospital calculated that whereas 500ml saline cost $1.50 to buy, it cost 1c to make. However, strict supervision and quality control are essential. No hospital should embark upon it lightly, or before they have enquired for possible alternative sources from neighbouring hospitals.

    Only the simplest solutions should be made initially. Normal saline, 5% dextrose, half-strength Darrow's solution in 2.5% dextrose, or Ringer's lactate (Hartman's solution) can all be made without difficulty. In addition to a suitable autoclave, a still, with a capacity of 5 litres an hour, operated by electricity or over a kerosene pressure stove, will be needed. Also the necessary 500ml glass bottles, rubber stoppers, screw caps and aluminium overseals. Only *freshly distilled* water should be used. Full details as to how to manufacture intravenous fluids, with some modifications possible in small hospitals, are set out clearly in *Primary Anesthesia*, edited by Maurice King (18). See also p112.

3. *Some essential solutions* can be made which are often hard to obtain commercially. As quantities required are small, one hospital may make them and supply to several in the area. The solutions are usually made in 50ml bottles, and the bottles capped like vials with a special device. A bottle opener should be used for removing these caps. Do not let staff ruin scissors on them. The solutions may include:

    sodium bicarbonate 4.2% or 8.4% (Note, this has a short shelf-life)
    potassium chloride 1 mmol/ml
    dextrose 50%
    mannitol 10% or 20%.

Fluids containing sodium, chloride, lactate and dextrose can also be made for peritoneal dialysis (19).

4. *Making or prepacking tablets.* The time required to make one's own tablets from powdered preparations is rarely cost-effective. It is better to buy commercially made tablets in large packs, and spend time pre-packing into smaller bottles for issue to departments, or into even smaller packs for convenient issue direct to patients to cover common prescriptions.

For example, at WGH Ilesha the following patient packs were prepared:

Diethylcarbamazine citrate (DEC)	21, 42 and 84 tabs
Ferrous sulph co	42 tabs
Folic acid 5 mg	7, 14 and 28 tabs
Isoniazid 100 mg	28 and 42 tabs
Phenobarbitone 30 mg	6 tabs
Thiazina	28, 42 and 84 tabs
Yeast 300mg	14 tabs

Each hospital will be able to select and prepare for its own most common prescriptions.

Supplies for other departments

The pharmacist may also be able to assist in obtaining the supplies needed by other clinical/technical departments, in consultation with their departmental heads. These include the laboratory, theatre, wards (for procedures), central sterile supply department (CSSD) and radiology. Storage of their supplies may be done together with drugs in one central stores, or they may be located near their own department. Stores for linen and food are likely to be elsewhere under the matron or caterer; stores for stationery and records, and for general maintenance will be under the hospital manager or engineer.

The laboratory

The needs of the laboratory will depend upon the staff employed, and the scope of service they can give. In most small hospitals this will be just the basic testing of blood, urine, stools, CSF, sputum and pus exudate, together with a simple blood bank service. Most doctors would be delighted to have more highly qualified staff who can add such items as serum electrolytes, electrophoresis, and some simple bacteriology and histology. Each section requires its own workbench, if not its own room, so the laboratory should always be built with a growth point which can allow for further expansion. The growth of the main laboratory at WGH Ilesha from one to four rooms is shown (see Figure 9.2).

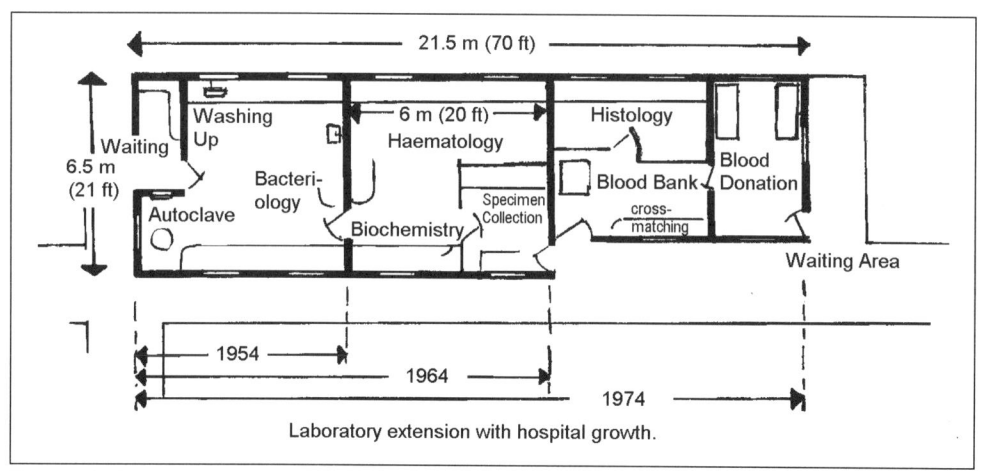

Figure 9.2: *Laboratory plan.*

Screening

Caution should always be exercised before allowing laboratory tests to be incorporated into routine screening procedures for all patients. The capacity of a small laboratory can quickly become swamped, and the staff demoralised. Routine haemoglobin (or PCV) estimations and urine albumin and glucose tests for ante-natal patients may be fully justified, particularly if assistance is given by the midwives, but routine stool tests on every child with a loose stool, for example, seldom are. The finding of parasites, many of them harmless commensals, does not necessarily contribute to better management. Selective testing when clinically indicated, gives a better service.

Essential reagents

The realisation of a need for a study of essential drugs on the pharmacy side has been paralleled by a study of *essential reagents* on the laboratory side. Hogerzeil and Hops (20) surveyed all the church hospitals in Ghana. 23 hospitals (79%) responded to their questionnaire, and from that they were able to find the 25 most common tests performed, and the 40 essential reagents or test strips/tablets required, with the approximate quantities needed per 30,000 out-patient consultations (see Appendix 5). In coming to their conclusions the authors decided that:

> 'Key features of the selected methods should be simplicity, reliability and low cost, involving the smallest number of steps possible and a minimal amount of equipment. The reagents should be stable and have a long shelf life. Materials and equipment should, ideally, be adapted to hot, humid or dusty climates.'

The recommendations were made with expert advice from such books as Monica Cheesbrough's *Medical laboratory manual for tropical countries.* (21)

On two matters in the Ghana scheme there was a variety of advice and particular choices were made.

1. *Estimation of haemoglobin.* The cyanmethaemoglobin method using the Lovibond colorimeter was chosen because of its accuracy, and because the chemicals it uses are stable.

   (NB. Where there is a constant supply of electricity with stable voltage, the EEL colorimeter is even better. It requires very little maintenance, and the photoelectric cell is long lasting. Again some centres prefer not to measure haemoglobin levels, but the packed cell volume (PCV) using a micro-haematocrit centrifuge.)

2. *Use of reagent strips and tablets.* Although relatively expensive these were chosen for the estimation of blood glucose and urea, and presence of bile and urobilinogen in urine, because of their convenience and sufficient accuracy. Pursuing the idea of limiting the number of essential reagents it was noted:

   > 'Using strips for these four tests reduced the number of necessary chemicals from 44 to 28 . . . Strips are simple, reliable . . . and may be cut lengthwise to halve their cost.'

   The basic chemical methods are an advantage only if the hospital is a training centre for laboratory assistants.

Equipment
Studies have also been made to work out the basic equipment needed for a small laboratory, and readers may find help from such sources as:

- King M. *A medical laboratory for developing countries* (22)

- Topley E. *A community laboratory service as part of health care* (23).

Blood transfusion service

In small hospitals this is normally run as part of the laboratory, preferably with a small pair of rooms set aside for the purpose. This allows blood donors to have a secluded couch away from the cross-matching desk and other laboratory activities.

The use of Eldon cards for grouping and cross-matching is convenient but expensive. The essential reagent list allows for Anti-A, B and D grouping sera which provide the same sera at a fraction of the cost.

Sterile, disposable plastic blood bags should be used in preference to blood transfusion bottles. These have to be sterilised in an autoclave before use, then washed and re-sterilised after use, a difficult and time-consuming process.

In an emergency it is perfectly possible to give blood donated, grouped and cross-matched on the spot and without interim storage. However some means of storing blood is desirable. A suitable domestic refrigerator may be all that is available, but a purpose-made blood bank refrigerator, with graphic temperature monitoring attachment, and alarm warning for power failure or cut out, should be obtained if possible. An automatic voltage regulator on the power supply to the refrigerator is advisable, particularly if the average voltage during peak use periods is, say, only 210 volts, when the apparatus is designed for 240 volts.

> Some abdominal emergencies which result in internal bleeding, without contamination (for example, ruptured ectopic pregnancy or ruptured spleen) can, of course, be treated with autogenous blood transfusion. Since it is the patient's own blood collected from the peritoneal cavity, and transfused back into a vein, no cross-matching is required at all (44).

HIV testing

As the HIV epidemic continues to spread around the world no country can afford not to have laboratories equipped for HIV testing. This is particularly important if blood transfusion is part of the service, and donors have to be screened. The definitive tests by Western Blot or Enzyme-linked Immuno-absorbent Assay (ELISHA) are too expensive for use except in major centres. More economical methods, which are nearly as good, are being developed and tested under developing country conditions. One is the Abbott Test Pack 1&2, which has the advantage of an integral control as part of each test. Another is the HIVCHECK.

> Work in Nyankunda, Zaire, together with a team in Edinburgh, has shown that HIVCHECK 1&2, of Orthodiagnostics, is sufficiently accurate with a sensitivity of 87.0–96.3% and specificity of 99.3–100%. A single test 'block'

costs US$4.50. However, in areas where the sero-prevalence is known to be low, say 4% or 5%, it is possible to test five sera together on one block. If the result is negative, all are negative. If the result is positive, all five have to be re-tested to see which one of them is positive. The sensitivity and specificity is still as good, and the cost per patient is reduced to 50 cents. However, as the general prevalence rises, the test has to be modified. At 6% prevalence, four sera can be done per block. If the prevalence is up to 20% only two sera can be done per block (24).

Standardisation and control

Many factors can affect the accuracy of laboratory tests, and where possible, arrangements should be made for periodic visits to be made from a central laboratory to check the instruments and reagents in use, and the accuracy of the readings. The hospital should endeavour, in turn, to do similar checks on any laboratory work being done in primary care facilities in the area served.

Equipment for the theatre, ward procedures and CSSD

Surgical instruments and sundries

The doctors, and the surgeon in particular if there is one on the staff, will have a special concern for the equipment in the operating theatre. Full lists of all the instruments needed for the theatre of a small hospital can be prepared. There should be a stock of spare instruments to cover all those in very frequent use – artery forceps, toothed dissecting forceps, scissors, and needle holders. Suture needles and scalpel blades are generally used for a while, so are not quite classed as expendables. Suture materials and other surgical sundries require constant re-ordering to keep stocks up to date.

It is an advantage to have several complete sets of instruments for common operations, such as hernia repair, laparotomy and caesarian section if the hospital can afford this. Sets can then be pre-packed and sterilised in the CSSD, and be ready for immediate use in an emergency.

Drugs, equipment and gases for anaesthesia are generally subject to re-order by the pharmacist, in consultation with whichever doctors are responsible.

Ward procedures

Equipment for injections, urinary catheterisation, naso-gastric aspiration, intravenous cannulation, removal of sutures and so on, is best kept in a surgical and medical sundries store by the pharmacist. Many of the items made of rubber or plastic do not have a long life in the tropics and quantities kept in stock should not be large.

Few hospitals can yet afford to have a syringe service which is entirely disposable, but the advancing AIDS epidemic may make this compulsory in due course.

Supplies of gauze, wool, bandages, pads and other dressings may be ordered, stored and issued by the pharmacist, though the matron may cross-check all ward and departmental requisitions.

Central sterile supply department (CSSD)
The age of disposables has not yet reached the developing world because of economic factors, and sterilisation of instruments and dressings by boiling, steam under pressure or dry heat is still the common procedure. Initially the theatre, maternity, wards and clinics may each do their own, but the advantage of centralisation is in due course likely to be accepted.

A CSSD may continue to be run in association with the theatre where the main hospital steriliser is likely to be. The scale may be small, with a couple of assistants doing it all under the supervision of a theatre sister, or it may need to be a large department employing many full-time staff.

Instruments for all common major operations (if possible) and all common procedures for the wards and casualty department are prepared according to agreed lists, and wrapped in two layers of linen cloth prior to being autoclaved.

> An alternative wrapping which was found effective at WGH Ilesha was silicone parchment, a paper used in the baking industry for lining bread and cake tins. It is resistant to heat and water, and yet allows super-heated steam to penetrate the package. The layers do not congeal together, and the paper can be reused many times over.

When a pack is to be used, the outer wrapping is undone by an unscrubbed nurse. She is careful not to touch the inner wrapping. The scrubbed nurse or doctor can then pick up the inner wrapping, and open the pack onto a sterile trolley. All the requirements for the operation are included, except for antiseptic fluids which have to be poured into the gallipots provided.

After the operation the instruments are then gathered together and checked for completeness against a standard list. Any item missing must be found, or its loss reported at once to the sister in charge. Theatre and CSSD staff sign the book when the pack is complete. It is then double wrapped once again and prepared for resterilising. A strip of sterilising tape is applied to the outside. This will change colour after exposure to steam at 15 pounds pressure for the required length of time.

After autoclaving, the sterile packs are stored on shelves easy of access to the theatre, and maternity department, and also to the ward nurses coming for packs for ward procedures. Again, all packs being returned from the wards after use must be scrupulously checked for missing items, and duly signed for by both ward and CSSD nurses.

Radiology

Radiology is a relatively expensive diagnostic tool, but clinically worth every penny. Care should be taken to secure the right equipment for the work to be done, with regular supplies ensured, and discipline maintained to limit the use of X-rays to that which is strictly necessary.

Equipment, and accommodation for it

Most hospitals begin their radiology service with a 30 milliamp portable X-ray machine, and a small department in one room. It is possible to do basic chest radiography, and skeletal X-rays sufficient for 90% of the needs of a district hospital with such a machine. In selecting a machine the most important factor is reliable servicing from the supplier. Contracts for annual or twice yearly visits are not cheap, but essential. Enquire also about emergency repair calls.

As a hospital grows, with increasing demands for more specialist investigations, then a larger X-ray department will probably be required in order to house a 100 or 250 milliamp machine. The opportunity can then be taken to include patient changing rooms, an office for reviewing the films taken, and a records office for film storage (see Figure 9.3).

Figure 9.3: *X-ray department plan.*

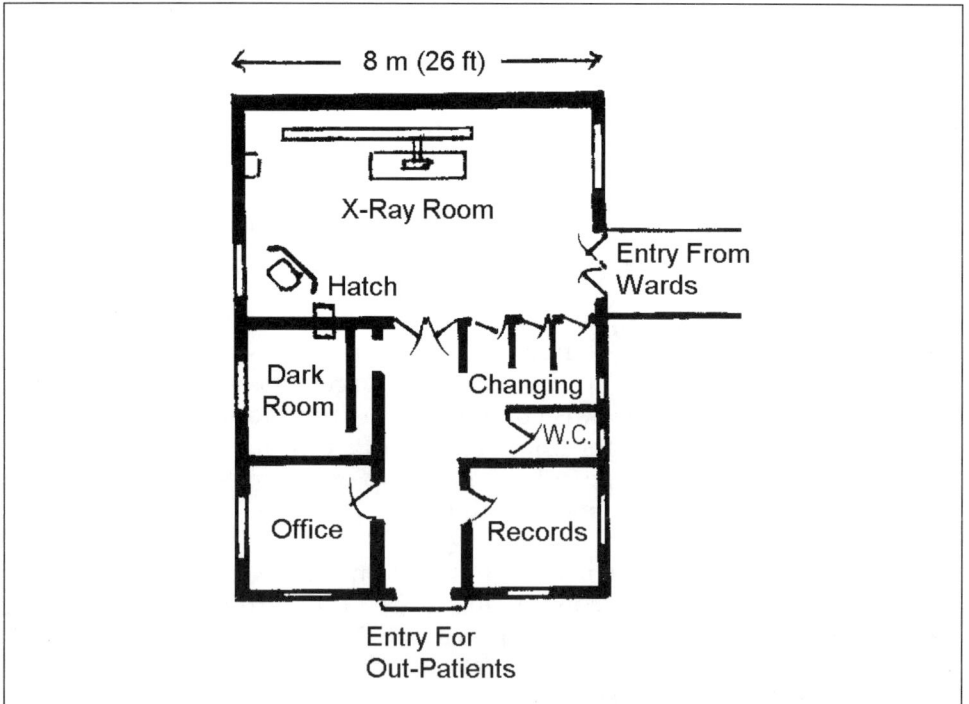

The X-ray department should not be too far from the mains inlet, or source of emergency power, and should be connected to it with a heavy duty cable of not less than 2.5 sq mm thickness for a portable machine, and preferably 6 sq mm for a large machine. Otherwise the voltage drop when full power is required for an exposure will be too great.

The dark room should be approached through a light trap, with walls painted black, but the dark room itself should have light coloured walls and ceiling. W de Rhoter (25) writes in *Radiology in a rural hospital*:

> 'The best illumination is made by a safe light pointed at the ceiling for diffuse illumination of the dark room, and a second safelight above the developing tank. Safelights often consist of an iron box, containing a 15-watt lightbulb and a filter in front which only lets through the 'safe light'.'

Then de Rhoter warns against putting in, say, a 40-watt light bulb (globe) which may give off too much heat, causing the filter to deteriorate and peel, allowing white light into the dark room. 15-watt bulbs can generally be obtained in the pigmy size with the normal bayonet fitting.

In the dark room there should be a dry bench for storing film and loading cassettes, and a wet bench beside the processing tanks. Over the dry bench there should be a hatch into the X-ray room, with light-tight doors each side, only one of which can be opened at a time. Cassettes can be loaded with fresh film as soon as the exposed film has been taken out, and placed in the hatch without danger of white light entering the dark room. Loaded cassettes can then be taken from the X-ray room side whenever needed, and without entering the dark room.

At least two cassettes of each size should be provided. For the most part 300 x 350mm (12 x 15 inch) is the largest needed for chests in developing countries, but some departments like to use the 350 x 430mm (15 x 18 inch). For each cassette size there should be six frames for processing.

Supplies
Supplies of film, and the chemicals for processing, can be ordered by the pharmacist, and stored centrally. X-ray film needs storage in 'cool, dry conditions', which are not easy to provide in the tropics. It is therefore best to order in small quantities, labelling the boxes with the date of arrival. The oldest boxes should be issued first.

A spare pair of intensifying screens for each size of cassette should also be kept in stock. These are expensive, but it is essential to replace screens in cassettes as soon as artifact shadows start to appear (see Figure 9.4) due to stains on the screen surface caused by disintegration of the fluorescent material (26). Always aim at good quality films.

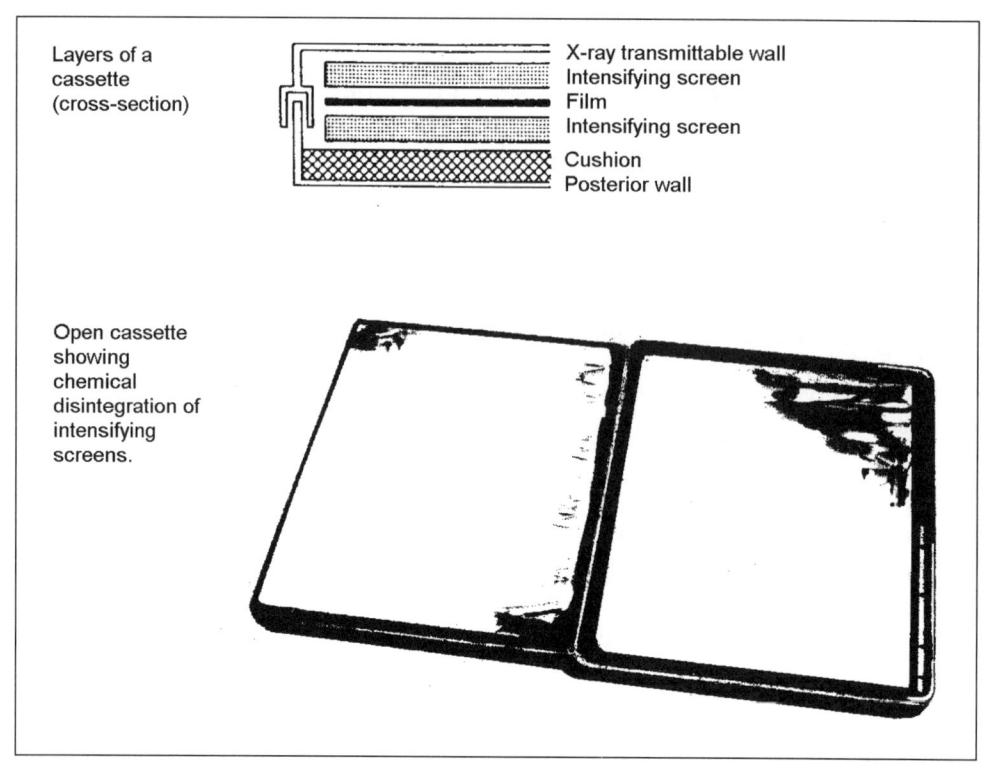

Figure 9.4: *Faulty intensifying screens which can cause poor quality radiographs.*

Essential radiology

Just as a district-level hospital may have a policy in relation to essential drugs for prescribing, and essential reagents in laboratory work, so too there should be a policy of 'essential radiology'. X-rays may be expensive, but can be so valuable if used wisely. WHO now advocates a 'basic radiological system' (27).

1. *Chest X-rays.* These may account for 50% of all films. A lateral is hardly ever indicated, and should never be ordered routinely. Pulmonary tuberculosis can be most cheaply diagnosed by sputum testing. An AP film usefully indicates the extent of disease at the start of treatment. A repeat film at three months, together with other parameters of improved weight and well-being, can confirm therapeutic progress. No further repeat films are necessary except at six months and 12 months. Chest X-rays of little children with suspected tuberculosis are of limited value, expecially if taken with a low power portable machine. The exposure time has to be relatively long, and children cannot hold their breath to stop chest movement. The image is always slightly blurred. Regular weighing, and the use of a growth chart, are a better means of monitoring progress.

A chest X-ray is not necessary to confirm a diagnosis of acute lobar pneumonia, or pleural effusion. Clinical signs, or a pleural tap, are quite sufficient.

2. *Fractures.* Limb fractures with obvious angulation or displacement do not always need a pre-reduction X-ray for diagnosis. Reduction and immobilisation can often be done first, and radiology limited to a post-reduction film.

   Fractures of long bones must have an AP and lateral view taken, but this should normally be done on the one film, blocking off the half not being exposed with lead sheet. X-ray of the skull should be done sparingly. Clinical assessment is far more important.

3. *Spine and abdomen.* A good AP view of the spine can be taken with a portable machine, so long as a fixed grid is used. The thickness of the body makes lateral views of less value.

   Straight abdominal X-rays are of limited use, whatever machine is used. X-raying the abdomen in late pregnancy for twins should never be done with a portable machine. The body is too thick, and the required exposure too long to be safe.

4. *Contrast examinations.* These should be limited to intravenous pyelogram and barium swallow, unless expert radiological help and a large X-ray machine are available.

As the use of X-ray examination will always be subject to a doctor's order, it should not be difficult for the medical staff to meet and draw up their own definitions of essential radiology along such lines as these.

Ultrasound

Diagnostic ultrasound is being introduced into developing countries. It is particularly valuable in obstetrics, and in general abdominal conditions, where it may prevent unnecessary laparotomies.

A general purpose ultrasound scanner, without Doppler or other specialised facilities, is suitable for the small hospital. Equipment with a curved linear transducer is recommended, and it should work off DC or AC of varying voltages. Surge protection should be provided. Arrangements for checking function (resolution and sensitivity) at least once a quarter, and for full servicing, should be assured before acceptance (28).

To minimise possible damage, do not carry the machine around. It is best to keep it in a room set aside for the purpose, with a couch, changing cubicle, and a toilet accessible. Running costs are less than with an X-ray, since there are no very expensive spare parts like X-ray tubes to consider. All that is required is the image-recording material, lubricant coupling-gel for the skin, and trained personnel – and this last point is the most important.

Initially it will be doctors who must learn the technique, and the interpretation of results. At least one month, and preferably six months, with an experienced sonographer is necessary to achieve reliability.

Despite these constraints, rural mission hospitals in Nepal, for example, have found that ultrasound machines have proved their worth, and even provide a considerable income for the hospitals.

Rehabilitation services

Physiotherapy
Every hospital has patients who need physiotherapy, particularly those involved in accidents requiring several weeks admission, such as patients with fractured femur, on skin or bone traction, requiring quadriceps drill, ankle exercises, and assistance with mobilisation and walking as soon as the bone is clinically united. In the absence of a physiotherapist the doctor and ward nurses will have to spend time teaching and encouraging the patient in what to do. Failure to pay attention to this part of the treatment will prolong the admission time, and may leave some permanent disability.

When a physiotherapist can be employed, this will add greatly to the effectiveness of hospital services, speeding up discharge of acute cases, preventing complications like pulmonary embolism, bed sores, ankle drop or muscle disuse atrophy, and providing follow-up for those discharged. The range of conditions that can be dealt with on an out-patient basis will be widened. The physiotherapist can, and should, do much for in-patients by going round to them on the wards, working closely with the doctors and nursing staff. However, an adequately equipped room, accessible to both in-patients and out-patients should be added as soon as possible. The emphasis should be on equipment which can be made from local materials, and with proven value for the most common problems. See Platt & Carter's *Making Health Care Equipment* (42).

Provision of splints, crutches, callipers and artificial limbs
A local carpenter and blacksmith, or the hospital's maintenance workshop, can provide most of the wooden or Thomas's splints, crutches made from a split sapling or bamboo, and other simple walking aids needed by patients recovering from injury, if given the necessary designs and sizes. See Werner's *Where there is no doctor* (29).

Workshops producing callipers, below-knee prostheses or special shoes with moulded insoles are likely to be confined to centres serving a large area, or with a particular demand such as for patients with the complications arising from leprosy. Neighbouring hospitals may refer cases for help, and such centres will be sustainable if the demand is sufficient. Furthermore, outreach from such workshops may develop into a *community-based rehabilitation service,* serving disabled people who have never come to hospital. This is a rapidly growing contribution to better health for many who may have given up hope (30).

Occupational therapy
Only hospitals with sufficient long-stay cases requiring stimulating activity or re-education can really make use of a full-time occupational therapist, but part-time service could be of help. Occupations taught will be based on local skills, and therefore use local materials.

A hospital with good technical facilities, wisely used, will attract staff keen to learn. The demand for training programmes will have to be considered. Hospitals should have a positive policy towards their training role in relation to all departments.

CHAPTER 10

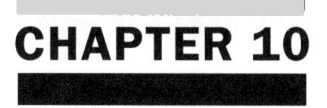

Training

Staff advancement strategies

Learning by experience
When staff are initially appointed they come for the job; they come to give service. They learn the work required of them from their supervisor and fellow workers and, hopefully, they learn to do it well. As experience is gained, whether as a gate-keeper or ward orderly, records clerk or theatre assistant, midwife or medical officer, they become valued members of the health team.

So long as good work is recognised, praise given where it is due, and salary increments added each year, or at the points agreed in the letter of appointment, the worker may be quite content. He has a measure of job-satisfaction. The health-related work itself, and the respect which it earns him or her from the community, may be quite sufficient. However, this should not always be taken for granted.

Promotion prospects may be limited
After a given number of years a 'bar' to annual increments is reached, and the worker realises, perhaps for the first time, that the workers in the next grade up have had the benefit of additional education or training which he or she has missed. In some cases promotion beyond a bar can be given on the basis of additional years of experience, or exceptional work record, on a scale personal to that one worker. For example, a laboratory assistant may require a school certificate, or its equivalent, to become a laboratory technician, but if his skills and character are outstanding he may be promoted senior laboratory assistant at the same, or even higher salary. However, the technician may be able to get into training to become a laboratory scientist and eventually earn an even higher salary.

Further training for higher educational and technical qualifications is the key to promotion. Not every staff member has the temperament or ability for increased responsibility. Promotion beyond a person's capacity can be a disaster. But those who have aspirations and genuine ability should be given every encouragement, and rewarded with promotion when higher qualifications have been achieved.

This is not always easy in a small institution recruiting independently. Senior and supervisory posts are strictly limited. The person who is now better qualified may have to be patient if there is no vacancy in his/her place of employment, or make an application elsewhere. However, if the employer knows he may lose a valuable worker this may lead to a reappraisal. The medical administrator should anticipate such situations, and try to clear the way.

In a government institution the person who is ready for promotion often has to accept transfer to another hospital. This may involve less waiting than in the private or voluntary agency hospital, and is one advantage of the system. Pension eligibility for the years of service spent working with the government is cumulative wherever that service may be given. The drawback lies in the disruption of home and family life caused by such transfers, and problems such as unavoidable breaks in the children's education.

If promotions are given in an institution, regardless of the needs of the establishment, till all labourers become 'head labourers', and all nursing sisters become 'matrons', that is evidence of a breakdown of administrative control. This tends to happen in times of national economic recession, when all staff are short of money. Administrators may see it as a way of giving financial relief irrespective of the work to be done. Ultimately it is a recipe for chaos.

Advancement through training

It should be accepted as a principle that all staff are entitled to achieve their fullest potential. Training may be through a wide variety of avenues. These include:

- individual initiative involving outside educational bodies,
- personalised training on the job,
- and participation in formal hospital-based training programmes.

Individual initiatives

The ambitious staff member will get on with his own training whatever be the policy of the hospital or employing authority.

This may take the form of:

1. Private study, and taking national examinations open to external candidates; such as subjects in the General Certificate of Education, or Royal Society of Arts typing and shorthand grades.

2. Applying for a place in another institution, such as a teacher training College, and asking for a scholarship, or sponsorship, or possibly just leave of absence without pay, with the job held open. It may not be possible to meet such requests financially, but they should not be met with hostility or indifference. Permission to have time off to sit an exam, or attend a school selection interview, should be granted if sufficient notice has been given to arrange for the person's duties to be covered.

Personalised training

There is no doubt that individuals given personal training by a senior member of staff can achieve high levels of competence in a limited sphere. They may have been appointed to the staff at a lowly level through lack of education, and this may have been more because of missed opportunities than any lack of intelligence. Many hospitals have come to value greatly the work of such people classed generally as medical auxiliaries. The cleaner in the X-ray department learns to produce excellent X-ray films. The ward maid learns to run the children's ward milk kitchen. The theatre assistant learns to do the eyelid operation for the entropion of trachoma patients. Such use of medical auxiliaries is widespread, and their service is a valuable asset to the health team.

The limitation of such service is that it can generally only be given under the supervision of a qualified person, who ultimately takes full legal responsibility. The auxiliary is also limited to that one hospital in the exercise of his or her particular skill. Further promotional opportunities are likely to be excluded.

Hospital-based training programmes

These may include schools for training nurses, midwives, enrolled nurses or nursing aides, laboratory assistants or technicians, pharmacy assistants, medical assistants, and pre-registration doctors. In some countries, for example Nigeria, it may include a role in postgraduate medical training in general practice, obstetrics or surgery.

Whereas such programmes may, in the past, have been pioneered by hospitals on their own initiative, in order to produce well-trained staff for themselves, and, incidentally, for the country, they have now, for the most part, been made subject to government regulation. This ensures that equal standards are reached by each class of personnel. They can be entered on a register and given official recognition within the country, and in some cases internationally.

Government regulation carries with it the need for all students to reach an agreed level of education before being considered for entry. Hospitals opening training schools have to be large enough to fulfil certain requirements in facilities and staffing, and be prepared for inspection before approval.

Bonding

There is a tendency for managements in all sectors, private, voluntary agency or government, to impose a legal obligation on all those who have received financial help while training to give so many years of service in return. There is a natural justice in this, and it is widely done. However experience has shown that it can be counter-productive, and medical administrators should approach the idea of bonding with caution.

A legal bond is what it says it is, a bond; and bonds are a restriction on freedom. The bond may be applied with the best of intentions, to provide service where it is sorely needed, and to compensate a hospital, or a government ministry, which has paid out, and maybe taxed the patients or the public in order to cover the training costs. The staff member who has benefited should come back to serve.

But when he or she comes under bond it is often with a sense of resentment. The service given is from compulsion, and not from free choice, and all too often the attitudes of such a staff member are poor, and the full value of their new training is not felt. Because they feel disgruntled they do not make good members of the health team, and the morale of all suffers.

> It was the practice in the early years of the WGH Ilesha Nursing School to require all student nurses to sign a two-year bond to stay on as staff nurses after completing the training. They were expected to be unmarried on admission to training, and to delay marriage until completion of bond, so that they could be resident at the hospital, and take their turns on all duty shifts, day or night, without the responsibilities of a family.
>
> It was undoubtedly the marriage restrictions which the girls found most irksome, but the very idea of bonding led to ill feeling which marred relationships. As soon as it was possible the legal bond was lifted. The emphasis then was on attracting the best graduates from the school each year into full-time service with the hospital. This proved mutually beneficial.

What is true for nurses is true also for doctors, nurse tutors, administrators or technicians – for any and for all given financial help in training. Legal bonding should be avoided, or kept to a minimum. Close relationships should be maintained during training, and vacation jobs or elective postings in the hospital encouraged. Every effort should be made to *attract* staff back into service after completion. Some may not return, but those who do will come with good motivation, and provide the right kind of leadership within the health team.

The essentials of a training policy

The two key features should be:

- *Those who have skills should be willing to teach, sharing their knowledge with those under their supervision.*

- *Staff at all levels should have the opportunity for advancement.*

Fulfilment of these in a busy service hospital may be easier said than done. Each group of staff presents a different challenge.

Labour staff and artisans
Skilled labour

General labour staff should have many opportunities for learning special skills, mainly on a personal basis. What they can do should never be underestimated.

1. *Gardeners.* Those who keep the compound tidy may learn some simple horticulture – the names of common flowering bushes, how to prune, how to cut hedges, how and when to take cuttings, and the need for watering till roots have struck deep. Naturally this is only possible if there is one member of staff who has already acquired this knowledge. Alternatively a member of the labour staff may be seconded to a neighbouring institution, where the gardens are well kept, to learn there.

   Respect for established trees is something that has to be taught, and also the need to plant more in open spaces, with protection for young saplings from goats and sheep. If areas of grass near to buildings are to be maintained as lawns, simple cutting with a cutlass is likely to be too slow. The operation of a rotary mower is another skill to be learned.

2. *Ward attendants.* Within the wards, and related departments such as hospital kitchen and laundry, there are many special skills to be learned on the job from supervisors. The need for training in how to wash vinyl tile floors has already been mentioned (see p113). The skills of hospital cooks and laundrymen are generally learned on the job while an attendant. Those taken on as ward maids may learn to assist the nurses as nurse-aides in the care of patients, preparing weaning foods or milk formulae for babies, weighing in the welfare department/under-fives clinic, or in the giving of nutrition demonstrations. Members of labour staff may have limited education, but they have experience of life. Many are parents, and respected members of their local communities. They have a valuable capacity for acquiring further skills.

Artisans

Carpenters, painters, plumbers, mechanics, electricians, and any other artisans on the staff, should be allowed to use the local apprenticeship system, if there is one.

At WGH Ilesha the system worked as follows:

> A senior artisan, such as the head carpenter, requested permission from the hospital to have an apprentice. If the load of work to be done could possibly justify an extra pair of hands this was allowed. The artisan then chose his apprentice who was granted apprentice status in the hospital and given a basic wage. He worked with his master in the hospital workshops for the three years or so, as stipulated by the local community and their artisan guilds. If the master was then satisfied as to the competence of his trainee, he was 'given his freedom' with traditional ceremonies, and allowed to leave the hospital and set up on his own in the town. The artisan might then request permission for a new apprentice to be taken on.

Senior artisans generally have the option of taking government recognised 'trade tests' which give them a national standing, and eligibility for a higher salary according to government grading. Civil service appointments in state hospitals depend on the passing of trade tests. School leavers can attend trade schools or technical colleges which give them the essential practical training for the trade tests under qualified instructors.

Drivers

Training and experience sufficient to pass a driving test and obtain a driving licence, are likely to take place before being employed. The hospital may require further evidence of competence, and the right attitude to driving, before entrusting a driver with hospital vehicles on his own (see p.119). Those who show interest and ability should be encouraged to acquire the skills for repairing and maintaining a car, and to take a trade test to become a driver-mechanic. They will then be better equipped to do routine maintenance on hospital vehicles at base, and to cope with emergency repairs which may be required on the road.

Clerical staff

Typists and secretaries

Further training for clerical assistants will come in the many jobs which have to be done, and through individual initiative. Higher speeds in typing and shorthand may be attempted in nationally organised RSA examinations, and time off for these should be allowed if due notice is given, and hospital business not seriously disrupted. Secretarial and administrative institutes also run correspondence courses which may attract the ambitious to sit their exams. These can be a key to promotion, especially in public service. If one typist can receive training in *audio-typing* this can be of great assistance to a medical superintendent, or other senior administrator, who find they can best answer mail after hours by dictating onto a personal tape-recorder.

Accounts clerks
There are many grades of book-keeping and accountancy which can be studied for on an external basis. Some staff should be encouraged to take such training, particularly if given provisional responsibility as accounts clerks. From these may come one or more who can take on the post of senior cashier or the full responsibility of accountant.

Medical records staff
Clerical assistants may begin as card clerks, and interpreters, and they may achieve considerable skill on the job. They need to have right attitudes, as well as knowledge and skills, so that they can deal with anxious patients with sympathy and understanding. After long experience they also learn all the techniques for finding lost cards and case-files, because they know the records so well.

The specific skills required for medical records can be acquired through the technical training of a medical records officer in some countries. It may be wise at times to release staff for such a training if they have the requisite educational qualifications for entrance. They will learn new, and probably better methods of medical records keeping, some of which can be introduced on their return, though rarely all. Changing records systems is not easy (see 68).

Computer training
When the money is available, and the hospital infrastructure adequate (see p32), there is no doubt that computers will find their place in many departments, and training in their use will be essential. Many hospitals have started with a computer in the accounts department, and discovered how useful it is there (see p45). The same machine may be used for *word processing*, and the typing staff allocated a period of time each day to use it for letters. There are many advantages, including the ease of correcting errors before a final print-out is made, and in the use of stock letters for frequently required replies, for example in dealing with applications for employment or training. A different name, address, and one or two details, can be quickly added to the basic text, and the letter sent off with the minimum of delay. In time, the administrative office may require a word-processor full time.

Staff in the technical departments
Laboratory
Many hospitals have to be content with a small laboratory staffed with laboratory assistants trained on the job, or at a neighbouring hospital.

Further individual training may be given in particular techniques by one of the doctors, or through personal study of one of the manuals of training prepared for tropical hospitals, which have already been mentioned (21,22).

The opportunity to train laboratory assistants more systematically may come with the appointment of a more senior laboratory technician or laboratory scientist who can run a course for a small number of students based on the hospital laboratory. In some countries these can be given recognition as an accredited qualification.

With increased facilities it may be possible to train for the higher qualification of laboratory technician, with recognition from a national institute or the London Institute of Medical Laboratory Technology. Such a level of training is only possible in hospitals with larger laboratories which include some bacteriology, biochemistry and histology in the service given.

Pharmacy

Those who assist the pharmacist in giving out drugs to patients may be known as dispensary attendants or pharmacy assistants. In most hospitals they are taught on the job by the pharmacist, or person acting in that capacity. When a department becomes big enough, and particularly if some manufacturing is involved, it may be possible to run a small in-service training school for hospital employees, and perhaps a few others sponsored by other hospitals.

For the public service the government may run schools for pharmacy assistants. Initially such staff may work in rural clinics, but they have the prospect, after gaining the requisite years of experience, of being upgraded to senior pharmacy assistant, and being put in charge of a pharmacy unit in a large health centre or a district hospital. They may carry a responsibility similar to that of a pharmacist, but be under the indirect control of a chief pharmacist in the capital.

Professional pharmacists are, of course, trained in schools of pharmacy attached to a university, but may receive some of their practical training experience in district hospitals. They have the option of setting up legally in the private sector, and it may be difficult to persuade them to continue in hospital work.

Nursing and midwifery
Nurse-aides and practical midwives

Informal programmes in small hospitals in developing countries are still common, and they serve a useful purpose, but more and more they are giving way to national programmes under the regulatory control of a nursing and midwifery board.

Enrolled nurses
A cadre below the level of a full professional nurse is still accepted in countries such as Kenya and Ghana. The educational entry point is lower, the training period only two years instead of three, and the content more practical with less science. The qualification is registerable, but they are expected to work under the control of registered nurses or midwives.

Registered nurses and midwives
The board in each country lays down the educational entry point, syllabus for training, and the standards required for hospitals to be used for training. The emphasis is moving towards a collegiate style of training, where most of the teaching is done by nurse tutors and clinical instructors in the nursing school, and only limited periods of time are spent 'in block' on the hospital wards receiving practical experience. Gone are the days when student nurses can provide a major part of the nursing service.

Nursing schools run by the government may be institutions quite separate from any hospital. It is appropriate that they should be self-governing, subject only to the chief nursing officer in the ministry of health. Students from the school are 'posted' for agreed periods to large government hospitals for practical experience. While there they naturally come under the authority of the hospital matron and the ward or departmental sisters to whom they are responsible.

Difficulties may arise when nursing schools have been started as an integral part of small hospitals, where all the nurses, whether qualified or still in training, come under the authority of the matron all the time. If the nursing school seeks to be independent of the hospital in such a setting, it can lead to strains. A degree of self government can be allowed to the school, but the overall responsibility of the matron for the nursing service needs to be maintained. While the students are in school, the matron devolves her responsibility on to the principal tutor and the school staff, but when the students are on the wards of the hospital they are fully under the matron and her nursing officers.

There does have to be close working cooperation and frequent consultation to be sure that what the school teaches, and what the hospital practises, are in conformity. Practical experience then reinforces lecture room instruction. For example, the type of ward trolley for administration of drugs to patients on the wards should be reproduced exactly for training the nurses in the school. Students will then have no difficulty in providing assistance to the ward staff nurses on their drug rounds. Should the method used on the wards be at marked variance with what has been taught in the school, the practical experience will simply cause confusion.

Doctors

The professional training of doctors takes place, of course, in medical schools and large tertiary care teaching hospitals, but there are ways in which the district and provincial general hospitals can be involved. Experience of primary care is generally included in the medical school curriculum during rotation to the department of community health, but exposure to secondary care in low technology general hospitals is often very limited or absent altogether. Yet in the medical service of most developing countries only 10% of hospital beds are likely to be in tertiary care specialist hospitals. Ninety per cent are in the general and maternity hospitals. A different range of clinical work is being done in these, often to quite a high standard. If students and young doctors can meet some of the senior practitioners who have made their career in secondary care, their eyes may be opened to the clinical interest and worthwhileness of such a career for themselves.

General hospital involvement with physician training may be through:

- contact with medical students,

- taking doctors just qualified for their internship year or a period of rural national service,

- or, in some countries, through approval for postgraduate training and having doctors on the staff as registrars.

Medical students

1. *Group postings.* Some medical schools have seen the value of sending small groups of medical students to a neighbouring general hospital, where one of the doctors has been accepted as an Associate Lecturer and is able to demonstrate innovative ways of meeting wide clinical demand with limited means. Such links with medical schools should always be encouraged, though extra work for the staff on the spot may be involved.

In 1959 medical students from Ibadan medical school were first sent to WGH Ilesha for a week of their senior paediatric clinical posting to be taught by Dr David Morley. Initially they had to be housed in rooms in the private patient block, and have their meals in the nurses' dining hall. A year later a special grant was obtained from a commercial source to build a students' hostel, with a common-room/dining-room and kitchen attached, so that special provision could be made for them. A varied programme of rounds in the busy children's wards, work in the under-fives welfare clinic, visits to the research village at Imesi-Ile and attachment to the mobile sisters of the Save the Children Fund, who visited homes in the smaller villages, provided a valued experience. More than half the paediatricians in Nigeria today are those who first saw the possibilities of such a career during that posting.

2. *Individual elective postings.* Medical schools in many countries allow their students to take one to three months off during their fourth or fifth year to study whatever aspect of medical care they may elect to take an interest in. Rural general hospitals may thus receive requests from medical students of a neighbouring medical school, or from another country entirely, asking if they can come for their elective. Hospitals which can accept them, singly or in pairs, invariably benefit from their keenness to learn and willingness to do whatever job is given to them. The students themselves receive an unforgettable experience which may affect their approach to medicine for the rest of their lives.

One or two students can sometimes be housed and fed with a member of staff, or can be allowed to use an empty flat for accommodation with part feeding with others, and part self-catering on their own. One doctor on the staff should take responsibility for arranging their programme, but should not take all the burden himself. He should involve others but serve as coordinator. Students coming from overseas will need special help, including instructions as to how to cope with immigration formalities, and currency exchange, the climate and special health precautions. It is often wise to see that they are met at the airport with a hospital vehicle to ensure an easy introduction to the country. Hospitals which frequently have medical electives may produce a duplicated information sheet to send to students in advance. This will probably need updating from year to year as conditions change. An example is given in Appendix 5.

After qualification
1. *Pre-registration internship.* All national medical councils responsible for the medical registration of doctors require doctors who have just qualified to do a year of further practical clinical work under supervision before receiving full registration. This is the 'pre-registration year' or year of 'internship'. This may be done in the teaching hospital, rotating through the departments of medicine, surgery, obs/gynae and paediatrics, or it may be in approved general hospitals with sufficient departmentalisation to provide the necessary experience.

2. *National service.* In some countries, recently qualified doctors are also required to do a period of national service, providing medical care in rural areas or less popular fields of work, such as police clinics or tuberculosis treatment centres. In Nigeria the year in the National Youth Service Corps, which is obligatory for all university graduates, immediately follows the pre-registration year. When these young doctors are put to work in a small district hospital, with one or two senior colleagues, the experience can be very valuable. They have much to give, and much to learn also.

When they are put to work entirely on their own in a local government health service, supervising a few far-flung rural clinics and primary health centres, they may find the experience daunting or even frightening. It is as if they are thrown into the deep end of a pool. They either sink or swim. Some just 'work out their time'. Others do remarkably well, and discover a new dimension to health care in the preventive and promotive field, with the occasional curative problem to keep them on their toes. Community identification and community support become very real. Medical superintendents in district hospitals in the area have a great responsibility to give them whatever help they can.

Postgraduate training
1. *The specialities of surgery, obs/gynae* and so on are normally taught to SHO/registrars at the big teaching hospitals. However, a few of the larger general hospitals, which develop strong units in one or other speciality, may find they can meet the needs of the national university or postgraduate college which gives accreditation. In Nigeria there are such hospitals with approval for obs/gynae, and others which could well apply for approval for surgery, ophthalmology, or dentistry for at least part of the four to five year residency.

2. *General practice.* General practice/family medicine has been accepted as a clinical discipline in the developed world since 1950. In Britain, for example, most of the medical schools have departments of general practice. The postgraduate programme of preparation for membership of the Royal College of General Practitioners (MRCGP) is called 'vocational training'. Two years of this is in approved posts in specialist hospitals – paediatrics, accident and emergency surgery, obstetrics, geriatric medicine, and so on. In the third year the trainee works in a National Health Service general practice where the GP principal has been approved as a trainer.

After satisfactory completion the trainee may then sit the MRCGP examination. Subsequent service is entirely outside hospital-based medicine in the field of primary care, 95% of which is provided by physicians. General practice involvement in hospitals is very limited, though there are some community hospitals in which GPs have a place in areas not well served by so-called district hospitals. The latter are all fully departmentalised and staffed by specialists. Community hospitals are the exception rather than the rule.

In most developing countries general practice still includes a proportion of hospital-based secondary care, in hospitals which have not yet become fully departmentalised. The general practitioner in this setting, or the general duty medical officer as some may prefer to call him, sees a great variety of clinically undifferentiated patients, and covers his own basic general surgery, and abnormal obstetrics. His work spans both primary and secondary care, and it may be undertaken in a government district hospital, a voluntary agency or private hospital, or in a university staff medical centre or general out-patient department. Such a GP generally has limited technology at his disposal, and accepts that there are many cases he must refer to specialist colleagues for tertiary care. On the other hand he knows he must share much of the primary care, particularly in rural areas, with nurses, midwives and other community health care personnel working in associated primary health care centres and clinics. To them he has to be teacher, administrator, general practice consultant, and supporter in every way.

It is this form of 'tropical general practice' which was accepted as a clinical discipline in Nigeria in 1970, though it was not until 1979 that a faculty board for general practice was formed under the auspices of the National Postgraduate Medical College of Nigeria. The college had faculty boards for surgery, physic, obs/gynae and all the main specialities, and the training for these was centred primarily on the teaching hospitals where the academic clinicians and the high technology were available. The new faculty of general practice was given full parity with the others, but it was agreed the training should be centred primarily on the general hospitals and primary care centres.

All training programmes of the college are for at least four years, with a primary examination in the sciences basic to the particular speciality taken at the start, and a final examination in two parts, the part I after two years of the programme, and the part II after a further two years. This includes the presentation of a dissertation on a subject approved by the appropriate faculty board. Examinations for all faculties are conducted under the authority and supervision of the postgraduate college, and successful candidates are made Fellows of the Medical College (FMC) in the appropriate discipline, FMCS for surgery, FMCP for physic, FMCOG for obs/gynae, and so on.

When the training programme was started for general practice in 1981 a similar structure was accepted, partly so that the Fellowship in General Medical Practice (FMCGP) would both be, and be seen to be, of similar status to the fellowships in the other specialities.

A closer look at the general practice training objectives
The *aims and objectives* of the programme have been set out as follows:

'The aim is to provide an advanced vocational training for the doctor who wishes to follow a career in general practice, whether in clinic, or comprehensive health centre, or as a general medical officer in a small hospital. He will be a frontline medical practitioner.'

Such a doctor should be:

a) generally clinically competent over the range of medical care defined in the curriculum, whether such care takes place in the consulting room, maternity department, operating theatre or in the community

b) able to integrate clinical knowledge from the various disciplines, and make an initial decision on every case presented to him

c) concerned to see each patient as an individual, and yet part of a family and community with social and cultural characteristics

d) ready to keep good records which promote continuity of care. He should be particularly concerned to be expert in early diagnosis

e) one who appreciates the doctor's role in health education, counselling, promotion of family planning, and all aspects of preventive and public health

f) experienced in receiving referrals from the primary care team, and cooperation with them, and also in making appropriate referrals to the consultant specialists, and learning from mutual interaction

g) knowledgable about administration and maintenance of the health care institution and its technical infrastructure, i.e. water, light etc'.

Details about the programme have been set out at some length because it is the medical administrators in small or medium-sized general hospitals who are most likely to be involved. It is these hospitals which have been inspected in Nigeria by the Faculty Board in General Practice and approved by the College for Part I FMCGP training.

Inspection of proposed training hospitals
In Nigeria this is undertaken by two GP fellows, who submit a report to their faculty board. *The criteria for approval* for Part I training are listed as.

1. At least two senior doctors on the staff of consultant grade, or qualified ten years, who are in sympathy with the GP training programme and willing to teach a registrar attached to them.

2. Reasonable buildings, and infra-structure – water, light etc.

3. A strongly supportive nursing service, and adequate technical facilities.

4. Good medical records.

5. Housing for a registrar, and consulting room space in the out-patient department.

For the Part II FMCGP the criteria are similar but only one senior doctor is required, preferably one who is a fellow of the postgraduate college, and who is prepared to act as trainer. There is a greater emphasis on rural or urban *primary care*. Smaller hospitals are accepted, many of them private hospitals that reach the standards required. Further details about the responsibilities of medical superintendents and trainers in such training hospitals, Part I or Part II, are included in Appendix 6.

As the syllabus includes organisation and management of health services, a selection of likely examination questions of the type which might appear in the FMCGP are included at the end of this book (Appendix 9).

International acceptance
Other developing countries have begun to develop similar programmes where 'tropical general practice' includes both secondary and primary care. The West African College of Physicians started a faculty of general practice in 1987, and may develop training in Ghana and other West African territories.

Nepal began a university and district hospital-based programme in 1987, and others have followed – Malaysia in 1990, India (under the Christian Academy of Medical Science) in 1990, and Zambia in 1994. Interchange of information is being maintained between them by the London-based organisation AIM (Action in International Medicine, c/o Department of Primary Health Care, Whittington Hospital, London N19 5NF, UK), which is particularly concerned with the promotion of district health systems. Further information can be obtained from that source.

There are similar developments in some industrialised countries which have large areas of sparse population. In Australia a Faculty of Rural Medicine has been formed within their College of General Practice to prepare doctors who have to be responsible for small hospitals in the 'outback'. A special curriculum has been prepared for those in the 'rural stream' of the general Family Medicine Programme (FMP) training. The four-year training will have two years at basic level, and two years at advanced level, and during the latter trainees will be required to 'major' in surgery, anaesthetics or obstetrics. WONCA, the world organisation of family physicians/general practitioners has a Task Force monitoring these developments.

Hospital chaplains and counsellors
Doctors are frequently conscious that, though their patients present with physical complaints, they need to look deeper to find the cause. Sometimes it is a straightforward anxiety or reactive depression, but in others there is

a strong cultural or spiritual disturbance due to fear, guilt or a sense of evil influences at work. Such patients need more than simple reassurance or tranquillisers. There is a place for training hospital chaplains or counsellors to assist the doctor, on a full or part-time basis.

Some church-based hospitals have run short courses for ministers in training at related theological colleges or seminaries. The period spent at the hospital under the supervision of the chaplain and medical superintendent introduces them to some aspects of modern medical care, and gives practical experience in relating to sick patients and the ways that counsellors can help to restore hope, and begin to understand the deeper needs of those who face the crisis of sickness. Sympathetic medical superintendents can do much to facilitate such work. The need to understand the cultural and spiritual background of Muslims and those who adhere to traditional beliefs, and to cater for their problems in relation to sickness, is equally important. Prayer is common to all at such times.

The special needs of patients with AIDS, and of the relatives who have to face the likely death of their loved one within six months of diagnosis, has added a new dimension to this need. Some hospitals set aside a special ward, and employ a full-time counsellor for this problem alone. Patients generally wish to die at home, especially those with a rural base, and Chikankata Hospital in Zambia has shown how a 'home care team' can advise on managing the terminal illness, and encourage the community to come to terms with the HIV epidemic (31).

The hospital should not be divorced from the community and its social life. It should have a strong interest in the people it serves and a concern for the primary health care services in the area.

CHAPTER 11

Primary Health Care Outreach

New attitudes are needed

The hospital is not enough
It is important that the doctor in charge of a small general hospital should work to achieve high clinical standards and effective back-up services. He hopes, as time goes by, to build up a good team of staff at all levels. This is the 'therapeutic community', and through it the patients who come for attention find fresh hope.

But this is not enough. What of the patients who do not come?

The hospital is set in a community, and those within 10 km radius may receive a full range of care. Those outside that radius are likely to come only for the direst emergency, and they may often arrive too late. Should the hospital doctor simply take the attitude, 'That is just too bad'.

And what of the patients who come with disease which could easily have been prevented – the girl who comes with tetanus due to contamination of a guinea-worm sore on the leg, or the child with pertussis whose parents did not live near enough to any centre giving triple antigen? Or the man with cholera contracted through drinking polluted water from the creek nearby? Can the doctor be so cure-orientated that he fails to see the need for preventive health care accessible to all?

> William Foege in 1970 wrote(32):
> 'A medical centre can become a mecca of quality medical care – but what is the price? If $100 would save a life, we are easily content to say the cost of saving a life is $100. But if that $100 had been invested instead in providing safe water supplies, or better nutrition, and if it would have saved ten lives instead of one, then the cost of saving one life is not simply $100, but is $100, plus nine deaths.'

Attitudes do have to change. The hospital-based doctor must be concerned with the primary health care network in his area, as stated in Chapter 1.

There should be orientation to the community

This is easier said than done unless additional help can be obtained.

> It was in 1955 at WGH Ilesha that the doctor in charge of the children's ward was so appalled at the high mortality among the children admitted, paticularly in those with severe malnutrition, and the complications of measles, that he suggested to his two medical colleagues,
>
> 'Why do we not spend half our time out in the villages, to provide preventive care and early treatment for these children, and give up half our time on the wards?'
>
> The sentiment was admirable, but 'easier said than done'. His colleagues pointed to the tremendous volume of work waiting in the wards, and the out-patient clinics, and said it was not possible to care for all the present patients in less time. They were already overworked. To spend half time in the villages was only possible with additional help.
>
> And then the help came. We were more fortunate than most! Dr David Morley was one of the first paediatricians to come to Nigeria. He had part support from a research grant from the West African Medical Research Council. His project was to do a village longitudinal study and find out the common causes of morbidity and mortality in children under five years of age. Within five years the concept of under-fives clinics had been born, the growth chart established as an invaluable means of monitoring children's health, practical midwives trained to provide the initial clinical care for all children up to five years, both curative and preventive care being offered in the same consultation. A census in the research village after five years showed that the mortality in the 0– 5 age group had been halved. The new concepts were introduced both into the hospital and into the related village maternity centres. Attitudes throughout the hospital began to show a far greater orientation toward community health.

The challenge to look outside the gates of the hospital at the needs of the community may be met with no more than pious platitudes 'Yes, we quite agree. Prevention is better than cure. We will think about it...tomorrow. In the meantime there is a patient with strangulated hernia waiting...'

We all know the feeling. So, to be practical, what can we do?

Steps which can be taken
Cooperation with community leaders
Consult with them to find out what are their felt needs. See in what way the hospital can help to fulfil these. Share with them your own problems. A 'Friends of the Hospital' community support group, meeting each month, may be a useful link.

> In Eruwa township in Nigeria, the chief of the town spearheaded such a group for their local government district hospital. It met monthly, and at Christmas the chief and town leaders visited the wards, gave token presents to the in-

patients, and a meal for the staff in the PMO's consulting room. Money collected from the group provided a small emergency fund for repairs to the hospital, grants to patients, for example when stranded far from home, and a revolving fund for purchase of anti-snake venom at a time when the central stores was short of it. The farming community felt the need for this was vital.

Cooperation with other health facilities in the area

Tour round and make a map of other health facilities in the area – maternity homes, health centres, clinics or dispensaries, whether under the local government, voluntary agencies or private practice. Get to know the midwives and other health workers. They may be lacking in professional supervision, and be glad of occasional help. Assistance with the repair of equipment, such as sphygmomanometers, will be appreciated. Supply of drugs to local government centres from the hospital pharmacist, if it can be arranged, may be more efficient and economical. Advice on the cases that should be referred to the hospital can be given.

> In 1966, at WGH Ilesha, the obstetrician was concerned at the serious overloading of the maternity ward of 26 beds, handling 100 deliveries a month, at a time when most women stayed in for five days. Several private maternity homes were identified in the town, most of them staffed by nurse/midwives trained at the hospital who were now setting up on their own. Six homes were inspected, found to be of good standard, and thereafter given supervision from the hospital.
>
> Cases found at the hospital ante-natal clinic to be progressing normally, with no at-risk factors, were given the option of delivering at one of the private maternity centres. Fees there were not high. Problem patients were booked for hospital delivery. The total deliveries at the hospital were cut by 10% over the next two years, despite the growing population. Standards at the maternity centres were improved, and referral to the hospital of any difficult cases they encountered was prompt, and accompanied by a proper referral letter.

Provision of new primary care facilities in under-served areas

Although the state may have accepted, in principle, that complete coverage of all the population should be provided, the achievement of this in practice is difficult. The hospital may become aware of under-served areas, or of villages with particular health problems like guinea-worm or hyperendemic onchocerciasis, through a run of seriously ill patients coming from those places. Alternatively the village community elders, or school headmaster, may approach the hospital directly to open a branch clinic. Such requests should be looked into carefully, and the appropriate response given.

1. *Provision of a mobile clinic.* Regular visits by a doctor or nurse will certainly help to gauge the real need, and some help can be given on each visit. However, the service given only touches the surface of their problem. A

full-time health worker on the spot, however limited his or her training, is likely to be of far more long-term value. Mobile clinic vehicles rarely justify their expense.

2. *Setting up a branch clinic.* Some requests for a new centre are justified by real need and an unacceptable distance from any other health facility. Other requests are more due to petty rivalries between adjacent villages. Village A has a centre, but village B people, 1 mile away, would not demean themselves by going to village A for anything. They must have their own place. Such requests should usually be turned down, and efforts made to bring about reconciliation between the feuding communities. At times, owing to population size, or natural factors like a stream between the two villages which gets flooded in the wet season, a second clinic can be justified. The inter-village rivalry can be turned to good effect by spurring community effort to get a simple building put up, a well sunk for water-supply, and a candidate put forward for training as a clinic attendant.

Always visit a village from which a request comes and make sure your map of the area is complete, and covers services provided by government, voluntary agencies and private sector. It is surprising how often one source of service ignores another, and two clinics appear virtually side-by-side.

Do not take on another centre unless you can provide proper supervision. This may be by a doctor or a nurse, or a trained community health supervisor. The new centre may have to be fitted into an existing schedule of out-station visits, and there is a limit to the number one person can cover. Distance, and the nature of road communication, is also a factor. Never take on a centre which is too far for a convenient day visit, there and back.

Training for primary health care
1. *Village health workers* (VHWs). Much can be achieved through training part-time village (or primary) health workers. These are mature men or women, chosen by their village community, and given a very simple training as near to their homes as possible. It is a mistake to bring them a long distance to a hospital centre, where they cannot keep an eye on their families and farms, and where conditions may be strange. For this type of work it is the trainers who should travel furthest. A mobile team of health educator, nurse, and driver/general assistant, with occasional medical back-up, will be needed for such work. A major village, with smaller settlements round it, is chosen as the temporary education centre. Perhaps a school building can be used, or the village chief's compound.

In the training at Idere in 1984-6, pioneered by staff of the College of Medicine Ibadan, it was found possible to teach farmers, petty traders, drivers and others to manage 10 simple aspects of primary health care. These covered 80% of the health problems in the village. The trainees did not have to have completed primary schooling, or even be literate. Education was in their vernacular, using stories, proverbs, dramatisation and simple line drawing pictures. Classes were held at the week-ends, when people normally left their farms, or closed their trading stalls, and covered a period of three months, ending with a verbal test, and presentation of certificates to those successful. The primary health workers formed their own association, with further supplementary subjects being taught (see figure 11.1).

It is hoped that those trained will continue with their usual occupation, receiving financial support from their communities for the hours spent on health work. They are not professionals and it should be possible to multiply numbers despite the relative poverty of a rural area.

Figure 11.1. Subjects which may be included in a village health worker training scheme.

Ten elements of primary health care taught to village health workers in Idere, Nigeria.
1. Malaria, treatment and prevention
2. Diarrhoea and oral rehydration therapy
3. Onchocerciasis
4. Guinea-worm
5. Child nutrition, and ante-natal care
6. Cuts and wounds, and burns
7. Environmental: water, latrines and composting
8. Farmers' health: snake-bites, poisoning, schistosomiasis, hookworm disease; and motor-cycle safety
9. First aid; fractures
10. Duties of a primary health worker; health education; essential drugs

* * * * *

Supplementary subjects taught at subsequent PHW Association meetings
11. Acute respiratory infections
12. Family planning
13. Prescribing practices
14. Simple physiotherapy

Once sufficient village health workers have been trained for one major village, the mobile training team can move on to another, after ensuring a system of continuing supervision for the VHWs left to do the work. This may be from a local government maternity centre or primary health centre in the area, or an extension worker based at the hospital.

Many books are available to help those planning such work; for example, *Where there is no doctor* by David Werner (29), and its companion volume, *Helping health workers learn* (33). *Where there is no doctor* is available as a special edition for Africa, and also in Arabic, Spanish and Portuguese. A Chinese edition is being prepared.

Occasionally, candidates put forward for training turn out tobe already accepted by their community as *traditional healers or birth attendants.* Every effort should be made to encourage them, since, with the extra skills learned, their work will be the more effective. If the traditional healer is prepared to share any of his secret knowledge of useful local herbs, the whole group will benefit. Dangerous traditional practices, such as putting the soles of the feet of a convulsing child in the fire, can be discussed in the group and firmly discouraged. Such teaching may get through to where it is most needed. Special courses for TBAs (traditional birth attendants) have been widely established, and their usefulness in some communities is well known.

2. *Community health assistants* (CHAs). An alternative approach is to train school leavers in the basics of health care, giving them a fairly comprehensive course. These will then be full-time workers, requiring a salary, accommodation and a career prospect. In most countries such schools are run under government auspices, but in some they have grown up alongside voluntary agency hospitals as their contribution to developing good primary care coverage in the region served.

Entrants are secondary school educated, and they are given a course of 1 to 2 years, depending on pre-test ability. They are taught some clinic-based duties, like assistant nurses – recording temperatures, keeping simple records, weighing children and filling in a growth chart, and administering medicines. They are also taught community-based duties, like health inspectors – health education, hygiene, care of water supplies and so on. They are allowed to do some primary clinical consultations under the supervision of nurses, guided by a bulky volume of standing orders.

A new emphasis within the hospital
New attitudes towards primary care outreach and towards community health may be reflected in many changes *even within the hospital.*

Introduction of growth charts for children under five

These have been referred to in Chapter 5 (p79). They should be used for all children attending that part of the hospital out-patient department set apart for the under-fives clinic. The charts should be 'home-based'; that is, retained by the mother, and brought on each occasion the child is in need of care. If growth charts are also used by neighbouring primary care centres, the mother should be encouraged to bring the chart issued from wherever she first attended. That should be asked for, accepted and used, rather than issuing another. Excellent integration of service and continuity of care is provided in this way. It is the best form of child referral from primary to secondary care. When the child is due for return from hospital to health centre, the chart should be updated, and suggestions for follow up added to the child's card.

If children are weighed on every visit, whether for a routine check-up ('well-baby visit'), or because of illness, the growth curve on the chart will give the most valuable indication as to the child's progress. A steadily rising curve shows adequate nutrition, but a flat or falling curve may indicate nutritional deficiency even before obvious signs of malnutrition have developed. It may also indicate a set-back due to acute or chronic infection, requiring closer examination, and possibly laboratory investigations. Such incidents of infec-

Figure 11.2. The growth chart in use.

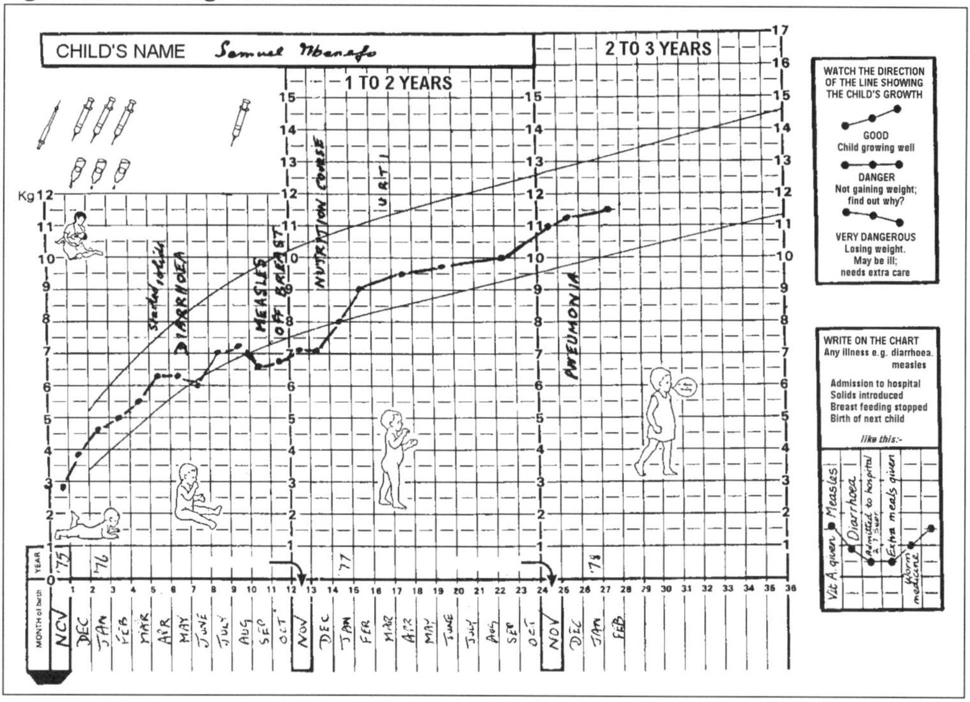

tion, and other milestones (for example, 'off breast-milk'), should be written on the chart in the column for the month (see figure 11.2).

Full instructions on the use of the chart can be found in such books as *See how they grow* by D Morley and M Woodland (34).

The growth chart is as much a clinical tool as a health education tool, and more valuable than any stethoscope.

The introduction and use of the growth chart involve several steps.

1. *Obtain large stocks of the chart.* If the government or UNICEF provides them free, well and good. Otherwise they must be bought or printed locally. Calculate the number required per year from the estimated population served by the hospital. Twenty per cent are likely to be under five. If the population served is 100,000, that means there are 20,000 children in that age group. Not all will come at once, so it may be sufficient to start with 10,000 charts, and add 2,000 more each year. Do not try starting with 1,000 only.

   A standard specimen chart, printed in black on white card, can be obtained from Teaching Aids at Low Cost (see page 239). A printer can use these on an off-set litho or similar machine to produce as many as required. Ask him to use a light ink (green or brown), on a coloured card (yellow is attractive), rather than black on white, and to be careful that the printing back and front is accurately centred, so that when the folds are made the panels come in the correct place on both sides.

2. *Polythene envelopes will be required in equal number.* If these cannot be obtained from official sources, and have to be ordered from a manufacturer, the specifications required are 140mm x 300mm x 125 microns (5 x 12 x 0.005 inches).

3. *Printing under-fives clinic record cards locally.* These should be lined on both sides and of similar dimensions to the growth chart, so that they will go in the polythene envelopes. These are for writing up notes of complaint and treatment on each visit.

4. *Provision of weighing scales.* Many hospitals have scales for weighing newborn babies in the maternity department, and scales for weighing adults, but nothing suitable for weighing toddlers. Two types are now available:

    a. A spring balance with a dial face. Model 235 PBW can be obtained from UNICEF, or by ordering from CMS Weighing Equipment Ltd, 18 Camden High Street, London NW1 0JH, UK. Price about £25.

b. A spring balance with linear indicator which can be read direct on to the growth chart. This new development, the direct recording scale, can be obtained from TALC, complete with suspension cord, 30 growth charts, a plastic sling for a sitting or lying child, and instructions for use, for £15.

5. *Setting up the scales.* Suspend the scales from a hook in the ceiling or above a doorway, or with wire looped over a roof beam, and brought down to about 1.5m (5 feet) height. Use a piece of bicycle inner tube between the suspension cord or wire and the hook of the scales. This will act as a 'shock-absorber', and reduce oscillation of the needle on the scales when a child is restless and bouncing about. If you have no sling, then a tray, made from local materials, suspended below the scales, makes the weighing of small infants easier. The scales must be duly adjusted to zero after adding the weight of the tray (see figure 11.3).

6. *Arrange to divide the general out-patient clinic,* if this has not already been done. All children under five should be routed to a separate desk for registration of repeat visits (see p81), and for weighing and charting of the weight. This should be completed *before* the process of consultation begins. A ward orderly, or clerical assistant, may be trained to do this, and to be the receptionist for the patients each morning.

7. *Assign a community health assistant or nurse to permanent out-patient duty in the under-fives clinic.* Train her to see all the children in this age group, take the history, interpret the weight chart, advise on nutrition, and treat simple conditions, referring the more seriously ill to the doctor. Instructions should be given as to when the mother should return with the child:
    monthly for the first two years,
    three-monthly for the next three years, and
    at any time when the mother is worried, or the child is obviously sick.

If the numbers attending are too many, add another community health assistant (CHA) or nurse, if space for another consulting desk can be found. When well-practised, one nurse should be able to handle 50 to 100 cases in a day.

It is not advisable to try to organise a separate 'well-baby' clinic except for those coming for a specific immunisation (see below). Many mothers who think their child is well do not recognise early sickness, such as anaemia, or marginal malnutrition; in any case they are likely to think up some complaint in the hope of getting a bottle of medicine to take home. Conversely many mothers misinterpret minor symptoms in their children as serious illness, when the children are really perfectly well. *See both the sick and well together.*

Inner tubing 'Shock absorber'

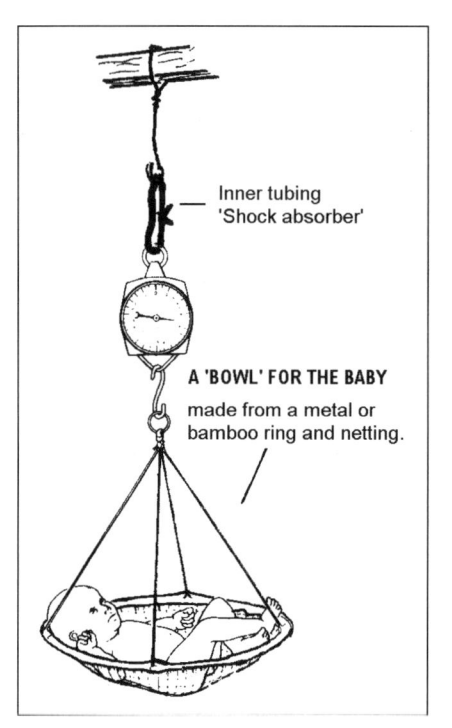

A 'BOWL' FOR THE BABY made from a metal or bamboo ring and netting.

It is always much appreciated if the CHA or nurse has a few of the more commonly used medicines in pre-packaged quantities on her consulting desk. These can be handed straight to the mother as she gets up to go. She will not then have to go and join another long queue at the pharmacy, and can return straight home.

Infertility clinic and family planning
The same clinic provides help for the woman who wants to stop having children, and the woman who wants another child, but is unable to conceive.

1. *Infertility.* Many hospitals are already besieged with women troubled by primary or secondary infertility. The social stigma attached to an inability to conceive drives them to any and every avenue from which help may

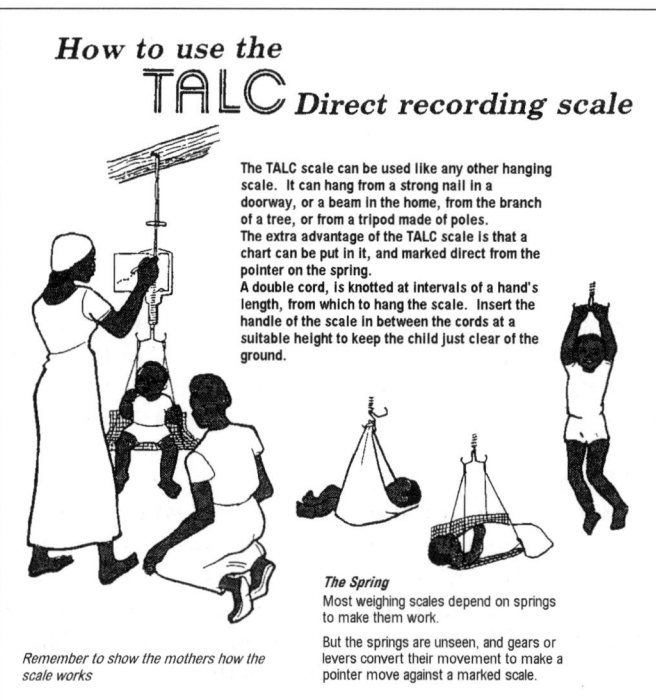

How to use the TALC *Direct recording scale*

The TALC scale can be used like any other hanging scale. It can hang from a strong nail in a doorway, or a beam in the home, from the branch of a tree, or from a tripod made of poles.
The extra advantage of the TALC scale is that a chart can be put in it, and marked direct from the pointer on the spring.
A double cord, is knotted at intervals of a hand's length, from which to hang the scale. Insert the handle of the scale in between the cords at a suitable height to keep the child just clear of the ground.

Remember to show the mothers how the scale works

The Spring
Most weighing scales depend on springs to make them work.
But the springs are unseen, and gears or levers convert their movement to make a pointer move against a marked scale.

Figure 11.3. *Spring balance scales (left) with dial face; and (below) TALC direct-reading weighing scales for under-fives clinics.*

come. The problem is a curative one, so part of the traditional hospital service.

2. *Family planning.* If, by turning left instead of turning right on entering the clinic, women can equally ask for advice and help for contraception, there will be ease of access without any embarrassment. The clinic may be run by a nurse/midwife, with additional training in contraceptive techniques, and access to a doctor for cases needing referral. She should be competent to advise on the use of oral contraceptives, and barrier methods, and be able to do a vaginal examination and judge the safety or otherwise of inserting a Lippes loop. She should also be able to recognise the cases that can be motivated to use the Billings technique, judging the non-fertile days in the menstrual cycle by the viscosity of the cervical mucus. Careful records should be kept in conjunction with the supervising doctor.

Contraceptive supplies are likely to be available from the state, or the national branch of the Family Planning Association. If supplies have to be bought from commercial suppliers this may make regular compliance by users more difficult because of cost. Where AIDS is a problem, free condoms may be available for those in at-risk groups.

Provide immunisation services within the hospital
Every hospital and health centre should be involved with immunisation.

1. Children from the under-fives clinic for their routine BCG, DPT, oral polio and measles immunisations. Some will have been already covered if the government has an expanded programme on immunisation (EPI).

2. Ante-natal mothers for their two or three doses of tetanus toxoid during pregnancy.

3. Contacts of patients with open tuberculosis requiring BCG.

4. International travellers requiring yellow-fever vaccine. The hospital may be authorised to issue and stamp international certificates of vaccination.

Notification of infectious diseases
Most countries have an agreed list of notifiable diseases, and when these are encountered in the hospital, information should be passed on regularly to the local health office. It will be their responsibility to pass on notification of particularly serious diseases to the state headquarters, and they in turn are statutorily bound to pass on notifications of yellow-fever, anthrax, plague, and cerebro-spinal fever, for example, to the World Health Organisation in Geneva.

Notification should therefore be done conscientiously, and close contact maintained with the local health office in order to give any necessary assistance. For example, a case of bite by a possibly rabid dog may require immediate notification by messenger, so that measures can be taken at once to find and destroy the dog responsible. Cases of typhoid fever, or of cholera, may show a clustering in a certain area, and cooperation from the hospital may help to trace a possible source or carrier.

Health education

Health education will be a major function in the primary care outreach services, but it should not be overlooked that the hospital itself has an ever-changing population wide open to health education too. Those who are recovering from sickness, their relatives who come visiting, and all who attend out-patient clinics, are already sensitised to health matters, and likely to be very receptive to advice given as to how to become, and remain healthy.

Many hospitals have large waiting halls in the out-patient department and under-fives and ante-natal clinics. Health talks given to those who have been registered and are waiting to be called in for consultation are generally well received. The presentation should, of course, be at a level the patients can understand, and should make use of stories, and pictures as aids to understanding.

Nutrition talks and food demonstrations may be organised for the mothers of undernourished children. Other special groups such as patients with tuberculosis, hypertension, diabetes or alcoholism may also be catered for, and courses organised for those who want to give up smoking.

Manpower and money for community health work

The new attitude to primary health care must be reflected in the administration, and its priorities. Plans for primary care outreach, and a new emphasis on community health, will have very limited effect if there are no staff who can give time to such work, and no additional financial resources.

Volunteers

If strong encouragement is given, much can be achieved in many communities by volunteers. In some situations this has been extended into the hospital, with volunteers visiting patients, comforting the lonely, and, with some appropriate training, assisting with health education and counselling. However, this can only happen with a dedicated supervisor (37).

A community health leader

The first requirement is one senior member of staff who is totally committed to outreach work. He or she may be a doctor, a health sister or a community health officer, and should be assigned to the work either full or part-time.

Whatever happens the person is likely to have to spend many extra hours on the job, in the evenings and at week-ends. Leadership qualities are needed. The staff in the Ludhiana community health programme in north India say that such work is for 'the second miler' – for those prepared to do a full day's work *and more*, that is, to 'go the second mile'.

The community health unit, or coordinating office

It is desirable that such a leader be given a base in the hospital from which community health activities within the hospital, and outside it in the villages, can be coordinated. Additional staff can be appointed to this unit – health educator, food demonstrator, community health assistant, clerical officer – as the requirements of the programme dictate. The unit will also need its own vehicle and driver to cover commitments outside the hospital.

In Nigeria, hospitals approved for training general practice registrars need such a unit, under the supervision of a doctor with particular expertise in community health, in order to provide some of the essential training in the FMCGP curriculum, Part I. Trainees can be attached to the unit for a period of six to eight weeks. As the syllabus says:

> 'During this period, through home visiting, attendance at out-stations, and sharing in health activities, the registrar will develop his ability to function effectively in the field of primary care, in cooperation with other members of the community health team. The posting should instil a thorough appreciation of the importance of community obstetrics, family planning, under-fives clinics, nutrition, immunisation, notifiable infectious disease and health education. Of all the rotational postings community health may be the most difficult; yet it is the most important if the general practitioner is indeed to be a front-line doctor'.

Financial resources

It is essential that additional resources be obtained for community health developments. You cannot charge patients for health education talks or displays. Primary care outreach services are generally to the poorest, who can least afford to meet the costs involved. They can pay something, perhaps to cover the bare cost of drugs, but the costs of staff involved and their transport will have to be met in other ways.

The community health unit will therefore need independent funding, and this can at times be obtained from additional grants from voluntary associations such as the Rotarians, or from international aid agencies. The hospital itself should allocate an agreed proportion of its budget to community health.

The principle should be agreed that the budget allocated and grants obtained, are irrevocably committed to the work of the community health unit, and that shortages on the curative side should not be met by cutting back on the preventive. It will need a strong commitment by the medical superintendent and the hospital board to see that this principle is fulfilled.

There are critics who say that curative services will always swallow up available cash, leaving preventive services to suffer. Therefore preventive services should be entirely divorced from the hospital. This is a pessimistic view. The dangers may be there, but they can be overcome if attitudes within the hospital have changed. When a hospital can actively contribute to the promotion of better health in the community, there is likely to be more rapid progress because the essential unity of health care has been preserved.

Starting a new project

Each community health project is different. There is no single right pattern to follow. Each community has its own peculiar needs. Each project leader has his or her own gifts and vision. Resources available may vary from an adequate sufficiency – to virtually nothing One can never be sure what opportunities may present. Just let the promotion of community health be the ultimate objective.

If there has been no primary care outreach before, then one should call for aconsultative visit from someone with experience. Each country has its own expertise; for example, the Christian Health Association of Nigeria (P O Box 6944, Jos, Plateau State, Nigeria) has a full-time primary health care coordinator, who is prepared to visit any voluntary agency hospital, either alone or with a group, to advise on how primary care might be developed. The approach is likely to be: 'Let us go to the people, talk with their leaders, find out what they consider their priority needs, then let us see what can be done.' He might also advise on other centres, with similar situations, to which visits could usefully be made, and suggest agencies to whom application might be made for additional project funds or personnel.

The needs are there, and there is always something which can be done. Once community health involvement has started, it may take diverse forms.

Illustrations of diversity
WGH Ilesha – early days
The story of developments at Ilesha is worth telling. It came in stages.

1. *Primary care centres in the district.* These began over 60 years ago. The first trained midwife was posted to Imesi-Ile village in 1934, 25 miles from the town, the last 10 of which had to be walked along a bush-path through the forest, then up to the higher rocky land where the village was situated, and a pastor and a few teachers were there to welcome her. Medically,

she was alone, yet she learned to cope magnificently and the people learned to trust in the health care she offered. Eventually a motor road to the village was completed. In 1956 that village was chosen for the longitudinal research project on childhood mortality, nutrition and growth, conducted by David Morley and Margaret Woodland. It was also the site of the first field trials of measles vaccine in the world, following its development by Enders in America.

From that one centre grew a chain of fixed maternity and child welfare centres nine to 30 miles distant from Ilesha, staffed by one or two midwives, and a helper. They gave simple emergency care to all, ran under-fives clinics, gave good ante-natal care to the expectant mothers, and delivered up to 30 babies a month. The people in the villages served were happy; village health committees were not organised, but the local pastor voiced community concerns. Environmental health services were provided by the local government.

2. *A mobile team.* In 1964 there came a surprise addition to the primary care services when a unit of the Save the Children Fund was established at Ilesha. It was run in close cooperation with the hospital, but managed separately by its own administrator. On another compound an office and four residences were built, and garage space for four landrovers. The purpose was to carry health and nutrition education into the homes of the people throughout the district. Initially the SCF sisters picked up the children being discharged from the hospital children's ward after being cured of kwashiorkor. They, and their relatives, were carried back home, often to people who had despaired of seeing the children alive again. The welcome was naturally warm, and good rapport established. The mother of the formerly sick child became the one to teach others. Homes were open everywhere to 'the sisters with the car', and over 40 village meeting points were established. After 10 years the project was handed over to the local government. The project was expensive in vehicles and staff, but it showed what could be done, given the resources and the will. To assist its coming was an opportunity not to be missed.

Baptist Hospital, Ogbomosho, Nigeria

This very successful general hospital wished to be more involved in community health. A previous scheme providing immunisations and nutrition advice to families in church congregations on a monthly visiting basis had ceased to operate. An orphanage, run by one of their nursing sisters on the outskirts of the town, was also doing excellent health and nutrition education, but the link with the hospital was weak. The hospital was popular as a centre for training general practice registrars, but it lacked an organised posting in community health. This requirement provided a useful stimulus towards setting up a *community health coordinating office (CHCO).* An expatriate doctor, with his boards in family medicine, and special interest in community health, was obtained as a volunteer for one year. The Ford Foundation gave a start-up grant. An office in the out-patient department was assigned to be the community health coordinating office, and the doctor set to work, with two junior staff to assist. Registrars were attached in rotation. Responsibilities of the unit included:

- liaison with the orphanage, and popularisation of its use of soyabean milk and other dishes

- survey of another village, preparatory to setting up a primary care centre there

- health education within the hospital, in the OPD, ante-natal clinic and wards

- support to the paediatric department in starting an under-fives clinic using growth charts

- liaison with the local government health office over notifications of typhoid, and other diseases; hospital transport was used in tracing contacts.

A Nigerian fellow in general practice was appointed after two years to head the CHCO and develop it further.

NKST Hospital, Mkar, Benue State, Nigeria

Concern for primary care came early. This very busy 250-bed rural hospital had a 75-bed maternity ward delivering 3,000 babies a year, and attached minimal care units for long-stay patients with leprosy or tuberculosis. From the 1950s onwards primary care developed, first with a mobile service, and then the establishment of stationary units, loosely attached to local village churches. The programme which came out of this provided, and still provides, an excellent model for the kind of balance which has to be kept between community participation, and supervision from the centre.

If a community requested help from the hospital, they were advised to build a simple first aid station (FAS) like a large village hut, in which deliveries could be done by birth-attendants, and simple treatments given by first-aiders. Local staff was trained for them at the hospital's school for medical auxiliaries. If the FAS prospered the local community was advised to collect funds to upgrade their centre to a dispensary, and to form a dispensary committee to administer it. The state government had to approve the site for building, and before starting there had to be housing for the community health assistant, and a well, latrine and refuse disposal pit. When ready, inspected and approved, the government appointed the CHA. If well supported, further up-grading to a maternity centre, with the appointment of a qualified midwife, was also possible.

By 1979, when there were 46 dispensaries and 24 first aid stations, the rural health programme (RHP) was given a separate administration from the hospital, though its headquarters were still in the same compound. The programme had its own pharmacy store providing the PHC essential drugs at cheap prices. These were sold at the out-stations at fixed retail prices which allowed a 10% mark-up at the FASs and 20% at the dispensaries. A full-time medical consultant was made director, with a team of supervisors who could travel round, and an administrator. The medical auxiliaries school was upgraded to be a full school of health technology, producing community health assistants for the programme, and for the state generally. The RHP continues to grow. Though it is independently funded and administered, it works alongside the hospital, and in close cooperation with it.

Initiating community health action

'There are two major ways by which hospitals can become more fully involved in community health. One is (as we have seen) to supervise a network of health centres. Another and more subtle way is to lead the community in the improvement of its own health, that is to initiate 'community health action'. Morley D (36).

Kwun Tong Hospital in Hong Kong illustrates this well
It is a city specialist hospital, built on reclaimed land and rises nine floors amidst a forest of tall buildings. It serves a population of 700,000 within a radius of one mile. The hospital authorities might well be forgiven if they claimed that curative services took up all their energies and resources. Why should a large hospital be concerned with primary care and community health?

1. *Community nursing service.* Concern for care in the community began, even before the hospital was fully completed, and beds were short. Early discharge for patients was arranged, and community nurses trained to follow up patients to their home, and continue dressings, medication and rehabilitation there. This service attracted state funding. Doctors went with the nurses, in rotation, and learned to appreciate their patients' home circumstances. They also achieved better communication with their nurses.

2. *Community health project.* This was set up, with its own director, who had her office in the hospital, and a staff of 60, including health educators, doctors and nurses, and carried preventive and promotive care for positive health right into the community. Health centres were established on

the ground floor of some of the high-rise blocks, and also a unit for the severely disabled, giving jobs within their capacity to spastics, paraplegics, or those with mental retardation. They were given piece-work rates for the components they put together, and earned more than the social security payment otherwise available.

All kinds of health education were promoted, including mutual help programmes for those with hypertension, anaemia, and arthritis. 'Sharing the happiness of health together clubs' were organised for the elderly, play groups for children with emotional problems, and campaigns run to help people stop smoking, using the Seventh Day Adventist's 'five-day anti-smoking course'. Visual acuity tests were offered in a park to pick out people who needed glasses, and health days held in the open using songs, music and dancing.

For all this no funding came from the government. All support had to be raised through special appeals.

In 1977 the medical superintendent wrote:

'We, in the project, believe that health care can be offered on three levels, the curative, the preventive and the positive.
- *Curative care* is mainly in the hospital, but is also in the health centres, and extended to homes through the community nurses.
- *Preventive care* is mainly in the health centres, and the community, but the hospital is by no means excluded. It is a demonstration model of a healthy community, and a centre from which supervision and training is given.
- *Positive health care*, defined as being concerned with growth and self-fulfilment of individuals and communities, is mainly in the community, and depends upon extension workers with no hospital commitment. Nevertheless the hospital remains the coordinating agency, and the headquarters of the whole project.' Paterson (37).

No hospital is too small to be involved in community health...and no hospital is too large
The medical administrator has a unique opportunity to promote better health services, both within the hospital and the community, and indeed within the nation at large.

CHAPTER 12

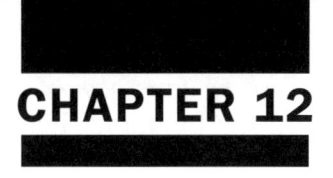

Wider Responsibilities

We have dealt at length with the doctor's administrative responsibilities in a hospital, and more briefly with his role in encouraging the hospital to play its part in spreading primary care to the surrounding community. The doctor may have still wider responsibilities at district or national level thrust upon him as the years go by. The community and the nation expect him to give a lead. He also has a responsibility to himself as a doctor, and to his family, and has to keep the balance between his public and private commitments.

District planning and national health administration

The realities of being in the public service

In the previous chapter the examples of primary health care outreach illustrated the diversity of options open to doctors working in hospitals with independent management as they respond to the needs of the community. Doctors in government may feel that such examples have little relevance to them. In the public service it may appear that all such planning takes place centrally, and the PMO in the peripheral hospital just has to fit into the national plan. There is truth in this; perhaps all too much truth. However, none will dispute that national plans work better if based on the genuine needs and aspirations of the districts.

There are books which describe the expertise needed for health planning and management at district and national level, in the context of the public service, and readers are referred to them for further study. *District Health Care*, by Amonoo-Lartson (4) has already been recommended. The World Health Organisation's book, *On Being In Charge* (38), is specifically for those in middle level management of primary health care.

The number of doctors who will actually be given the responsibility of medical officer of health for a district may be few, and at national level in the ministry of health those responsible are even more select. Those who do have the opportunity need proper preparation and training. They should learn to follow sound planning and management principles.

Defining the problem, and working from objectives

One must begin by surveying the field and finding out what is happening on the ground, so that problems which have to be overcome may be recognised. Practical objectives within the resources available have then to be defined, and the strategy for achieving them worked out. The tasks which have to be done should be clearly allocated to the units responsible within the district, or, at ministry level, to the appropriate divisions within the ministry, and then on down. The plans are put into effect, and each year the feed-back from the periphery enables evaluation to take place, which in turn may lead to modifications in the objectives, or in the resources required, and ultimately in the overall plan (see Figure 12.1).

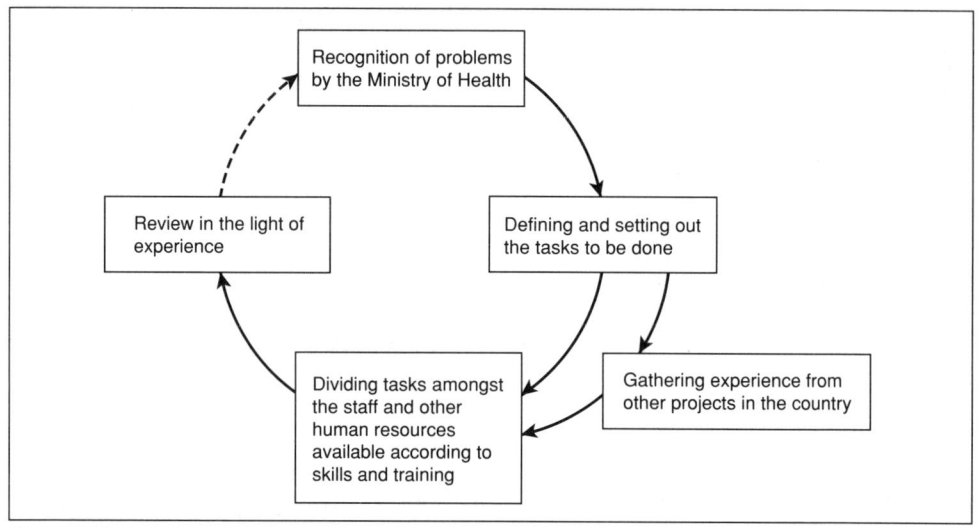

Figure 12.1: *Matching needs to resources.* (From Amonoo Lartsen (4)).

It is recognised that, ideally, this management cycle should operate at the district level in public service. The district PMO should be patient if he finds that ideals are not always followed, and most decisions appear to come down ready made from above. His chance may come.

Setbacks can occur

The best national plans may fail through inadequate knowledge of conditions at the grass roots, or through the conservatism and narrow prejudice of local politicians, or indeed through the greed and graft of unscrupulous contractors. Furthermore, the dramatic changes in the economic situation of a country may suddenly cut expected resources to the bone.

> The Federal Ministry of Health, Nigeria, following enlightened opinion from the World Health Organisation, produced an excellent development plan for 1975–80 which made provision for comprehensive health care services based

on a basic health services scheme, which would bring coverage to the whole nation.

Each of the 19 states was to have a school of health technology to produce the new style of community health worker at the levels of aide, assistant, supervisor, and, with university help, the community health officer. Initially 450 basic health units were planned, each to serve 150,000 people, and to consist of:

- 1 Comprehensive health centre (CHC) with 30 beds, theatre maternity unit, lab and X-ray
- 4 Primary health centres (PHCs) with 12 beds, feeding into the CHC
- 20 Health clinics around each PHC.

Financial stringency caused a scaling down to 285 units, but when the price of oil fell, and the oil boom evaporated in 1977, the plans were cut to only 19 units, one for each state, and most of these were never properly completed. The training of community health personnel went ahead, but the CHAs when qualified had to fit into the old style of local government maternity centres and dispensaries, if they found jobs at all. Only in recent years has that situation begun to change.

Vision for the future

It is a good exercise in medical administration to work out what one would like to see, even though one may have no opportunity or power to implement the plan. The exercise itself gives one a better sense of what should be the priorities.

In 1979 the Nigeria Medical Association requested a number of people to make their input to a 'blueprint for rural health services', to be presented to the government, and the author was among them. Trying to produce an overall plan was challenging, and in the doing of it many of the principles put forward in this book began to come together. As the remit was for rural services, no plans for the tertiary level specialist medical services were included. Attention was directed to the secondary and primary care levels only.

A blueprint for rural health services
1. The *objective* was set out as follows:

   'Our aim should be to provide good base hospitals in all our rural townships, around each of which should be a network of rural health centres and dispensaries, integrated with the hospital. Around each rural health centre or dispensary should be an even greater network of part-time voluntary village health workers, controlled by their own village communities, and working on a basis of self-reliance. They would deal with the simple remediable or preventible health problems which account for 80% of the disease in the community' (see Figure 12.2).

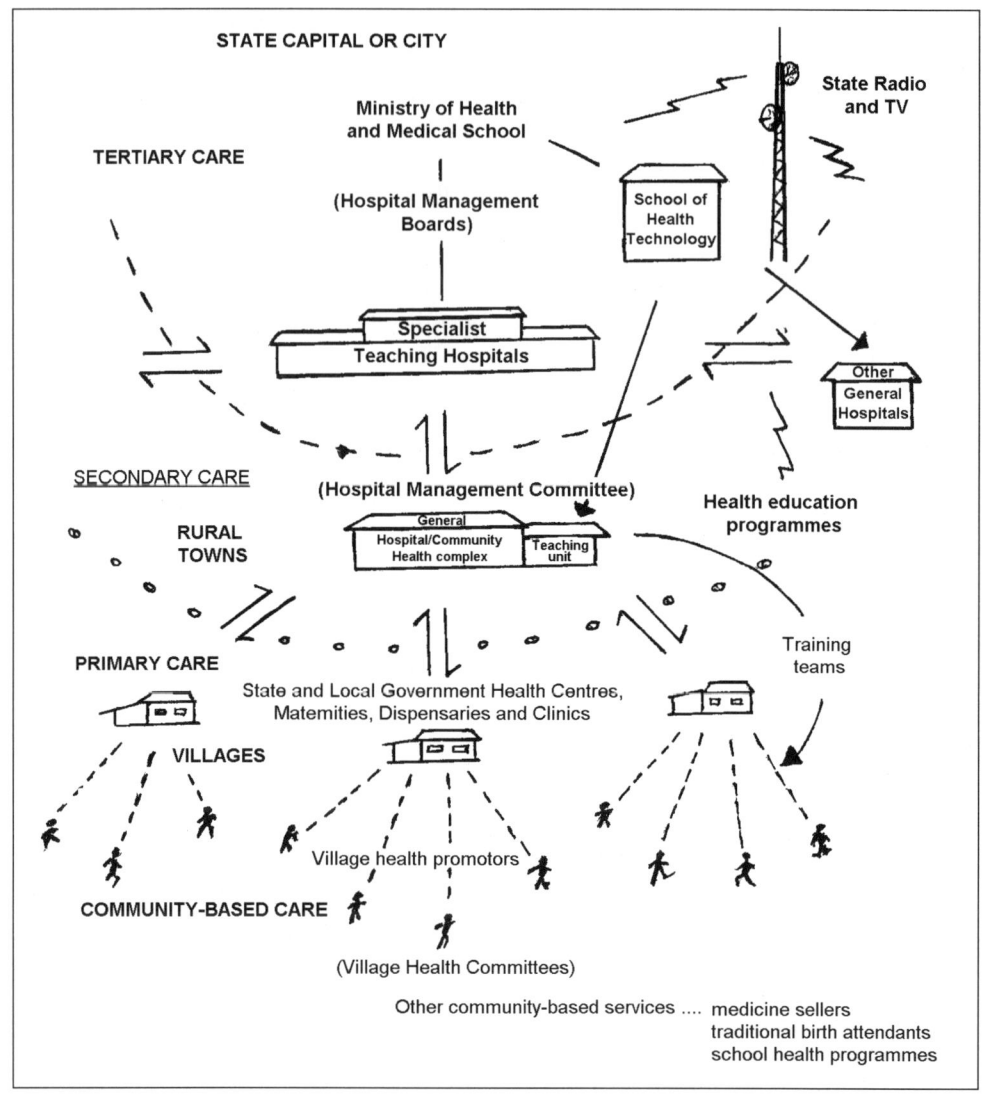

Figure 12.2: *Blueprint for rural health services; organisational diagram.*

2. *The secondary care level*

The district general hospital, with its surrounding health centres, is usually given little prominence in plans for the national health care system, and yet it can be the key. As the World Health Organisation says,

'This may be the lowest level of the health system that is in communication with central government, as well as being the highest level in direct contact with the communities.' (39).

The blueprint continued:

'The base hospital must be properly run, with a PMO fully in charge, chairing a district health management committee, which also coordinates the primary health care services in the area, and the environmental health office too. One doctor would be part-time in the hospital, and part-time available to give any necessary support to the PHC services.

The hospital should have a financial allocation from the centre, and a local bank account with the PMO and the hospital secretary as signatories. Finance should be at least sufficient to cover running costs, and preferably junior staff salaries as well. The hospital should have its own maintenance unit and quota of artisans.

Houses or flats for all key hospital staff should be made available on or near the hospital compound, particularly where hospitals are in rural townships. This makes it possible to ensure a basic infrastructure of water and light for all, and encourage a good spirit of working together.

There should be cooperation with other general hospitals in the area, including those of voluntary agencies.

3. *Doctors for the rural areas*

    Medical staff policy should place the emphasis on generalist doctors for District general hospitals. There is, of course, a real place for a surgeon or an obstetrician to be appointed, so long as they are willing to take their share of general on-call duties. All doctors can then deputise for each other in providing a 24-hour service. No hospital should have less than two doctors, and numbers should generally be increased at a ratio of two for every 50 beds. Larger numbers are unnecessary.

    Doctors should be encouraged to make their career at this level by allowing them to do postgraduate training for a fellowship in general medical practice, where this is available. Without this they will tend to move away to specialist hospitals in order to further their career, or else opt out into private practice. General hospitals of adequate standard can themselves be training centres, and thus have GP registrars during their training years as well. Doctors on rural national service may also be available in a junior capacity.

4. *Primary care level*

    Primary health care services should be grouped in networks around general hospitals, and not run separately by local government. They should have their own budget, distinct from that of the hospital, but be responsible to the same district health management committee. Drugs should be supplied to PHC centres by the hospital pharmacy, and there should be an integration of record systems, particularly in the use of growth charts by children under five. The records held by the mothers for their children could then be used at any of the PHC centres, or when referred to the district general hospital.

Around each of the primary health care centres there should be a network of village health workers, supported by their own village health committees. Training for VHWs would be provided by the district through a mobile health team of nurses and health educators, and with the support of a doctor when required. Supervision of the VHWs trained would be provided by the health staff at the PHC centre around which the VHWs were clustered.

The VHWs would provide liaison with other sources of health care in the community – the medicine sellers, the traditional healers, and heads of families, and teachers in the schools.

Environmental health staff would also have their work coordinated at district health management committee level, where one of the doctors would be medical officer of health.'

International opinion

Enlightened international opinion can undoubtedly have a beneficial effect on national health administrations. Since the Alma Ata Declaration of 1978, pressure for improved primary health care has been universal. At times this has seemed to play down any important role for the district hospital, on the assumption that it consumed too great a proportion of the resources, and was only concerned with curative care.

However, the proper place of the first referral hospital at the apex of the primary health care system was given strong emphasis by Dr Halfdan Mahler, former Director General of the World Health Organisation, at a conference in Karachi in 1981. He concluded his key-note speech there by saying:

> 'A health system based on primary health care *cannot*, and I repeat, *cannot* be realised, cannot function and simply cannot exist without a network of hospitals . . .'

But he also made clear that 'hospitals have to change their ways' and be more outward looking. 'Front-line hospitals', as Dr Mahler preferred to call them, should be providing secondary care *in support of* primary care. A major conclusion of the conference was that each of these hospitals should have a 'department of community health' to encourage primary health care in the hospital's catchment area, and to press for an increasing proportion of the hospital's budget to be spent on that.

The district health system
From all this has come the well-defined concept of the District Health System in which the community-based primary health care services of a given district are considered *together* with the first referral hospital providing secondary care – one integrated system. For this to work well it is also agreed that there should be considerable decentralisation of powers from the centre to the district, for example in the use of locally collected hospital fees (see p.14). The proper role of low-technology secondary care hospitals in rural and urban districts has also been set out clearly by WHO (35). This includes recommendations on staffing, equipment and operative procedures to be covered.

The WHO's Division for Strengthening Health Systems has been pressing the concept of the district health system in many developing countries. Implementation in Ghana has already gone far. Zambia is trying it in pilot districts. Nigeria has put all primary health care under the authority of Local Governments, and is now encouraging the thirty State Ministries of Health to upgrade secondary health care, with decentralisation of authority to the districts. Liaison between secondary and primary services is seen as essential, but may not be easy to implement given the dual loyalties at district level. In the Philippines, control of secondary care is being given to provincial Governors, and primary care to town Mayors, again raising the problems of dual control within the district health system.

The man at the top
The Minister of Health in each country will ultimately have the responsibility for guiding the development of health services, and securing a reasonable proportion of the gross national product for the health sector.

However, we all know that no one person can work miracles. Patience is needed. Resources in most developing countries are desperately limited. In general, population growth continues, and food production is not keeping pace. Economic prosperity is delayed. The man at the top may have unparalleled opportunities. He also knows more directly than most the constraints under which the national administration works. In the meantime each one of us must do the best he can at our own level, and in our own situation.

Our responsibility as doctors in society

The influence we can bring to bear as medical administrators in our hospitals, and as leaders in society, depends much upon the respect accorded to doctors as members of a noble profession, dedicated to helping others. This is a legacy passed on to us from our medical forbears, and from our current seniors in the profession. It can be all too easily undermined through thoughtless individual or corporate action. It behoves each of us to do what we can to preserve the good name of 'doctor'. That name depends, very simply, upon our being 'good doctors' – and that may be taken in either its professional or in its moral sense.

Keeping up to date

What we learned in the five years of medical school is just a beginning, even though it enables us to earn a medical degree. Knowledge fades fast, and if the quality of care we give is to be maintained and improved, our growing range of experience must be supplemented by *continuing medical education*. This is particularly important for the district medical doctor who has to be responsible for such a wide range of service. It is also particularly difficult, since he is away from the academic stimulus of a teaching hospital, and the burden of work may be heavy, but *he neglects it at his peril*. There is nothing more likely to undermine his authority than to gain the reputation of being medically out of date. Learning must go on throughout our working lives.

The methods which may be used are many

1. *Regular reading of journals.* Relevant magazines and journals are many. Some are free on request by doctors in developing countries. Others are on subscription.

   Medicine Digest. Monthly, free, from 11/12 Bouverie Street, London EC4Y 8DP, UK. Readable abstracts. Always useful.

   Children in the Tropics. Bi-monthly, free, from International Children's Centre, Chateau de Longchamp, Bois de Boulogne, 75016 Paris, France (in French, English or Spanish).

   Africa Health. Bi-monthly, free, from FSG Communications Ltd, Vine House, Fair Green, Reach, Cambridge CB5 0JD, UK. Good clinical and news articles.

   Tropical Doctor. Monthly, from Royal Society of Medicine, 1 Wimpole St, London W1M 8AE, UK. £25 annually. Uniformly excellent.

   East African Medical Journal. Monthly, from Kenya Medical Association House, Chyulu Road, P.O. Box 41632, Nairobi, Kenya. A long record of good original articles.

2. *Books.* The number of books, specifically written for doctors in district-type hospitals in the developing world, is increasing yearly. Most are available in soft covers, many at subsidised prices, though even these may appear high when local currencies in developing countries have been devalued.

   A few examples are given:

Medicine in the Tropics, (Eds) A W Woodruff, S G Wright. Churchill-Livingstone, London, UK.

Primary Diagnosis and Treatment, D E Fountain. Macmillan, Basingstoke, UK.

Clinical Tuberculosis, J Crofton, N Horne, F Miller. Macmillan, Basingstoke, UK.

Practical Care of Sick Children . . . in Small Tropical Hospitals, P Deane, G J Ebrahim. Macmillan, Basingstoke, UK.

Primary Surgery, Vol 1. Non-Trauma, (Ed) M King, OUP, Oxford, UK.

Primary Surgery, Vol 2. Trauma, (Ed) M King, OUP, Oxford, UK.

Primary Anaesthesia, (Ed) M King, OUP, Oxford, UK.

Obstetrics and Gynaecology in the Tropics, J B Lawson. Arnold, UK.

Principles and Practice of Community Health in Africa, (Eds) G O Sofoluwe, F J Bennett, UPL, Ibadan, Nigeria.

Nutrition for Developing Countries, F Savage King, A Burgess. OUP, Oxford, UK.

Every doctor should develop his personal library, as opportunity offers, adding to it from time to time according to his particular interests. Important suppliers are:

The World Health Organisation, which has published a whole range of books for the district level doctor – apply for a list through the WHO national office. Sometimes groups of books are offered at a discount.

Tropical Health Technology, 14 Bevills Close, Doddington, March, Cambridge PE15 0TT, UK – for both clinical and laboratory technology books.

AMREF, P.O. Box 30125, Nairobi, Kenya – a useful source for those in east and south-east Africa.

Undoubtedly the best cheap source of books, and other teaching aids, world-wide is:

Teaching Aids at Low Cost (TALC), P.O. Box 49, St Albans, Herts AL1 5TX, UK. Only books within a limited price range are stocked. Anyone may write and ask to receive the current list and prices.

If the personal purchase of books proves difficult, an alternative is to plan for a small *hospital library* to serve medical, nursing and other health staff. In some countries the *Tropical Health and Education Trust* in London, has provided a gift pack of about 40 books precisely for such libraries. The books, selected by Professor E H O Parry, are all highly relevant to the secondary and primary care of developing countries. *TALC* has a recommended pack of 17 books for such a library, currently costing £85 (including postage and packing), but goes further in offering invaluable advice on how to organise and run the library. It is all too easy to accept books and lock them away in a cupboard for safety, then find the books are not being used, so this is important.

Suggestions about making shelves with planks and bricks (or concrete blocks), simple cataloguing of the books, and ideas for control of lending, are outlined. A small users committee may need to decide about penalties for books that are spoiled, or not returned when they should be. Encouraging respect for library books takes time. Ask TALC for advice.

3. *Attendance at day conferences*, or medical workshops. Occasional opportunities for these may present themselves, and they should be taken whenever it is possible to get away. Papers by those with special expertise, and the chance to ask questions, provide a good forum for learning.

In the UK every major city now has a postgraduate medical centre, with a regular programme of meetings. General practitioners in the National Health Service have to attend a given number of such meetings each year, and can claim a refund from the government for travel and overnight expenses. Similar facilities should be developed in every country.

Working for higher degrees

Most doctors will work for a higher qualification if given the chance. For all tertiary care specialties, that means a return to the teaching hospital, or even a period of some years abroad. Subsequent return to a district hospital in their own country will then be unlikely.

However, a new type of postgraduate training specifically to prepare doctors for district hospital work, is becoming available in some developing countries (see p208). This is a branch of general practice, but is hospital-based, and includes more general surgery and operative obstetrics than in the usual form of general practice common on industrialised countries. Such programmes also emphasise community health and the management of both hospital and district health service. The doctor who qualifies as a MD (General Practice) in Nepal, Fellow in General Practice (FMCGP) in Nigeria, or District Health Specialist (M.Med(DHS) in Zambia, is more likely to make his career at district hospital level. Such doctors will be excellently placed to help their peers keep up to date through continuing medical education. They will also be trained and motivated to undertake useful lines of research arising out of their clinical work.

Clinical research
Personal observation
The 'good doctor' will keep his eyes open to learn from his day-to-day experience. Though pressed for time, he will try to keep reasonably satisfactory medical records. The clinical variety may be bewildering, but in due course he may come, for example, to recognise new patterns of presentation emerging which merit careful observation and research. He will naturally look up what he can in the textbooks or journals, and discuss his ideas with anyone he can find with specialist knowledge. The outcome may be a pilot project with a more detailed questionnaire, and eventually a controlled trial which can show whether the original observations were significant or not.

Shared projects
Alternatively a specialist from a nearby teaching hospital may request him to cooperate in a project for which the small hospital or clinic can provide the necessary patients for a particular trial. The work will be shared and publication of results done jointly.

Either way, more detailed observation will be made and the quality of medical care will be advanced.

Research is not limited to specialists
As Sir James Mackenzie said nearly 70 years ago:

> 'Whole fields essential to the progress of medicine will remain unexplored until the general practitioner takes his place as an investigator. The reason for this is that he has opportunities which no other worker possesses – opportunities which are necessary to the solution of problems essential to the advance of medicine.'

The late Dr Dennis Burkitt used to assert that every doctor in charge of a rural African hospital is *a world expert on the diseases in his area*. He may be far from the academic stimulus of the teaching hospital, but if he has eyes to see, and an enquiring mind, he may have insights and understanding which could be of benefit to the whole field of medical care.

Sharing in the work of professional associations
Inevitably, as time goes by, the doctor will find himself drawn in to one or other of the professional associations. Some of these are primarily medico-political, some purely academic, and some a mixture of the two. It is important that the district doctor plays his part in these, when time allows, rather than leaving them to be run entirely by the city-based physicians or specialists. He may feel reluctant to get involved, but his viewpoint should be represented and should be respected. If he has a concern for the good name of the profession it is through such associations that it can be voiced.

Medico-political organisations for the whole profession

In most countries the medical profession has one representative association or union through which it can speak to the government and make representations when necessary. Whether it be, for example, the Ghana Medical Association (GMA), the Kenya Medical Association (KMA) or the Nigeria Medical Association (NMA), doctors from all branches of the profession, including general practitioners and district doctors, play a part. When the government wants to draft a new national health policy the national medical association is invited to submit its proposals. When crises occur it is the national medical association that is the voice of the profession in negotiating with government. Through their annual conferences in each country the profession monitors current problems and new developments, and speaks out to make the views of doctors known. Mutual assistance is given on a regional basis, for example for much of Africa, through the Confederation of African Medical Associations and Societies (CAMAS). All doctors should join their national body and be prepared to bear office when so called upon.

Associations for groups within the profession

1. *Hospital doctors,* particularly at the house officer/registrar level, often feel vulnerable to bureaucratic decisions taken at higher levels, and feel the need to organise. If financial cut-backs, for example, lead to inadequate provision of drugs and materials with which to treat the patients, it is usually the resident doctors who feel most strongly the patients' disappointment. In Nigeria, the National Association of Resident Doctors (NARD) has often reacted vigorously, to the government's displeasure, during times of economic recession. Doctors in peripheral hospitals may feel somewhat distant from such developments, but their position may not be at all dissimilar.

2. *Private doctors* may find they have to organise separately to standardise salaries in the private sector, and to control competition for retainerships and the like. Wise leaders among them know they must discourage a purely commercial approach, and encourage responsible service. Governments may, quite rightly, set standards for private clinics and hospitals, and the doctors need a united voice in negotiations. Many private hospitals are run to a first class standard, and provide a comprehensive health service. Some GP associations, such as the Egyptian Doctors' Syndicate, and the Association of General and Private Medical Practitioners, Nigeria (AGPMPN), have done much to promote postgraduate medical education in their discipline, with a curriculum tailored to the primary/secondary health care needs of the country.

3. *Specialist associations.* These are primarily academic in nature. Each speciality has its association, whether it be for surgeons, paediatricians,

community physicians, or whatever. The district doctor who has taken a postgraduate degree will enjoy sharing in the regular conferences that are organised. Although most of the contributions will be from lecturers and professors in the medical schools, there will be knowledge to contribute from the primary/secondary care angle which can be uniquely important.

Associations for voluntary agency health workers
The voluntary agencies provide a sizeable proportion of the primary/secondary level of health care in many countries, even though the national government undertakes overall supervision. Most of the agencies are church-related, Anglican, Baptist, Catholic, Presbyterian, Methodist, Seventh Day Adventist and so on, and their contributions have not always been well coordinated.

Governments have, in the past, found it difficult to negotiate with them. Now there are associations in most countries through which not only the doctors, but the nurses and administrators too, can get together. The Christian Health Associations of Sierra Leone (CHASL), of Ghana (CHAG) and of Kenya all provide a united voice. The leadership in such associations generally works very closely with government, and the medical superintendent of a voluntary agency hospital should always be ready to help where he can. These associations can play a constructive role.

The *Christian Health Association of Nigeria* (CHAN) works in a country of nearly 100 million people, and does much of its negotiation with government through its state branches. There are 31 states within the Federal Republic of Nigeria, and health is controlled at state level. CHAN has four main technical arms for assisting the 120 or so member hospitals.

1. *CHANPHARM.* A central drug buying and manufacturing agency supplies 50 of the most common primary care drugs to the hospitals (see Chapter 9).

2. *Primary Health Care Coordination Unit.* The CHAN PHC coordinator travels to the many secondary care hospitals and encourages development of PHC outreach through branch primary health centres and community-based village health worker programmes.

3. *Administrative and Management Project* (AMP). This gives training to middle level management, particularly those concerned with storekeeping and accounts.

4. *A task force on holistic health care* is concerned with hospital chaplaincy training, and with promoting study of spiritual healing and the ways in which traditional beliefs impinge upon the work of doctors and nurses in hospitals and health services (see Chapter 10).

Medical ethics
The dangers of corruption
All that has been written about good administration can come to nothing if a hospital becomes riddled with corruption. It may begin at the lower levels with the gateman extracting a fee for letting emergency patients in after hours, or patients finding they have to pay staff to get the medicines or injections ordered for them on the wards. If it also affects the pharmacy so that drugs begin to 'walk', or the junior doctors demand additional personal fees before doing essential operations, things are bad indeed. Corruption can be checked if the doctor in charge is himself honest, hard-working and incorruptible – and seen to be so. He may not find it easy, but discipline can be achieved, so long as those in the board of management or Ministry of Health are prepared to back him up.

Professional integrity
The Oath of Hippocrates is still taken to be binding on all doctors who enter the medical profession, though it dates from about 500 BC. It governs the doctor's relationship with his patients and with his colleagues. A re-wording in more modern language was adopted by the World Medical Association in 1948, the *Declaration of Geneva*, together with an International Code of Medical Ethics. The declaration includes a solemn pledge to consecrate one's life 'to the service of humanity'. Matters of personal integrity are implied, rather than spelt out. It reads as follows:

At the time of being admitted as a member of the medical profession:

- I solemnly pledge myself to consecrate my life to the service of humanity;
- I will give to my teachers the respect and gratitude which is their due;
- I will practise my profession with conscience and dignity;
- The health of my patient will be my first consideration;
- I will respect the secrets which are confided in me, even after the patient has died;
- I will maintain by all means in my power the honour and the noble traditions of the medical profession;
- My colleagues will be my brothers;
- I will not permit considerations of religion, nationality, race, party politics or social standing to intervene between my duty and my patient;
- I will maintain the utmost respect for human life from the time of conception;
- Even under threat, I will not use my medical knowledge contrary to the laws of humanity;

- I make these promises solemnly, freely and upon my honour.'

Those who accept the Christian faith may be prepared to go further in defining the personal integrity which is at the heart of medical ethics. In 1975 the Christian Medical Fellowship drew up a statement of 'Christian ethics in medical practice' (see Appendix 7). There is much in it with which those of other faiths would equally agree.

Social and family responsibilities
Social obligation
Doctors are frequently requested to allow those who are 'high-ups' to be seen first. Generally a strictly observed 'first come, first served' policy works best. The poorest and most marginalised person in the community has as much right to his place in the queue as the wealthy contractor, school principal or town chief. In some hospitals a special clinic can be organised for such 'senior service' people, and they pay extra for the privilege. Where that is not possible the doctor may be able to use some discretion in allowing those with limited time off, such as school principals, to be seen early. The community may also be embarrassed if their chief, or their minister or malam, is kept waiting, and occasional privileged entry will be generally accepted.

Doctors who come to work in their own home area will have the particular problem of the extended family and clan, all of whom will expect priority treatment. Some doctors refuse to serve their own community precisely because of such anticipated strains, which can be a cause of deep misunderstanding and resentment from the very people who should be most supportive. Should the opportunity be accepted to come home to work, education of the extended family should be undertaken even before arrival. Problems may well continue, but if gradually overcome, the doctor who works in his own area can actually achieve much more. He knows his own community so well.

Personal health
The doctor has a duty to take off sufficient time to be with his family, and to relax or take exercise. A game of tennis, squash or badminton, or hoeing up the yam heaps on a farm behind the house can all provide the short bursts of real exertion which promote physical fitness.

Moderation in diet and in alcohol consumption are obvious essentials to keep down the weight, and possible hypertension. Alcohol not only affects the liver, but all the systems of the body and the unborn child too. The Royal College of Physicians, London, in its 1987 report on the medical consequences of alcohol abuse (40), gives evidence that alcohol impairs the sex life as well. The College puts the danger level at two to three glasses of wine per day, or 1 to 1.5 pints of beer.

Many doctors use a car more as a status symbol than out of necessity, even for quite short distances. Excessive dependence can take away the chance of some walking exercise and accelerate the onset of obesity. Driving, after even the smallest amounts of alcohol – and long before 'drunkenness' becomes apparent – is, of course, particularly hazardous, and has been the cause of the tragic early demise of too many young doctors. The conditioned reflex reaction to danger is critically slowed and the emergency stop comes just too late.

The smoking epidemic is gaining ground in developing countries (41) just as the devastating effects of cigarettes on the lungs and heart are being fully realised in the west. The doctor can do much through education of his patients, and encouragement of national measures, to control tobacco use – but not if he is an inveterate smoker himself.

Stress is not always avoidable in the doctor's work. Difficult decisions, broken nights, and the dispiriting effect of the occasional failure and tragic death in a patient for whom one has struggled – these are what the job is made of. The queue in the out-patients may seem interminable, but the discipline of a short mid-morning coffee break, and a chat with colleagues, is an excellent anti-ulcer regime. The doctor must be able to get his meals with reasonable regularity, and get enough sleep. These are the measures to keep stress within bounds.

The family home, and children's education

The 'front-line doctor's' job is a very demanding one, and it taxes those who undertake it to the limit. A happy marriage is, of course, the greatest source of strength, stability and inner calm amid the stresses of the job.

The arrival of a family can add to this stability if both parents understand how to handle children. If not, the peace of the home can be sadly disturbed. Some couples feel that the only solution is to move to the city, where they can find a good nursery school for a fractious child, little realising that the solution may lie more closely to hand.

In Nigeria, the doctors training for the FMCGP, and expecting to serve in small townships as front-line doctors, raised the problem, very naturally, of schooling for their own children. The issue was taken up by suggesting they should think of themselves as 'front-line parents', and prepare accordingly. Some thoughts along these lines were prepared which began as follows:

'Children are born into a family, with father, mother, brothers, sisters and other relatives. Caring for children is the responsibility of both parents, and education begins at birth. Young babies are played with and stimulated, but as they become toddlers and there is another baby in the house, they are often left to their own devices – 'Go and play . . . you are troublesome'.'

Parents are often embarrassed because they honestly do not know how to help and train their children. They need to know:

a) how the child develops in the early years – physically, socially, psychologically and in terms of mental growth

b) that one child may differ in its needs from another

c) how they can interact with the children, helping and yet allowing them to develop at their own pace in their own way

d) as children grow older, what they can do at home to supplement nursery school and primary school.

Good child care practices do not always come instinctively. What mother-in-law says or grandpa thinks is not always right. Much can be learned from modern educational practice. This whole area is of supreme importance, particularly for doctors aiming to make a career in a relatively remote area, but, in practice, for those in the city as well. Child care can be just as bad there, if not worse. Guidelines for front-line parents are given in Appendix 8 and further reading suggested.

A concluding thought

There can be few careers in medicine which can exert, on the one hand, such great pressures to try and do too much, and yet, on the other, give such genuine job satisfaction.

To be a 'front-line doctor' is not an easy option, and the one who takes on the challenge may well feel he needs a strength greater than his own. Many have found help in Reinhold Niebuhr's well-known prayer:

> 'God grant me the *serenity* to accept the things I cannot change,
>
> The *courage* to change the things I can,
>
> And the *wisdom* to know the difference.'

APPENDICES

Appendix 1

Constitution of the community hospital

I. NAME
   The name of the hospital shall be the .... Community Hospital.

II. PURPOSE
   The purpose for which the hospital exists is to provide comprehensive health care to the community without discrimination as to ethnic origin, party or religion, and to provide training for health personnel.

III. CONTROLLING BODIES
   A. The Hospital Management Board, subject to
   B. The .... (a higher body) .... representing the .... Community.

IV. HOSPITAL MANAGEMENT BOARD
   A. *The Board shall consist of fifteen members*
      5 from the .... community appointed by .... (of people having some understanding and concern for health matters, and broadly representative of all sides of the community – men and women, church and mosque, traditional rulers and business leaders).
      3 from the .... College of Medicine appointed by .... (only relevant if cooperating with a university)
      2 from .... Local Government, appointed by the Chairman
      2 from the State Government appointed by the State Health Management Board
      3 hospital officers, the Medical Superintendent, the Matron and Hospital Secretary

   B. *Officers of the Board:* these shall consist of a Chairman and a Secretary.
      1. The Chairman – shall be appointed by the traditional leader in Council from among the five community representatives he appoints to the Board;
      2. The Secretary – shall be elected triennially from among the members of the Board. He shall keep the Minutes of Board Meetings, conduct Board correspondence, and, in consultation with the Chairman, issue the notices calling meetings of the Board; and do all such things as are necessary for the better execution of his office.

   C. *General Meetings:* the Board shall meet every six months at .... Notices, with copies of the agenda prepared in consultation with the Medical Superintendent and Chairman shall be sent by the Secretary to all members not less than twenty-one days before the date for which the meeting was called.

   Emergency Meetings of the Board may be called at the request of the Chairman and Secretary, or at the written request of five members of the Board. Notice of Emergency Meeting, with the business to be considered, shall be delivered by hand to all members not less than five days before the date for which the meeting is called. Decisions taken shall be subject to approval at the next General Meeting.

D. *Quorum:* six members shall form a quorum at a General Meeting for the purpose of transacting business.

E. *Functions*
   1. Control and define the general policy of the hospital.
   2. Accept and adopt the Annual Statement of Accounts, and the Budget.
   3. Appoint the Auditors.
   4. Receive the Annual Report from the Medical Superintendent.
   5. Appoint the Hospital Officers – the Medical Superintendent, the Matron and the Hospital Secretary.
   6. Approve the appointment of Senior Staff and confirm their dismissal.
   7. Appoint an *Executive committee* consisting of the Chairman, the three Hospital Officers, and two others, to hear, and to act on urgent matters between the Board meetings.

      On Establishment, the Executive shall;
      determine the fixed establishment, and review as necessary; consider rates of pay and conditions of service, and make recommendations to the Board;
      appoint senior staff, subject to confirmation by the Board, and deal with all other staff matters.

      On Finance, the Executive shall;
      authorise the opening of bank accounts in the name of the Hospital; examine the Annual Statement of Accounts and Budget, and Auditor's Report, and make recommendations to the Board; examine tenders for capital works approved by the Board, and award contracts.
   8. Appoint other such committees as may be necessary for the good management of the Hospital, and determine the terms of reference.
   9. Have power to recommend amendments to this Constitution. These shall be tabled at one Meeting, but not voted on till the next. A three-fourths majority of the members present and voting shall be necessary to confirm the amendment.

V. BYE–LAWS
   1. The Officers of the Hospital shall have the following responsibilities:
      (a) *Medical Superintendent.* He shall be a person with registrable medical qualifications, and appropriate experience. He shall be the Executive Head of the Hospital, and shall see to its efficient and satisfactory administration. He shall, however, delegate the duties specified which fall within other departments.
      He shall be the recognised correspondent for the hospital on all official matters.
      He shall be responsible for the admission, proper treatment and discharge of all patients.
      He shall make recommendations to the Executive and/or Board for all matters to do with Senior Staff, other than those of the nursing service.
      He shall appoint and dismiss all other employees.
      He shall commence, carry on or defend all actions and proceedings concerning the Hospital.
      (b) *Matron.* The Matron shall be a person with registrable nursing and midwifery qualifications. In consultation with the Medical Superintendent she shall be responsible for the satisfactory administration of the Nursing Service in the hospital.
      She shall be the recognised correspondent with official bodies on matters concerning the Nursing Service.
      She shall, in consultation with the Medical Superintendent, make recommendations to the Executive and/or the Board for all matters to do with qualified staff of the Nursing Service.
      She shall be responsible for the discipline and care of the nurses, and all auxiliary staff attached to the Nursing Service, including maids and cleaners.

She shall be responsible for the general cleanliness of the hospital, and for the care of linen and nursing supplies.
(c) *Hospital Secretary*. He shall be a person with a training in administration (or accounting), and suitable experience.

He shall, in consultation with the Medical Superintendent, be responsible for the general and financial administration of the Hospital, and will see that proper accounts of all hospital moneys are maintained.

He will be responsible for the ordering of supplies, other than drugs ordered by the Pharmacy section.

The Maintenance staff shall be responsible to him for the maintenance and repair of the buildings, equipment and vehicles, and for the general upkeep of the hospital and grounds.

He shall, in consultation with the Medical Superintendent, appoint junior clerical and labour staff, and, in consultation with the appropriate head of section, junior technical staff.

He shall conduct such correspondence as the Medical Superintendent may assign him.

2. Voting.
Subject to the exception noted below:
- each member of the Board shall have one vote
- the Chairman shall exercise his vote with the other members voting
- in case of a tie vote the motion is lost
- there shall be no voting by proxy.

Exception:
The Hospital Officers on the Board shall not vote on any matter concerning the appointment or dismissal of Hospital Officers. When the status, salary and allowances, or personal conduct, of a Hospital Officer comes up for discussion, the Officer shall be privileged to make a statement concerning the matter, and then shall withdraw.

3. Quorum.
Unless otherwise stated then not less than half the members of any committee or subcommittee in the Hospital shall form a quorum for the purpose of transacting business.

4. Absentee members.
If a member of the Board fails to attend three consecutive meetings without reasonable excuse, a replacement shall be called for.

5. Right of appeal.
Any member of the Senior Staff shall have the right of appeal to the Hospital Management Board against any decision of the Hospital Officers taken against them. Junior staff have right of appeal to the Executive.

Appendix 2

Policy for cleaning and decontamination of equipment or environment

Modified from *Control of Hospital Infection: a practical handbook.* E J L Lowbury *et al*, Chapman and Hall, London, 1981.

Equipment or site	(1) Routine or preferred method	(2) Acceptable alternative or additional recommendations for infected patients
Ampoules	Wipe neck with 70% alcohol; do not immerse	
Bed–frames	Wash with detergent and dry	After infected patient use a phenolic
Bed–pans	If possible wash in machine with heat disinfection cycle, or use disposables	Patients with enteric infections. If (1) is not possible, empty, wash and use phenolics. Individual pan for infected patient
Bowls (surgical)	Autoclave	
Bowls (washing)	Wash and dry	For infected patients use individual bowls and disinfect on discharge, by heat or a phenolic
Cheatle forceps	If possible, do not use	If used, autoclave daily and store in fresh phenolic solution
Crockery and cutlery	Handwash by approved method	For patients with enteric infections or TB use disposables or heat disinfect
Floors (wet cleaning)	Wash with detergent solution: disinfection not usually required	Known contaminated and special areas, use a phenolic
Furniture and fittings	Damp dust with detergent solution	Known contaminated and special, areas damp dust with a phenolic

Infant incubators	Wash with detergent and dry with disposable wipe	Infected patients, after cleaning, wipe or spray with 70% alcohol or hypochlorite solution
Mattresses and pillows	Water-impermeable cover, wash with detergent solution	Disinfect with phenolic if contaminated
Mops (wet)	Rinse after each use, wring and store dry; autoclave periodically	Soak in hypochlorite solution for 30 min, rinse and store dry
Nail brushes	Use only if essential	A sterile nail brush should be used for all clinical procedures
Razors	Disposable, or autoclaved	Phenolics or 70% alcohol
Sputum container	Use disposable only if possible	Non-disposable containers should be emptied with care and autoclaved
Thermometers (oral)	Individual thermometers, wipe with 70% alcohol, store dry; terminally disinfect as (2)	Collect after round; wipe clean with phenolic, or 70% alcohol for 10 min; rinse, wipe and store dry
Thermometers (rectal)	Clean with 70% alcohol and treat as above	
Toilet seats	Wash with detergent and dry	After use by infected patients, or if grossly contaminated, use phenolic, rinse and dry
Trolley tops	Clean first then wipe or spray with 70% alcohol	Clean first then use phenolic and wipe dry
Urinals	Use washer with heat disinfection cycle or use disposables	Use phenolics: if a tank is used it must be emptied, dried and refilled at least weekly
Washbasins	Clean with detergent Disinfection not normally required	If contaminated use hypochlorite solution

Appendix 3

Model list of essential drugs

Extracted from the Technical Report Series 825, *The use of essential drugs*, World Health Organisation, Geneva, 1992. (Seventh Revision).

Explanatory notes
Many drugs included in the list are preceded by a square symbol (❏) to indicate that they represent an example of a therapeutic group and that various drugs could serve as alternatives. It is imperative that this be understood when drugs are selected at national level, since choice is then influenced by the comparative cost and availability of equivalent products. Example of acceptable substitutions include:
- ❏ Codeine: other drugs for the symptomatic treatment of diarrhoea such as diphenoxylate or loperamide or, when indicated for cough relief, noscapine or dextromethorphan.
- ❏ Hydrochlorothiazide: any other thiazide-type diuretic currently in broad clinical use
- ❏ Hydralazine: any other peripheral vasodilator having an antihypertensive effect.
- ❏ Senna: any mild stimulant laxative (either synthetic or of plant origin).
- ❏ Sulfadimidine: any other short-acting systemically-active sulfonamide unlikely to cause crystalluria.

Numbers in parentheses following the drug names indicate:
1. Drugs subject to international control under (a) the Single Convention on Narcotic Drugs (1961), and (b) the Convention on Psychotropic Substances (1971);
2. Specific expertise, diagnostic precision, or special equipment required for proper use;
3. Greater potency or efficacy;
4. In renal insufficiency, contraindicated or dosage adjustments necessary;
5. To improve compliance;
6. Special pharmacokinetic properties for purpose;
7. Adverse effects diminish benefit/risk ratio;
8. Limited indications or narrow spectrum of activity;
9. For epidural anaesthesia.

Letters in parentheses following the drug names indicate the reasons for the inclusion of *complementary drugs*:
A. When drugs in the main list cannot be made available;
B. When drugs in the main list are known to be ineffective or inappropriate for a given individual;
C. For use in rare disorders or in exceptional circumstances.

* When the strength is specified in terms of a selected salt or ester, this is mentioned in brackets; when it refers to the active moiety, the name of the salt or ester in brackets is preceded by the word 'as'.

Drug	Route of administration, dosage forms and strengths *

1. Anaesthetics

1.1 General anaesthetics and oxygen

diazepam (1b, 2)	injection 5mg/ml in 2-ml ampoule
ether, anaesthetic (2)	inhalation
halothane (2)	inhalation
ketamine (2)	injection, 50mg (as hydrochloride)/ml in 10-ml vial
nitrous oxide (2)	inhalation
oxygen	inhalation (medicinal gas)
❑ thiopental (2)	powder for injection, 0.5g, 1.0g (sodium salt) in ampoule

1.2 Local anaesthetics

❑ bupivacaine (2,9)	injection, 0.25%, 0.5% (hydrochloride) in vial injection for spinal anaesthesia, 0.5% (hydrochloride) in 4-ml ampoule to be mixed with 7.5% glucose solution
❑ lidocaine	injection, 1%, 2% (hydrochloride) in vial injection, 1%, 2% (hydrochloride) + epinephrine 1:200 000 in vial injection for spinal anaesthesia, 5% (hydrochloride) in 2-ml ampoule to be mixed with 7.5% glucose solution topical forms, 2–4% (hydrochloride) dental cartridge, 2% (hydrochloride) + epinephrine 1:80 000

1.3 Preoperative medication

atropine	injection, 1mg (sulphate) in 1-ml ampoule
chloral hydrate	syrup, 200mg/5ml
❑ diazepam (1b)	injection, 5mg/ml in 2-ml ampoule
❑ morphine (1a)	injection, 10mg (sulphate or hydrochloride) in 1-ml ampoule
❑ promethazine	elixir or syrup, 5mg (hydrochloride)/5ml

(see WHO booklet for the complete list)

Drug	Route of administration, dosage forms and strengths *

2. Analgesics, antipyretics, non-steroidal anti-inflammatory drugs and drugs used to treat gout

2.1 Non-opioids

acetylsalicylic acid	tablet, 100–500mg
	suppository, 50–150mg
allopurinol (4)	tablet, 100mg
colchicine (7)	tablet, 500µg
❑ ibuprofen	tablet, 200mg
❑ indometacin	capsule or tablet, 25mg
paracetemol	tablet, 100–500mg
	suppository, 100mg
	syrup, 125mg/5ml

2.2 Opioid analgesics

❑ codeine (1a)	tablet, 30mg (phosphate)
❑ morphine (1a)	injection, 10mg (sulphate or hydrochloride) in 1-ml ampoule
	oral solution, 10mg/5ml
	tablet, 10mg (sulphate)

Complementary drug

❑ pethidine (A) (1a, 4)	injection, 50mg (hydrochloride) in 10-ml ampoule
	tablet, 50mg, 100mg (hydrochloride)

3. Antiallergics and drugs used in anaphylaxis

❑ chlorphenamine	tablet, 4mg (hydrogen maleate)
	injection, 10mg (hydrogen maleate) in 1-ml ampoule
❑ dexamethasone	tablet, 500µg, 4mg
	injection, 4mg (as sodium phosphate) in 1-ml ampoule
epinephrine	injection, 1mg (as hydrochloride) in 1-ml ampoule
hydrocortisone	powder for injection, 100mg (as sodium succinate) in vial
❑ prednisolone	tablet, 5mg

(see WHO booklet for the complete list)

Drug	Route of administration, dosage forms and strengths *

4. Antidotes and other substances used in poisonings

4.1 General

❏ charcoal, activated	powder
ipecacuanha	syrup, containing 0.14% ipecacuanha alkaloids calculated as emetine

4.2 Specific

atropine	injection, 1mg (sulphate) in 1-ml ampoule
deferoxamine	powder for injection, 500mg (mesilate) in vial
dimercaprol (2)	injection in oil, 50mg/ml in 2-ml ampoule
❏ methionine	tablet, 250mg (racemate)
methylioninium chloride (methylene blue)	injection in oil, 50mg/ml in 2-ml ampoule
naloxone	injection, 400µg (hydrochloride) in 1-ml ampoule
penicillamine (2)	capsule or tablet, 250mg
potassium ferric hexacyanoferate (II).2H$_2$O (Prussian blue)	powder for oral administration
sodium calcium edetate (2)	injection, 200mg/ml in 5-ml ampoule
sodium nitrite	injection, 30mg/ml in 10-ml ampoule
sodium thiosulphate	injection, 250mg/ml in 50-ml ampoule

5. Antiepileptics

carbamazepine	scored tablet, 100mg, 200mg
❏ diazepam (1b)	injection, 5mg/ml in 2-ml ampoule (intravenous or rectal)
ethosuximide	capsule or tablet, 250mg syrup, 250mg syrup, 250mg/5ml
phenobarbital (1b)	tablet, 15–100mg elixir, 15mg/5ml
phenytoin	capsule or tablet, 25mg, 100mg (sodium salt) injection, 50mg (sodium salt)/ml in 5-ml vial
valproic acid (7)	enteric coated tablet, 200mg, 500mg (sodium salt)

(see WHO booklet for the complete list)

Appendix 4

Essential reagents for rural medical laboratories

(H V Hogerzeil, M Hops. Tropical Doctor 1986; 16: 58-60)

Average number of laboratory examinations per 30 000 out-patient consultations (OPC)

Laboratory test	Average no. tests/30 000■	Recommended method(s)	Projected no. tests/30 000▫
Blood			
Haemoglobin	4300	Cynamethaemoblobin with Lovibond	10 000
Sickle cell	1400	Sodium metasulphite	1500
ESR	830	Westergren	1000
WBC count	1300	Acetic acid, Neubauer	1500
WBC differential	270	Leishman stain	250
		Giemsa stain	250
Thick film (malaria)	930	Giemsa stain	650
		Field stain	1000
Blood group	630	Anti A, B and D	1000
Cross match	450	Saline and albumin	600
Glucose	190	Strip: Dextrostix	250
		(alternative: modified Folin-Wu with Lovibond)	
Bile	190	Jendrassik-Groff-Powel with Lovibond	250
Urea	69	Strip: Urastrat	100
		(alternative: diacetyl-monoxime with Lovibond)	
Urine			
Albumin	2100	Sulphosalic acid	2000
		Strip: Albustix	1000
Glucose	1400	Tablet: Clinitest	1500
Sediment	1500	Microscopic	2000
Bile	210	Strip: Icotest	250
		(alternative: Fouchet test)	
Urobilinogen	110	Strip: Bilugen	150
		(alternative: Ehrlich test)	
Stool			
Parasites	2500	Saline and iodine	3000
Blood in stool	100	Tablets: Haematest	100
Cerebrospinal fluid			
Albumin		Pandy	100
Glucose		Strip: Dextrostix	100
Bacteria		Gram stain	100
		Ziehal-Neelsen stain	100

Laboratory test.	Average no. tests/30000■	Recommended method(s)	Projected no. tests/30000❐
WBC count		Acetic acid, Fuchs Rosenthal	100
WBC differential		Giemsa stain	100
Sputum	240	Ziehl-Neelsen stain	400
Pus, exudate	300	Gram stain	400

- ■ OPC= out-patient consultations, excluding prenatal visits and healthy under-fives, but including the average proportion of in-patients.
- ❐ The average number is a mean based upon 3.5 million treatment episodes in 21 mission hospitals in Ghana, 1981/82

Simplified standard package of essential laboratory chemicals per 30 000 out-patient consultations

Acetic acid, glacial 99.7%	32 ml	*Strips and tablets*	
Acetone	5 litres	Albustix strips	1000
Anti-A grouping sera	50 ml	Bilugen tablets	50
Anti-B grouping sera	50 ml	Buffer tablets	50
Anti-D grouping sera	50 ml	Clinitest tablets	1500
Bovine albumin 30%	60 ml	Dextrostix strips	350
Field stain A	25 g	Haematest tablets	100
Field stain B	25 g	Icotest strips	250
Fuschsin, basic, stain powder	50 g	Urastrat strips	100
Gentian violet	14 g		
Giemsa stain powder	4 g		
Glycerol	250 ml		
Hydrochloric acid	200 ml		
Iodine tincture	40 ml		
Leishman stain powder	0.5 g		
Methanol	10 litres		
Methylene blue, stain powder	0.5 g		
Phenol crystals	265 g		
Potassium cyanide	5 g		
Potassium ferricyanide	20 g		
Potassium iodide	75 g		
Potassium phosphate, monobasic	65 g		
Sodium citrate	20 g		
Sodium chloride	275 g		
Sodium metabisulphite	75 g		
Sodium nitrate	0.5 g		
Sulphanilic acid	25 g		
Sulphosalic acid	70 g		

Note: This is the version of the list in which reagent strips are used for blood glucose and urea, and for urine bile and urobilinogen, not the longer version using chemical tests.

Tables prepared by H V Hogerzeil and M Hops, (17).

Appendix 5

Notes for elective medical students from overseas

Prepared for those applying to come to the Ibarapa Community Health Programme, College of Medicine, University of Ibadan, 1987.

1. **Background to the Ibarapa programme**
    Ibarapa district (population about 150 000) is a rural area, 100 km to the west of the city of Ibadan within Oyo State. It contains two main townships, Eruwa and Igboora, each of about 50 000 inhabitants, five other towns and many villages. The area is picturesque with woodland savannah plains, broken rocky outcrops (inselbergs) around which the towns and villages cluster. The people are predominantly Yorubas and on their farms grow yam, cassava, maize, guinea corn and melons. The latter are something of a speciality and their local name 'bara' provides the origin of the name of the area 'Ibarapa'.

    In 1963 the University of Ibadan Medical School came to an agreement with the State Ministry of Health in Ibadan to organise a joint community health project in the area to promote the better teaching of community health to medical students, nurses and other health personnel. Whithin the University the Department of Preventive and Social Medicine is specifically responsible for the programme.

    The existing Government health facilities are the basis around which the teaching is organised. These consist of:
    1. A 36-bed district hospital at Eruwa
    2. A rural health centre and community hospital complex at Igboora
    3. Maternity centres and dispensaries in each of the seven major towns
    4. Local government health offices concerned with environmental health.

    The University has a network of village and neighbourhood based primary health care services to complement the static health facilities.

    At the rural health centre (RHC) site in Igboora the University has developed a campus consisting of a students' hostel, dining hall, staff residences and a suite of consulting rooms and records offices, and a teaching and research block consisting of tutorial and lecture rooms, library, laboratory and offices. In addition there is a branch of the University of Ibadan maintenance department responsible for the upkeep of the facilities. The transport office maintains a fleet of vehicles which conveys students and staff to outlying clinics, and maintains the link with Ibadan.

    All Ibadan medical students do an eight-week community health/general practice attachment at Igboora, coming in groups of 30 to 40. They are divided into six groups which rotate through postings in:
    1. Igboora Rural Health Centre;
    2. Health education and school health service;
    3. Maternal and child health;

4. Environmental health;
5. Eruwa Hospital;
6. Occupational health.

Each group also undertakes an original epidemiological research project and presents a seminar on topics of current interest.

Elective students may join in whatever aspect of the programme they wish, and thus get a general introduction to the type of rural health service available in Nigeria. At Igboora and Eruwa they can work in clinical, laboratory and child health services with the medical officers providing supervision. In the community they can provide health education, supervise primary health workers, make follow-up home visits, conduct environmental inspection tours and examine the health status of the local school children.

There is room for electives to develop programmes to suit their individual needs. Please inform staff of your special interests.

2. **Application procedure**
(Details are given as to the address of the Dean, to whom applications should be addressed; and those who should be copied. Advice is added as to what to say in the application.)

State the dates you want to come, and your willingness to pay any necessary costs. (Actually your main expenses will be food). Request reply by airmail but do not be too surprised if there is a postal delay.

3. **Board and lodging**
Accommodation at Igboora is of youth hostel type, of reasonable standard. Bring sheets, pillow–case, towel and toiletries. No charge is made except for food. The catering service provides adequate meals of Nigerian foods on a 'Pay as you eat' basis.

There is mains water and light – most of the time. Bring a torch for emergencies, and water heating coil (220-240v).

4. **Climate and health**
Igboora is about 130km from the coast, north of Lagos. The altitude is 155 meters above sea level, and generally rather hot. There is a dry season from October to March with temperature 32°C to 36°C , and a wet season April to September with temperature 27°C to 32°C. The best time to visit is between March and June, or in December when cool dry harmattan winds reduce heat.

General health hints
Water Tapwater, when available, in Ibadan and Igboora is generally safe. Elsewhere it is preferable to have water boiled and filtered.
Diarrhoea Learn how to make and use oral rehydration therapy.
Insects Insect repellant may be helpful on occasion.
Salt Always take more than you are used to. After heavy exertion and sweating a quarter teaspoonful of salt in an ounce of water tastes really sweet, because of salt depletion, and it can be washed down with a glass of plain water if you are in doubt.
Sun Tropical sun, especially between noon and 3 pm, can soon give ultra-violet radiation overdose, with headache, vomiting and weakness. You may adapt by a steady degree of increasing exposure. (Sun screen creams advised)
Cooling Surprisingly, this too can be a danger, especially at night, if no cover is retained over one's middle. A brisk diarrhoea next morning, possibly due to failure of fluid absorption by the bowel, is the usual result. Always keep a sheet over the abdomen even if legs and arms are exposed. At times a light blanket is needed.

5. **Entry visa**
   Entry visas are required. Telephone the nearest Nigerian High Commission, Embassy or Consulate for visa requirements and forms. An acceptance letter from the University of Ibadan will likely be among the requirements. Visa applications may be handled in person or by post.

6. **What to bring**
   a. *Clothing.* Hot weather clothing is the order. Cotton and polyester shirts and dresses, preferably drip-dry, are best. There are few occasions when students will need to dress formally, but at all times they should dress well. For women, trousers are fine on campus when off duty, but are not appreciated by the community. You may want to bring shoes for hiking or football, as our students often engage in these activities. Generally shoes or sandals should be comfortable, and allow your feet to 'breathe'. As a general advice, pack lightly. There is a laundry service available on a fee basis.

   b. *Camera film.* Bring enough to cover the elective. Film is available locally, but is expensive.

   c. *No text books* are needed if you are just staying at Igboora. There is a small but adequate medical library on the campus, and Ibadan students always carry an assortment of their own texts.

   d. If you do not bring *bed-linen* this can be hired at a small charge from the Administrative Officer in Igboora.

   e. *Torch and spare batteries* are useful during night walks, and because power cuts are frequent.

   f. *Money.* Bring travellers cheques.

7. **On arrival**
   Immigration formalities. These normally take time, but your patience is requested. Do not give your passport or other particulars to anyone except immigration officials who are in uniform posted behind the immigration counter. (Details are then given about foreign exchange and currency regulations pertaining in Nigeria at the time.)

   Travel from the airport. It is best to plan arrival in the morning or early afternoon. Travel by road from the airport at night is not recommended. If you must arrive after dark you should consider staying in a hotel until dawn unless you have specific arrangements or contacts to stay in Lagos that night. It may take one to two hours to clear customs and collect baggage. Official airport taxis can be booked at a desk across from the customs hall exit. Rates are fixed, and paid for, in advance.

   (Further details are then given about travel on to Ibadan and Igboora.)

   Please address any questions to .... (give the relevant name and address).

Appendix 6

Guidelines for general practice training hospitals

Faculty of General Medical Practice, National Postgraduate Medical College, Nigeria.

Guidelines for proprietors and medical superintendents of training hospitals approved for FMCGP residency training, Part I

Accreditation
A general hospital, or a generalist department of a teaching hospital, may apply for accreditation by the National Postgraduate Medical College through the Faculty of General Medical Practice, if the authorities feel that the criteria for recognition can be met.

Arrangements will be for inspection of the hospital by two Fellows of the Faculty, or senior doctors designated by the Faculty. Their reports will be conveyed to the Secretary of the Faculty Board, and the Board will place its recommendations before the Senate of the Postgraduate College.

Formal notification of approval will be sent to the hospital's Medical Superintendent or Principal Medical Officer, with a copy to the relevant hospital authorities, and to the Ministry of Health of the State in which the hospital is situated. The Medical Superintendent will be considered as the Supervisor of Training, or he may designate another interested member of his senior medical staff to act for him. Subsequent correspondence between the Faculty and the Hospital will be through the Supervisor.

Accreditation will be subject to review from time to time, to ensure that standards for training are maintained.

Appointment of a doctor for training
Doctors have to qualify, and complete a year of internship in a teaching hospital or other hospital recognised by the Nigeria Medical Council, before they can be registered with the NMC. They must then do a further year, usually the year of NYSC service, before they can start postgraduate training. They do start with a good grounding.

No doctors are 'placed' or seconded by the Faculty to an approved hospital. Intending trainees are given a current list of approved hospitals, and they are free to choose where they wish to apply. Applications, with *curriculum vitae* and names of referees will be sent to the proprietor of the hospital in the usual way, and appointment may be made after interview if the doctor meets the requirements of the proprietor, and shows himself to be in sympathy with the general aims of the hospital.

The doctor so appointed will, in teaching hospital terms, be designated Senior House Officer for his first year, and then Registrar (equivalent of Medical Officer II and Medical Officer I in Government terms. The term Registrar will be used subsequently in these Guidelines.

The Registrar should be given a letter of appointment for two years in the first place, to cover the Part I FMCGP training period. Though a trainee, he will be a full member of the hospital staff, subject to the usual hospital regulations and discipline, and expected to take a full share of routine and emergency clinical duties, with necessary supervision and cover by consultants or other senior medical staff. He will be reponsible to the General Practice Supervisor and/or Medical Superintendent, who will expect him to be punctual in following the hospital timetable or roster given to him. He will use his own time for furthering his private studies.

He should not take on a second job for financial gain, e.g. by attendance at a private practice nearby. A training hopital where this is known to happen is liable to have its accreditation reviewed, and possibly suspended.

It is the duty of the Medical Superintendent to notify the Faculty Board Secretary in Lagos of the date when any new Registrar is appointed and takes up his duties. This determines the date when the two year Part I training period is deemed to have begun. Copies of the letter should be sent for information to the Ministry of Health of the Registrar's State of origin, and the Ministry of Health of the State in which the hospital is situated; also to any other relevant sponsoring body, e.g. Armed Forces or Federal Government.

Also, if the Registrar resigns, or has to be dismissed, or leaves the Training Hospital for any reason, the Faculty should be informed, and his training will be deemed to have been discontinued until acceptable alternative arrangements have been made.

Salary and allowances
The hospital is free to make its own contractual arrangements with the Registrar, according to its ability to pay. However, the Federal Ministry of Establishment's 'rate for the job', negotiated by the Nigeria Medical Association, is usually followed. (Local details omitted)

Housing
Wherever possible the doctor's residences should be on, or very near to, the hospital compound, together with other senior staff, so that he may feel an integral part of the hospital community. As the doctor may be a family man, and in any case as full member of the medical staff, the residence should be of reasonable size (two or three-bedroomed), and preferably with hard furnishings provided (beds with mattresses, cooker, fridge, chairs, tables etc).

Leave entitlement
The Registrar's busy rotational programme may make it difficult for him to fit in annual leave, but he should be entitled to a month a year, by arrangement with the Medical Superintendent.

Any additional days for personal business matters, emergencies, sickness or casual leave, must be subject to the regulations of the hospital, and at the discretion of the Medical Superintendent.

Examination leave of one or two weeks for those who have to sit... Part I finals in Lagos, should also be allowed.

Settling in and starting work
The Registrar may be a local person, or he may have come from a distant state and may find the environment strange. Whatever the case the Medical Superintendent should extend a welcome in the usual way, and give necessary help in settling in. This might include a meal on arrival, loan of hospital linen till he gets his own unpacked, some advance of money on his first month's salary and advice on the best local markets and stores; introduction to a local bank, if desired; and, when there is time, a tour of the town and introduction to local community leaders, pastors etc.

Every hospital has its own way of doing things, and any handouts about the hospital, which may be available, can be of help in the Registrar's orientation: a plan of the hospital, usual time-table, staff-list, methods of organising duty-call, hospital formulary and up-to-date list of any items not available; also any currently accepted protocol for handling particular clinical problems; methods of prescribing, including any customary limitation on the number of prescriptions per patient; the hospital fee list (if charges are made), and the doctor's role in this.

The more complete such initial information giving can be, the less danger of misunderstandings through a 'communications gap' later.

Rotation of clinical duties
The Registrar has to cover all aspects of medical care, in accordance with the curriculum for Part I FMCGP. It is the duty of the General Practice Supervisor/Medical Superintendent to see that the clinical assignments given to the Registrar enable him to have sufficient experience to become clinically competent in the areas prescribed.

Some hospitals do not divide the clinics or wards on a departmental basis, and the training can take place on a fully generalised basis all the way through. Others have departmentalisation, partial or complete, and the Medical Superintendent must take the initiative in seeing that the Registrar moves around at regular intervals, to work with the various consultants. In some hospitals five two-month block rotations in a year may be arranged. Other hospitals prefer longer attachments of up to five months. Early attachments in surgery and obstetrics will enable the Registrar to cover a wider range of responsibility when taking general on-calls. Some flexibility is essential to allow for such contingencies as consultant's leave, staff sickness, the Registrar's own annual leave, and his personal interests and particular needs in relation to deficiencies in previous experience. Examples of rotational training programmes are given at the end.

Additional postings
Some hospitals can provide all that is required for the Part I FMCGP curriculum within their own compound or associated health facilities. For others some short postings to other centres (e.g. for ophthalmology or psychiatry) may need to be arranged. The responsibility for this lies with the General Practice Supervisor/Medical Superintendent, in consultation with the Registrar, and, if need be, with the Director of Training of the Faculty. The Registrar should not make the arrangements on his own. Such postings will usually be in the second year.

Normally, the hospital employing the Registrar will be responsible for paying salary during such periods of outside posting. If the hospital can develop sufficient facilities within the hospital, it may not be necessary for the Registrar to travel away, and the hospital will retain his services all through.

The experience of community health should, wherever possible be given in a primary health care programme organised *in relation to the hospital*. The posting may be given on an extended basis, e.g. on one day a week for 20 weeks, or on a two-monthly block attachment. If the hospital does not yet have any such PHC outreach, then an outside posting to an approved community health service should be arranged.

The log book
A clinical practice record book, or 'log book', has to be maintained by the Registrar. This will be provided by the Faculty, or the General Practice Supervisor/Medical Superintendent may have a local stock from which it can be supplied.

The book sets out the curriculum of types of cases to be managed, or operations performed, with room to insert the hospital number of cases for which the Registrar has been responsible. The log book should be in constant use, and so far as possible, kept up to date day by day, and not filled in ling after the event. It does not matter if the book comes to look worn in the process. As the Registrar fills up a section of similar cases he will bring his log book to the Supervisor, or departmental consultant to be 'signed up'. The Supervisor should do so if sufficient cases have been dealt with, and he is reasonable confident that adequate competence has been achieved. A spot check of particular hospital records, according to the hospital numbers entered, may be called for if felt necessary.

The Supervisor should examine the Log Book occasionally to see where there are still gaps, and should advise the Registrar on what can be done to fill them. It is recognised by the Faculty that diseases have different prevalence in the various parts of the country, so the Registrar will not be penalised if he does not see everything. The log book is, however, a valuable guide.

Study time
The Registrar will need time to keep his log book up to date, and to read his text-books and journals, and any duplicated materials sent from the Faculty. He will use his off-duty time for this.

Regular clinical meetings and tutorial sessions - weekly, fortnightly or monthly - can be a great stimulus to both Registrar and senior staff. Teaching ward rounds ('grand rounds') can also be used. Attendance by the Registrar at weekend Faculty workshops, particularly when held in their area, should be encouraged. A small medical library and tutorial room in the hospital can be a valuable focal point for the training.

Examinations
Part I Finals. College exams are held in May and November, usually in Lagos, and application for entry must be completed three months in advance. Application Forms have to be accompanied by the Registrar's Completion Certificate (or evidence of posting). his Clinical Practice Record Book, and a bank–certified cheque for the entrance fee, all of which are the Registrar' responsibility. He is also advised to bring personal diagnostic instruments (stethoscope etc) for the Clinical Examination; they can be provided if he does not.

Part II Finals. This comes after the Part II posting, at the end of the minimum period of four years for the whole residency training. On receipt of the Fellowship in General Medical Practice (FMCGP) the doctor is accorded similar status to other doctors who have done a specialty training, such as surgery or obs/gynae, in a teaching hospital.

The specialist general practitioner
The doctor who completes his four-year training, and achieves his FMCGP, is then well equipped for work in a secondary care general hospital, where he can serve as Senior Registrar I (SMO I) for one year, and then as Consultant GP, or PMO.

He will also be well equipped for work in primary care, e.g. as a doctor in charge of a district hospital or comprehensive health centre, or medical consultant for a rural medical service.

He is also free to set up in practice on his own, covering primary and secondary care, according to his facilities. He should be able to set high standards of care.

A voluntary agency hospital will find such a doctor is ideally prepared with clinical and administrative skills for a post of senior Medical Officer or Medical Superintendent.

In helping to train this cadre of doctors a training hospital is providing an invaluable service to Nigeria. The Faculty extends its thanks to the proprietors and the Medical Superintendent, General Practice Supervisor, and all involved in the training process.

The Faculty of General Medical Practice, and the National Postgraduate Medical College of Nigeria, will be pleased to help accredited hospitals in every way open to them.

Specimen rotations

Mkar Hospital, Benue State

Paediatrics	4 months
Medicine/mental health	5 months
Radiology	Every morning at daily X-ray reviewing sessions (all doctors)
Surgery (including sub-specialties)	6 months
Obs/gynae	6 months
General practice/community health	3 days every 2 months, visiting 2 dispensaries per day, spread over the 2-year period
Ophthalmology/ENT (alternate days)	1 month, sandwiched between other postings. (This will usually be an outside posting at a teaching hospital)

Eku Hospital, Bendel state

General practice/community health ⎫ Internal medicine ⎪ Obs/gynae ⎬ Paediatrics ⎪ Surgery ⎭	Five 2-month blocks each year, i.e. 20 months
Elective, to include minor postings	4 months
Clinic work in OPD	Registrars will be allocated a panel of patients for whom they will provide comprehensive and continuing care throughout the 2-year period.

Guidelines for trainers, FMCGP Part II (for centres not also doing Part I)

Introduction

We thank you for your interest in the FMCGP training programme. The Faculty believes your contribution could be important in the development of postgraduate medical education for high standards of general practice in Nigeria. We would like to share with you the aims and objectives of the programme and suggest various ways in which the trainer can best help to fulfil these objectives.

The kind of doctor we want to produce

The objectives of the FMCGP programme are set out in the first page of the Faculty guidelines, or 'Green Book'. This states:

'The aim is to provide an advanced vocational training for the doctor who wishes to follow a career in general practice, whether in clinic, or comprehensive health centre, or as a general medical officer in a small hospital. He will be a front-line medical practitioner'.

A more detailed description of the kind of doctor we want to produce then follows.

After passing a primary in basic sciences, the GP registrar first enters a Part I training hospital for two years, during which time he gains a high degree of competence in a broad field of medicine, surgery, obs/gynae, paediatrics etc, so that he is able to cope with a large proportion of cases presenting in an undifferentiated general practice clinic, and provide the necessary care, whether through medical treatment, operation, obstetric care or health education counselling. He is also taught to recognise those points at which cases should be referred for specialist help in a tertiary care centre. The log book, which he maintains through his two years of Part I, is evidence of the wide range of work which has been done.

The nature of Part II training
The GP Registrar now comes to Part II of his training. What are the particular areas of knowledge, and the attitudes and skills, which he still needs to acquire? In what way can the Trainer best contribute to this process? Let us consider what more the Registrar can learn.

1. *Knowledge.* Learning is a lifelong process, and even clinical knowledge gained during undergraduate training, internship and Youth Corps service, is still far from complete. The long experience of the trainer is a priceless asset, and if he works alongside the Registrar he will often have opportunities to pass on tips in diagnosis and management. The process may well be two-way. The more recently graduated doctor will have some advantages in terms of knowledge obtained from research, or new approaches to therapy, and the trainer can learn from his trainee, if he so minded. The stimulus of the learning process is mutually beneficial.

2. *Attitudes.* It is here that the trainer can have great influence. In the larger hospitals it is all too common for the care to be impersonal, and with little regard for the patient's family and the local community. If the trainer knows is local community well, and gives good personal care to his patients, taking into account their economic background, cultural factors, and stresses in family relationships, or their fears of 'outside influences', then the trainee will begin to adopt similar attitudes. Every patient wants a doctor who will take a special interest in him, or in whom he feels he can place his trust. This is the essence of general practice/family medicine.

3. *Skills.* There will still be many operations or procedures in the Part I syllabus where the Trainee was not fortunate to see sufficient cases during his two years. Some conditions only come up once or twice a year (e.g. dislocation of the jaw) yet the GP should be skilled in their care. Such learning of skills should continue through the Part II training.

   In addition, the skills involved in running a hospital – administration, finance, drug-ordering, staff management etc– are all areas in which the trainer should try to involve the trainee, to help him to gain some ability as a medical administrator.

The dissertation and case–book
In addition to continuing his practical in-service training, the Registrar also has to produce two books, a dissertation and a case-book. The dissertation has to be written on a subject approved by the Faculty, and considered to be of importance to the discipline of general practice in Nigeria. It also needs to be chosen in consultation with the trainer/medical director, since it must be possible to do the research within the limits of time and facilities available at the Part II centre. Additional consultant advisers from the nearest teaching hospital can generally be found to help. The title of the dissertation, and the name of the trainer, and one consultant adviser, should be registered with the Faculty. Letters of consent to supervise the project should also be obtained from the trainer and consultant.

The case–book is a series of case histories collected throughout the Part II posting. They should have all been handled by the Registrar himself, and should cover all aspects of general practice.

Characteristics of a Part II Centre
Accreditation for Part II FMCGP training has to be obtained separately from approval for Part I training. The two features which the Faculty looks for above all others are, firstly, a good Trainer, and secondly an emphasis on primary care, and what one may call 'a general practice approach'.

1. *The trainer.* The trainer will normally be the Medical Director of the hospital or health service programme. In most cases he/she will be a Fellow of the Faculty in General Medical Practice, but fellows of other faculties of the Nigerian College, or of colleges of general Practice of

other countries, and senior doctors of undoubted experience gained over many years of practice, are warmly welcomed as trainers too. The vital thing is that they should be committed to the FMCGP programme, seeing it as an important contribution to improving primary/secondary care medical services in the country. They should themselves be actively involved in day to day medical care, and prepared to have the trainee working alongside, with mutual interchange and sharing of ideas. Every effort should be make to impart:
- good consultation technique,
- sound clinical judgement,
- appropriate prescribing,
- legible and efficient record-keeping, allowing good continuity of care,
- insight into cultural and psycho-social factors, and the need for counselling,
- desire to encourage behavioural changes which will lead to prevention of disease; and to community action to improve the environment,
- a compassionate approach to the poor, those with chronic disease or disability, and to patients in need of terminal care.

2. *Primary care emphasis.* General practice in Nigeria spans both primary care and secondary care. During Part I, the training programme of FMCGP puts more emphasis on hospital-based secondary care, with just two months or so of primary care, During Part II this should, so far as possible, be the other way round, with more emphasis placed on the general practitioner's role in primary care. This will, of course, vary in different situations, and the Faculty recognises the need for flexibility. Primary care in a city clinic or health centre often depends solely on physicians. Primary care in a rural health service is provided mainly by the non–physicians of the primary health care team, with only occasional supervisory visits from a medical officer as a 'consultant generalist' in a supportive role. Between the two extremes are the rural hospitals where nurses and assistants treat or screen many patients, but where doctors play the major role, and provide primary and secondary care side by side. This is the common situation in the smaller district hospitals, whether government or voluntary agency. Can we distinguish a 'general practice approach' in each of these situations?

3. *The 'general practice approach'*
In a private hospital
Some hospitals are frankly specialist in orientation, and run on departmentalised lines as far as possible. It is not easy for such hospitals to accommodate FMCGP training at the Part II stage. The general practitioner in the set-up is usually the junior doctor sorting out cases for his consultant superiors.

However, some hospitals, though headed by a surgeon, or a physician, or some other specialist, are genuinely general practice orientated. Doctors on call take whatever comes, and clinics are not rigidly compartmentalised. It should be possible in such hospitals for a GP registrar on duty to admit, and provide continuing care for any patients, whatever the condition. If emergency surgery is required, for example, and the operation is within his competence (as attested by his Part I FMCGP), then he should be expected to go ahead. If there is a colleague on the staff with a surgical specialist qualification, he should act as 'consultant adviser' to the GP registrar, but not necessarily alter all the post-operative treatments ordered, and take over the case on the rounds next day. This would be one way of emphasising the 'general practice approach'.

In a rural health service
Here the doctor may be partly mobile, touring to a number of village centres manned by non–physician staff. In each situation he needs to see referred cases on arrival, teach the PHC staff to extend their knowledge and skills, check on administrative matter, drug supplies etc, and be a true friend and adviser to those working often in very isolated situations. This is the only form of general practice which most patients in remote rural places are ever likely to receive, and the Faculty sees it as part of its responsibility.

A Registrar on this type of Part II posting, may, with advantage, be allowed to live at a base hospital, taking his share of emergency call, and thus keeping up his secondary care skills too.

Completion
When a doctor has satisfactorily completed his minimum period of two years in a Part II centre he can have his Part II completion certificate signed and sent to the Faculty for endorsement. He will then be eligible to sit the Part II final examination, and may be released from employment in the Part II centre at a time mutually convenient.

The Faculty requests Medical Directors not to offer permanent employment to a Part II trainee on the staff unless a vacancy for another trainee can be declared open. Only in this way can we maintain the desired number of approved Part II centres.

Appendix 7

Ethics and religion

Christian ethics in medical practice

Introduction
Medical practice demands more from the doctor than the accumulated knowledge and technical skills handed down from the past. One who is a Christian will wish to be guided, in his personal relations and attitude to work by the ethical teaching of Christ as recorded in the Bible. Central in this stands His unequivocal and far-reaching summary of the moral law:

> 'Love the Lord your God with all your heart, with all your soul, with all your mind and with all your strength . . . and love your neighbour as yourself' Mark 12, 30–31.

Some implications of this principle for the doctor are outlined in the following affirmation. No Christian, however, can hope to meet such a standard except on the basis of his redemption and reconciliation to God in Christ, and by the power of the Holy Spirit in his daily life.

Christ further taught His disciples: 'I am come that they may have life, and have it more fully'. 'It is more blessed to give than to receive'. 'Freely you have received, freely give'. We are accountable to God in all we do and, therefore, we shall endeavour to conduct our private and professional lives in accordance with the standards of Christ.

In relation to human life
1. To acknowledge that God is the Creator, the Sustainer and the Lord of all life.
2. To recognise that man is unique, being made in the 'image of God' and that he cannot be healthy in body and mind unless he lives in harmony with the natural world around him, which he neither ignores nor exploits.
3. To promote a sense of vocation in the work by which men serve one another, and to honour and recommend the Creator's rule of one day's rest in seven.
4. To maintain the deepest respect for individual human life from its beginning to its end, including the unborn, the helpless, the handicapped and those advanced in years.
5. To uphold marriage as a lasting bond, being the divinely appointed means for the care of children, the security of the family and the stability of society.
6. To recognise that sexual intercourse is intended by God only for the marriage relationship and, hence to advocate premarital continence and marital fidelity.

In relation to patients
1. To give effective service to those seeking our medical care irrespective of age, race, creed, politics, social status or the circumstances which may have contributed to their illness.
2. To serve each patient according to his need, subordinating personal gain to the interest of the patient and declining to take part in collective action which would harm him.
3. To respect the privacy, opinions and personal feelings of the patients and to safeguard hid confidences.
4. To speak truth to the patient, as he is able to accept it, bearing in mind our own fallibility.

5. To do no harm to the patient, using only those drugs and procedures which we believe will be of benefit to him.
6. To maintain as a principle that the doctor's first duty is to his patient whilst fully accepting our duty to promote preventive medicine and public health.

In relation to colleagues
1. To deal honestly with our professional and administrative colleagues and to fulfil those just requirements of the state which do not conflict with these basic ethical standards.
2. To work constructively with colleagues in scientific research and in training doctors, nurses and paramedical workers, for the benefit of individual patients and the advance of health care throughout the world.

Other religions

In the late nineteenth and twentieth centuries many members of the world's great religions have been trained in western medicine. In recent times their numbers practising in English-speaking countries has greatly increased. Some of the religions of Asia have medical traditions stretching far into the past. There were certain codes, appropriate to the prevailing religion such as The Oaths of the Hindu Physicians (taken from the 'Susruta'), the Chinese code from 'The Canon of Medicine' (early Han dynasty 200BC-AD200), and 'The Five Commandments of Chen Shih-Kung' (early 17th century).

Reference to the literature of India, China and Islamic countries no doubt shows similar developments, influenced by the respective religions, professional and cultural outlook of the various peoples.

(Prepared by the Christian Medical Fellowship, UK.)

Appendix 8

Guidelines for 'front-line parents'

by Mrs J M Pearson

Education begins at birth

How you start is so important – so, first, a few thoughts on that.

As parents – together – make your own family rules; then keep them, and be sure the nurse-maid can keep them too.

'Let your yea be yea, and your nay be nay'. Never give an order unless you are prepared to see it is carried out.

You can often avoid confrontation, quarrels and boredom, by suggesting a diversion.

Avoid confrontation
You say, 'Don't!'. He says, 'I want to!' Avoid a battle by diverting his attention to something else.

You demand 'Come!' or 'Do!', and he says 'I won't!'. Only demand if obedience is important; otherwise say, 'Who will help?', or some other form of question. That is to say, ask in a way that the child will be happy to obey; then praise the one who helps.

Avoid quarrels
You can prevent them before they happen if your ears are tuned to the changing decibels of sound, by suggesting a diversion.

Avoid boredom
Catch them before they get into trouble. So much so-called 'wrong-doing' is because of surplus energy, natural curiosity, or lack of stimulus. Knowing your child helps – whether he needs physical activity to 'let off steam', or mental activity to engage his mind.

Make time to know and understand your children, so that they feel secure and loved within the family, yet have freedom to grow and develop. You will reap the rewards of continuing friendship and affection.

How to help your child at home
Pre-school education indicates the learning process in the years before proper school. It does not mean either that such education should be at school, or that it should be like school, with desks and formal education.

As stated by the United Nations Children's Fund:

> 'The vital stage in a child's development is from birth till the age of two, during which time he needs proper stimulation by techniques within the scope of parent or child care worker . . .

Stimulation is necessary ... up to the age of six, when formal education begins ...

'The mother is indispensable in the early months, and the father, as well as the rest of the family, must be increasingly involved.'

Unicef News 1981

Talk with your child – in the car, or at home, or wherever. Encourage observation and speech, recognition of colour, sounds, textures, smells, tastes, counting. Do not treat him as if he is not there.

Use pictures and stories. Encourage concentration for short periods when reading stories. Act or draw a picture afterwards. Let the child talk about pictures in books. Encourage him to chatter and make up stories, whether in English or the vernacular. You will want him to be fluent in both. Remember that 5 minutes concentration is enough. Then let them play.

T.V. Do not leave it on as a background noise. Watch definite programmes, and discuss them with the child.

Counting can be fun. How many spoons or plates? How many people in the room? Sharing or dividing can be learned naturally too. For example: There are 6 sweets to share between 3 children. How many each? They will give you the answer!

Practical hints on saving time for busy parents

Eating habits. Always insist on the following four points.

1. Having proper food at regular intervals. No food in between to take the edge off the appetite. No bribery with bits of bread!
2. Washing hands before eating.
3. Eating food sitting down only; no wandering around during meals.
4. Washing hands afterwards too – as soon as the child leaves the table.

Points 3 and 4 will save having to clear up bits of food dropped around the house, and having to wipe sticky furniture. It will keep always ants and cockroaches too. Visiting children will soon learn to copy the habits of the host family.

Tidiness with possessions; some practical suggestions
1. Have a box or cupboard for toys. Remember that toys, to a child, are not just the big or expensive items that have been bought, but small bricks, empty cotton reels, the 'treasures' collected by a child which are important to him. With imagination he can make things with them. Older children may graduate to a lockable cupboard or box, so that younger ones cannot break up special things, or models under construction.

2. Clearing up should be done by the child – but give him 5 minutes warning when possible. He may be immersed in a game of make-believe, or problem solving, and does not like to be disturbed, any more than you do. Quiet play on his own is an important part of a child's development – often referred to as his 'quiet growing time'.

3. Establish rules about biro or crayon or clay, so you do not find clay in the carpet, and biro over the walls.

For example
- Crayons and biro – always on paper. Encourage scribbling and free expression. This is important in learning control. Do not laugh at his work. Praise, and let him tell you what he has drawn.

- Chalks – always on a blackboard. See that there is one available, and a tin to keep chalks in.
- Plasticine or clay – always on a plain wood board. See that there is a board kept for the purpose, and a tin for storing material.
- Paint – preferably on big sheets of paper. Use up plain sides of used foolscap, computer paper or even cement bags. Again, encourage free expression. If you want children to paint only in a veranda area, or wherever, make your rule and stick to it.

These are simple rules – and you may think of others. They do save time for busy parents. If you have in mind appropriate diversions in case of need, you can keep children happily occupied on their own, while still busy yourself with other duties about the house. You do not have to be with the children all the time.

Once the family has its rules, visiting children usually fit in. When your own children say 'We do this in our house', it is much more effective than when told by the grown-ups. These things do work if all the family members agree and keep the rules, and parents remember to praise the children when praise is due.

A true story.
A nursery teacher was in a busy Lagos market, and noticed a mother trying to force medicine down a screaming child's mouth. The teacher sat on a stool, called the child over quietly, and asked the mother for the medicine.
'He always screams' she said,
The teacher talked quietly; the child took the medicine, and was handed back to the mother. She was silent.
"There is something you have forgotten,' said the teacher. 'He has obeyed you, and taken the medicine. You must now praise him.'
The mother did, and was rewarded with a wonderful smile from the boy.

Letter from a Nigerian mother, a doctor's wife in a rural area
'It is a pleasure to share my experiences with "Junior" with some other mothers.

The best thing is to have mother at home all the time, but this seems impossible, at least in present day Nigeria, so a mother should try to be home when the child needs her most; e.g. feeding times, bathing time and few hours for playtime. This is important for the mother/child relationship.
- Give all the love when you are there, but do not pamper the child.
- Watch what you say or do, because the baby may not be able to talk, but he understands your movements and things uttered.
- Encourage early learning – academic or play. Children do assimilate what you tell them at this stage.
- Do not give a child of two, for example, everything he asks for, even if you can afford it.
- Encourage mixing with other children in the neighbourhood, whether of lower, same or higher class. This helps the child to see things in their true perspective.
- Teach and encourage independence as much as possible, so that when mother is not there, the child can manage on his own.
- Children are very inquisitive, so be ready to answer questions – and correctly too!
- Greatest of all, teach a child to be God-fearing, be you a Christian, Muslim or a traditionalist.

To Parents – from their Children. Ten Don'ts.
1. Don't spoil me. I know quite well that I ought not to have all I ask for. I'm only testing you.
2. Don't be afraid to be firm with me. I prefer it. It makes me feel more secure.
3. Don't let me form bad habits. I have to rely on you to detect them in the early stages.
4. Don't correct me in front of other people if you can help it. I'll take much more notice if you talk quietly with me in private.
5. Don't make rash promises. Remember I feel badly let down when promises are broken.

6. Don't tax my honesty too much. I am easily frightened into telling lies.
7. Don't tell me my fears are silly. They are terribly real and you can do much to reassure me if you try to understand.
8. Don't ever think it is beneath your dignity to apologize to me. An honest apology makes me feel surprisingly warm toward you.
9. Don't forget I love experimenting. I couldn't get on without it, so please put up with it.
10. Don't forget how quickly I am growing up. It must be very difficult for you to keep pace with me, but please try!

E Mildred Nevill

Organizations which can help
Organization Mondiale pour l'Education Prescholaire (OMEP) has offices in Canada and the UK, and in various African cities. The UK address is:
   Ms Tricia David, Chairman OMEP (UK), Dept of Education, Westwood, University of Warwick, Coventry, UK. (Tel: (0)1203 523523; ext 2832).

It's aims are:
- to use every possible means to promote for each child the optimum conditions for his well-being, development and happiness in his family, and society.
- to promote education of parents and guardians as regards their responsibilities to children.
- to encourage the production of suitable toys, books and other educational materials for children.

The Pre–school Play groups Association (PPA) produces a useful series of play-based books for introducing the beginnings of maths, science etc to the under-fives. A full list can be obtained from:
   PPA, 61-63 Kings Cross Road, London WC1X 9LL, UK. (Tel (0)171 8330991)

Worldwide Education Service, (formerly PNEU) can help mothers to provide home-based primary schooling for their own children through supervised distance learning by correspondence. Address for enquiries:
   Ms Christine Stephenson, Worldwide Education Service, Home School, 35 Belgrave Square, London SW1X 8QB, UK. (Tel: (0)171 232880. Fax: (0)171 2595234)

Further reading
Baby and Child: from birth to age five, Penelope Leach. Penguin Books, UK, 1979.

Just Playing?: the role and status of play in early childhood education, Janet R Moyles, Open University Press, Milton Keynes, UK, 1989.

Time to Play in Early Childhood Education, Tina Bruce, Hodder and Stoughton, London 1991.

Working with the Under 5's, an in-service training pack. Open University, Milton Keynes, UK, 1991.

Under Five – under educated? by Tricia David. Open University Press, Milton Keynes, UK, 1990.

What Children Learn in Play-groups: PPA Guide to the Curriculum. Pre-school Play-groups Association, London, 1991.

Appendix 9

Specimen short essay type questions on medical administration

(. . . as might be used in the finals examination of the FMCGP, National Postgraduate Medical College of Nigeria, or other similar exam.)

1. Name by office three staff members in a secondary-care hospital whom you consider should form the basic leadership team. List their main duties.

2. You are a government doctor in a district hospital 100km from the capital city. A storm causes substantial damage to the roof of a ward. Enumerate briefly the steps to be taken to get it repaired.

3. What is an 'imprest account'? Briefly describe two situations in a hospital, firstly where such an account works well, and secondly where it results mainly in frustration.

4. Give four essential clauses you would include in a letter of appointment for a member of hospital staff. Explain each briefly.

5. Give three criteria by which a system of medical records may be evaluated. Describe their application briefly.

6. A 100-bed hospital can only afford to run a 10kva stand-by generator for emergency power. What policies in the use of electricity should the hospital have for:
   a. theatre lighting
   b. sterilising of equipment
   c. air conditioning
   d. cooking stoves in staff residences on the compound.

7. What is a septic tank? Draw a diagram and describe how it works. Name two things which may stop it working.

8. If a child has to be admitted to a children's ward, what provision should the hospital make for the mother, or other relative who comes with the child? Give reasons.

9. Describe briefly an 'essential drugs list'.

10. A medical student from a distant university applies to come for an 'elective period' to gain experience. How should the application be handled?

11. What do you understand by a village health worker? List six important items of health care which they can be taught to do.

12. List three common domestic or family difficulties a doctor may face if he serves in a rural hospital. Suggest ways in which he/she might overcome one of them.

Model answers to the questions

Short essay questions require brief, concise answers of 250 to 500 words only (one to two sides). These model answers are written in note form, identifying the key words an examiner may look for.

1. Medical superintendent, matron and hospital secretary – all equivalent titles acceptable.
   - *Med supt.* Usually designated the Executive head of hospital, responsible to the board. Official correspondent. Care of patients. Medical and technical staff. Legal affairs. Other functions as assigned by board.
   - *Matron.* Head of nursing service. Official correspondent for nursing matters. Discipline and care of nurses, and nursing students when in the hospital; also nursing auxiliaries and maids. Cleanliness of the hospital. Nursing supplies.
   - *Hospital secretary.* General and financial administration of the hospital. Annual statements and budget. Clerical and labour staff. Maintenance of the buildings and equipment. Supporting services In some situations the matron or hospital secretary may be the executive head, not the senior doctor.

2. A government doctor must act within civil service system. Usually no maintenance workers on the staff. So personally review the damage. Use initiative for interim protection. Send off report to the Board or Ministry in the capital. Await repair team. Move patients meanwhile. Alternatively, if authorised, call local contractors to make estimates. When one accepted, send for AIE. Sign completion certificate for contractor when work done so that he can collect payment from capital.

   Alternative systems, that are within other government procedural guidelines, also acceptable by the examiners.

3. Imprest account: money given in advance for minor expenditure; i.e. on loan, to be accounted for.
   - Works well when the advance is given from accountant to spending officer in the same institution. Advanced one day, accounted for same evening.
   - Causes frustration when advance given to spending officer working in a distant hospital. Little relation to actual needs. Unable to account for it till a month later. Usually overspent because of unexpected needs. Expenditure covered personally may exceed the next imprest given, i.e. spent before received.

4. Letter of appointment – state any four clauses from among:
   - Title of post and main duties, and hours.
   - Salary at start, increments, fringe benefits.
   - Length of appointment in first place, and means of extending it.
   - Probation period if any. Explain reason for this.
   - Annual leave and any allowances. Why necessary.
   - Pension or retirement gratuity, if included. Possible problems.
   - Means for terminating the appointment from either side. Natural rights, even of someone who has misbehaved. Must have notice, or cash to live on pro tem.

5. Three criteria for good medical records:
   - Economical and within hospital budget to maintain.
   - Concise but clear and not too bulky for easy filing.
   - Easily retrievable from file when patients return.

   Records are required in large quantities; use local printers, relatively cheap materials. Reorder well in advance before supplies are used up.

   Storage of large bulky records requires much space; keep cards small, encourage doctors to write neatly and with a small hand; only one tenth admitted so file in-patient charts separately. No need of bulky folders for every case.

Check retrievability, speed of finding OP cards, IP case sheets. Danger of losing continuity of care if new cards issued too easily when the old cannot be traced.

6. Emergency power supply is reasonable, but with little margin, so use following policies:
   a. theatre lighting, priority at all times; shadowless lamp, or multiple fluorescent tubes; emergency lighting also from batteries,
   b. sterilising; electric power convenient and clean, but expensive. May have to consider gas, if replacement cylinders no problem, kerosene pressure stoves or steam from firewood fuelled boilers.
   c. limit air-conditioning to theatre, X-ray or pharmacy stores, where essential. Improve ventilation and cooling of other rooms by fans, ceiling level vents or asbestos roofs, where possible.
   d. forbid cooking by electricity, except for electric kettle. Allow gas kerosene stoves, if cooking inside; or firewood if cooking outside.

7. Clear drawing of septic tank. Labelling to include: inspection chambers, outlet 4 inches lower than inlet, baffle, sloping floor, covers approx sizes; also soakaway pit or trench for effluent.

   Works by bacterial biodegradation of faeces in wet environment. Effluent safe, nearly odour free. Sludge needs to be removed every few years.

   Function may be spoiled by excessive water taps left running in to it; disinfectants, such as lysol, which destroy the bacteria in tank; too many users, tank full.

8. Mother should be allowed to come into hospital with child; assists in nursing, feeding; provides warmth and security.

   May have adult beds, for mother and child together; or mothers bring sleeping mats to put beside child's cot at night. Mother's shelter nearby the ward for daytime rest and food preparation.

   If mother not allowed, child suffers maternal deprivation syndrome. Long-term consequences for child. Opportunity for health and nutrition education of the mother missed.

9. Cost of pharmaceuticals very high. Need to economise and be sure essential drugs are available at a reasonable price. May be dealt with at national level, or at hospital level. An essential drugs list will:
   - avoid duplication of similar drugs; decide on one in each drug group
   - avoid excessively priced drugs; or use only under strict control
   - order drugs by generic name, where possible
   - exclude drugs with known dangerous toxic effects
   - exclude drugs of limited or no value; also all fake drugs.

   The essential drugs list should include a hospital policy for antibiotics, and their rational use; also a policy for antiseptics and disinfectants.

10. Application should be welcomed. Medical electives can be a stimulus to good care. They learn much, but also bring new ideas from medical school.

    Write back, give background information on the hospital or health service; state who will supervise; give details of how to get to the hospital, accommodation arrangements. If from overseas, hints on personal health care, and costs. Visa requirements etc. Arrange transport from main airport or city.

If many applications, prepare a descriptive leaflet which can be sent to all applicants.

11. Village health worker, not a full-time professional. A mature person, male or female, resident in the village, supported partly from own work, and partly by the community for services rendered. Village health committee.

    List of services will depend on what are the local felt needs. The six are likely to be from this list:
    - Malaria treatment, and suppression.
    - Care of mothers during pregnancy.
    - Knowledge of breast feeding and child nutrition.
    - Diarrhoea oral rehydration therapy.
    - First aid for wounds and burns, and simple fractures.
    - Family planning methods
    - Local endemic diseases, e.g schistosomiasis, guinea-worm, onchocerciasis, hookworm etc.
    - Safe drinking water, safe latrines.

12. Difficulties in rural medical service may include:
    - Lack of facilities in the home – water, light, furnishings etc.
    - Lack of work for wife
    - Lack of educational facilities for the family.
    - Distance from major urban centres for shopping, entertainment etc. Problem of roads, vehicles for transport,

    Facilities at home can be dealt with; ingenuity essential; e.g. collection of rain water, digging of wells, reserve water tanks; small generator for light; pressure gas lamps. Solar power for lamps and pumps in the future.

    Wife can perhaps assist in hospital, according to her skills.

    To overcome the lack of good school facilities, parents can learn to supplement their child's education, with books, educational toys, and spending time with the children themselves.

REFERENCES

1. A Wilmott. *God's way to successful management.* SIM, Jos.
2. S Srinivasan (Ed). *Management process in health care.* Voluntary Health Association of India, New Delhi, 1982
3. R hoffenberg. *Clinical freedom.* Nuffield Provincial Hospitals Trust, London. Quoted, *Lancet* 1987; **ii**: 1511
4. R Amonoo–Lartson *et al. District Health Care:* challenges for planning, organisation and evaluation in developing countries. Macmillan/ELBS, London, 1985.
5. M Jancloes *et al.* Financing urban primary health services: balancing community and government financial responsibilities; Pikine, Senegal 1975-81. *Tropical Doctor* 1985; **15**: 98–104.
6. Conference of Missionary Societies. *A model health centre,* 1975 (out of print). For an alternative, see *Design for Medical Buildings.* AMREF, P.O. Box 30125, Nairobi, Kenya.
7. J Elford. *How to look after a refrigerator.* TALC, St Albans, U.K
8. M King. *Medical care in developing countries.* OUP, London, 1966.
9. A Derrick. Photo-voltaic refrigerators and lighting systems for medical use. *Africa Health,* 1987; **9**: 9–11. Also see articles by Derrick and others in *Africa Health* 1988; 10: 5 and 1988; **11**: 4. And the book *Solar photovoltaic products.* IT publications, London 1989.
10. M J Burke *et al.* Sphygmomanometers in hospital and family practice. *Brit. Med J* 1982; **285**: 469–471.
11. G D Jacobs and S A Sayer. *Road accidents in developing countries.* Transport and Road Research Laboratory, Crowthorne, Berks, UK, 1983, Supplementary Report 807.
12. R. Feacham, S Cairncross. *Environmental Health Engineering in the Tropics.* Wiley International, UK, 1993.
13. Morgan P. *Rural Water Supplies and Sanitation.* Macmillan, London. 1990.
14. D C Morley. *Paediatric priorities in the developing world.* TALC, St Albans, UK, 1973.
15. G A J Aycliffe *et al. Chemical disinfection in hospitals.* Public Health Laboratory Service, UK, 1984.
16. S Athey. WGH Ilesha Hospital Report, 1974–75, Ilesha, Nigeria.
17. Solvik N. A drug delivery system for small hospitals. *Tropical Doctor,* 1990; **20**: 139–140.
18. M King (Ed). *Primary Anaesthesia.* OUP, London 1986 (and from TALC).
19. R Jeyarajah *et al.* Intermittent peritoneal dialysis. *Tropical Doctor* 1986; **16**: 13–17.
20. H Hogerzeil and M Hofs. Essential reagents for rural hospitals in Ghana. *Tropical Doctor* 1986; **16**: 58–60.
21. M Cheesbrough. *Medical laboratory manual for developing countries,* Vols I and II. Tropical.

Health Technology, Cambridge PE15 0TT, UK, 1990.

22. M King. *A medical laboratory for developing countries.* OUP, London, 1973.

23. E Topley. A community laboratory service as part of health care; in *Principles and Practice of community health in Africa.* (Eds) G O Sofoluwe and F S Bennett, 437–456. University Press Ltd, Ibadan, Nigeria 1985.

24. Wannan GJ et al, How many bloods will a HIVCHECK check? *Tropical Doctor* 1992, **22**: 151–154.

25. W de Rhoter. Radiology in a rural hospital, *Tropical Doctor* 1985; **15**: 29–31.

26. W de Rhoter. Quality improvement of radiographs. *Tropical Doctor* 1985; **15**: 72–82.

27. P E S Palmer et al. *Manual of radiographic interpretation for general practitioners.* WHO, Geneva, 1985.

28. World Health Organization. *The future use of new imaging technologies in developing countries.* Technical Report Series 723, Geneva, 1985.

29. D Werner. *Where there is no doctor* (Africa edition). Macmillan, London 1993.

30. AHRTAG. *Community Based Rehabilitation (CBR) News.* Appropriate Health Resources Action Group, 1 London Bridge St, London, SE1 9SG, UK.

31. G. Williams. *From fear to hope.* AIDS care and prevention at Chikankata hospital, Zambia. Strategies for hope. No 1. Action Aid/World in Need, 1990.

32. W H Foege. *Community medicine.* Protestant Christian Medical Association, Nairobi, Kenya 1970.

33. D Werner and B Bower. *Helping health workers learn.* Hesperian Foundation California, USA, 1982 (and from TALC).

34. D C Morley and M Woodland. *See how they grow.* Macmillan, London 1987.

35. World Health Organisation. *The Hospital in Rural and Urban Districts.* WHO Technical Report 819, 1992, Geneva.

36. D C Morley. *Some steps through which hospitals may become more deeply involved in community health care.* Contact 20, Christian Medical Commission, Geneva, 1974.

37. E H Paterson. *The Kwun Tong community health project.* Contact 28, CMC, Geneva, 1977.

38. World Health Organisation. *On being in charge.* WHO, Geneva, 1980.

39. World Health Organisation. *Health manpower requirements for the achievement of health for all by the year 2000 through primary health care.* Technical Report Series 717, WHO, Geneva, 1985.

40. Royal College of Physicians, London. *A great and growing evil: the medical consequences of alcohol abuse.* Tavistock Publications, London, 1987.

41. Uma Ram Nath. *Smoking: third world alert.* OUP, London, 1987.

42. Platt A and Carter N. *Making Health–care Equipment.* Intermediate Technology Publications, 103–5, Southampton Row, London WC1B 4HH, UK. 1990.

43. Awojobi OA, The hospital water still. *Tropical Doctor,* 1993; **23**: 173–174.

44. Poeschl U. Emergency autologous blood transfusion. *Update in Anaesthesia* 1992; **2**: 1–3.

INDEX

Accommodation *see* Staff housing
Account book ledger, 40, 41, 43, 45, 46
Accountant, role of, 35–38, 46
Accounting, leadership team, 30
Accounting practices, open, 26, 27
   audit, 46
   centralised, 28, 47
   closing the accounts, 41
   computerisation, 32, 34, 45
   for local government health service, 50
   'fudging', 27, 29
   in primary cealth care, 47–50
   private practice, 27, 30
   public accounting, 27
   ruling off, 36
   self-accounting, 29, 30, 31, 47, 50
   accounting systems, basic requirements, 30
   software, 34
Accumulated fund, 43
Administration, place of doctor, 2
   by physician, 6
   non-medical, 5
Voluntary agency, 17
Administrative meetings,
   departmental, 62
   training, 8

Administrator, hospital, 4, 5, 9,
   medical, qualities of, 6
   organisation of time, 7
Admission book *see* Medical records, in-patient register
Advertising job vacancies, 51, 52
Agenda, 21, 23
AIDS *see* HIV
AIE *see* Authority to incur expenditure
Air conditioning, 101
   see also Ventilation
Air vents, 147, 148
Almoner, 40
Aluminium, roofing material, 146
Ambu suction pump, 101, 111
Analysis book, 34 47. 48
Antibiotics, hospital policy on, 176
Aqua-privies *see* Sanitation
Artesian bore hole, 95
Artificial limbs, in-house manufacture, 194
Artisans *see* Hospital staff, labouring
Asbestos roofing material, 145–150
Assessment officer, 39, 40
Assets, 43–45
Audio-typing, 202
Auditor, role of, 45, 46
Auroscope/ophthalmoscope, maintenance of, 109
Australia, Faculty of Rural Medicine, 211
Authority to Incur Expenditure (AIE), 11, 13, 28, 31

Balance sheet, 43–46
Bank account, 26, 31, 45
   balance, 36,
   statements, 31, 36
   transactions, 36
Blockwork, open, disadvantages of, 148
Blood transfusion service, 187
'Blueprint' for rural health services, 233–236
Books, recommended for continuing education, 238–240
Budget, 46, 47
Building contracts, 163

Cash, book use of, 35–38, 41, 46

boxes, 32, 38
  in transit, 32
  insurance against loss, 32
  register machine, 37
  security of, 32
  transactions, 26, 32, 37
Cashier, role of, 32, 35, 37, 38
Castor wheels, maintenance of, 116
Central sterile supply department (CSSD), 188, 189
Cheque account, 31, 36, 38, 50
Chikankata Hospital, Zambia, 212
Children's wards, 168–171
Christian Health Associations,
  of Ghana, 180, 243
  of Kenya, 243
  of Nigeria, 180, 243
  of Sierra Leone, 243
Cleaning procedures, floors and walls, 113
Clinics, branch, 216
  family planning, 222, 223
  infertility, 222
  mobile, 119, 215
  under fives, 79–82
  vaccination, 223
Committees, disciplinary, 63
  management of, 21
  meetings, 21
  minutes of, 21, 24
  role of chairman, 22
  role of secretary, 21, 22,
  staff, 62
  voting procedures, 22
  work of, 21
Communication, radiophone, 122, 123
  telephone services, 121, 122
Community health,
  assistant, for under-fives clinic, 222
  co-ordinating Office (CHCO), 227
  leader, 224, 225
  officer, 4
  programmes, successful examples, 226–230
Community support groups, 214

Computer equipment, hardware, 33
  software, 33, 34
Computerisation, associated costs, 34
  for accounting purposes, 32, 45
  problems associated with, 32
  word processing, 203
Computers, training in use of, 203
Conflict situation, 62–64
Constitution, 18, 19
Contract appointments, 55
Bye-laws, 19, 20, 22, 55
  voting procedures, 19
Cooking equipment, 126, 127
Corruption, dangers of, 244
  financial, 25
Cost recovery, WHO recommendations, 15
Courier services, 121
Credit note, 40
Creditors, 39, 44
Culverts, 151
Curtains, 145

Dapsone card *see* Medical records, special clinics (leprosy) card
Dark room requirements, 191
Databases, 34
  see also Computers, equipment and Computerisation
Debtors, 39, 44
Democratic procedure, 21, 22
Departmental design *see* Floor plans
Depreciation, 45
Disciplinary procedures, 62, 63
Disinfectants, 176
Disposable equipment, 188
District health system, 237
District hospitals, WHO recommendations, 15
Doctors, personal and family well-being, 245–247
  training of, 206, 207
Drivers *see* Hospital drivers
Drugs *see* Pharmacy services
Earth leakage circuit breaker (ELCB),

153
Egbe, Nigeria (ECWA Hospital), 96
Eldon cards, 187
Electrical adapters, 155
    earthing, 153, 154
    insulation, 155
    plugs, recommended fuse rating, 154, 155
    wiring, 155
Electricity *see* Power sources
Enquiry desk/office, 121
Equipment of Charity Hospitals Overseas (ECHO), 180
Erosion, prevention of, 149
Essential drugs lists (EDL), 177
Essential reagents
Estimates (building), 163
Ethics, medical, 244, 245
Eruwa, Nigeria, 214
    water distillation plant, 112
Expenditure, 36, 38, 40, 41

Family planning clinic, 272
Fees, 11, 16, 45
    deposit, 39, 40
    rebates, 40
    reduction of in cases of hardship, 37
    single scale, 39
    unpaid, 39
    WHO recommendations, 15
Fences, perimeter, 162, 163
Finance, 11, 15, 16, 18, 25
    see also Cash, Fees
    private, 25, 45
    public, 25, 26, 32
    voluntary agencies, 30, 45
    WHO recommendations, 15
Financial resources for primary health care, 225
Fire prevention, 154
    fighting, 155
    hazard, 152, 155
    prevention, 152, 154
Firewood *see* Power sources
First aid station (FAS), 228

Floor plans, ante-natal clinic, 165–167
    delivery/maternity units, 167–168
    infants/children's wards, 168–169
    laboratory, 185
    neonatal and premature baby units, 170–171
    operating theatres, 167
    out-patient departments, 164–166
    pharmacy central stores, 181
    radiology (X-ray) department, 190
    under-five's clinic, 165–166
    waiting areas, 164
Formulary *see* Hospital formulary
Front-line doctor, aims and objectives of, 209, 210
Front-line parents, 246

Gas, bottled *see* Power sources
General Orders (GO), 11, 13,
General practice, postgraduate training in, 208, 209, 211
Generators, 102, 103
Growth charts, 79–82, 218–220
Guttering, collection of storm water, 97–99, 149, 150

Hardware, *see* Computer equipment
Health centre, 3
    education, 224, 229
    plan, 8
Herl stove, 126–127
Hippocratic oath, 244, 245
HIV, 212, 223
    counselling, 212
    testing, 187, 188
'Home-based' medical records, 70, 218
Hospital
    buildings, expansion and extension of 143–171
    orientation of, 144
    chaplains, 211
    counsellors, 211
    district, 7
    drivers, 119–120, 202
Hospital cont.

training of, 202
environment, landscaping, 59, 60
equipment, in-house manufacture of, 111–112
formulary, 175–177
library, 238–240
maintenance, 93–116
care of medical/surgical equipment, 107–109
equipment necessary, 106
painting, 114–115
preventive, 107, 116
staffing, 105, 106
structural repairs, 115
mission, 17
public service, 3
report, annual, 90, 91
role of doctor in 2
secretary, 3, 9, 10, 11, 13, 32
financial role, 46
staff, accountancy, 3, 4, 11,
training of, 203
appointment procedure, 51, 52
clerical, 3, 4,
training of, 202
committee, 62
community activities, 59
consultation meetings, 62
health, 61
housing, 56, 57
housing, furniture requirements, 56, 57–58
house inventory, 58
labourers, 3, 4, 201, 202
loans, 35, 43
stores, 174, 180, 181, 184
supplies, 173–195
support services, 117–141
vehicles, 117–119

Ice-plant hedging, 60, 149
Idere, Nigeria, 216
Igbo-Ora, Nigeria, 103
Ikole, Nigeria, 20, 49
Ilesha *see* Wesley Guild Hospital, Ilesha

Immunisation *see* Vaccination
Imprest account, 11, 28, 29
Incinerators, for waste disposal, 131
Income, 35, 40, 41
Income tax, 27
Infectious disease, notifiable, 223, 224
Infrastructure and maintenance, 93–116
Inspection chambers, 139
Intravenous fluid preparations, 183
Inventory, staff house, 58
Invertor, 33
    see also Solar power
IOU, 35
Irhuekpen, Nigeria, 49
Iron, corrugated roofing material, 145, 146, 150
Iseyin, Nigeria, 102

Job description, 55
Journals, recommended for continuing education, 238

Kaiama, Nigeria, 96, 97
Kerosene *see* Power source
Kitchen services, 123, 125–127
Kwun Tong United Christian Hospital, Hong Kong, 164, 166, 229

Laboratory services, 185
    basic equipment, 186
    essential reagents, 185, 186
    standardisation and control, 188
Laboratory staff, training of, 203, 204
Laboratory tests, request forms for, 76
Landscaping hospital grounds, 59–61
Latrines *see* Sanitation
Laundry services, 123–125
Leadership, 3, 5, 64, 65
Leadership, doctor's loss of leadership role, 5
Leadership team, 18
    basic requirements of, 3, 4, 5, 14,
Ledger *see* Account book ledger
Letter of appointment, 53

Liabilities, 43, 45
Light bulbs, 104
Lighting, 101
Lightning arrestors, 154
　conductors, 152, 153
Limited liability company, 17
Lotus software, 34

Maintenance, routine, 105–112
　castor wheels, 116
　hospital vehicles, 119
　medical equipment, 107, 108
　surgical equipment, 109, 110

Management, Government system,
　　advantages/disadvantages of, 11,
　change in, 13
　committee, hospital, 14
　district-level, 14
　government system of, 9, 10, 11
　personnel, 51
　private practice, 15, 16
　public service, 9
　structures, 9
Maternal deprivation syndrome, 168
Maternity home, 4, 7,
Matron, 3, 4, 9, 10, 20
　dealing with financial matters, 31, 38
　pharmacy supervision, 174
　responsibility for nursing discipline, 63
　supervision of kitchen services 125
　supervision of laundry services, 124
Medical associations, 242
Medical education, continuing, 238–240
Medical instruments, maintenance of, 107–109
Medical Missionaries of Mary, 5
Medical records, 67–91
　ante-natal clinic (ANC) cards, 77–79
　attendance statistics, 71
　changing the system, 68
　discharge summaries, 77, 89
　'homebased', 70, 218
　in-patient charts, 77, 84–88,
　in-patient register, 89, 90
　infant and children's clinic cards, 79–82
　maternity record cards, 78, 79
　out-patient card (retained by hospital), 74, 75, 89
　out-patient register, 70–72,
　out-patient registration card (retained by patient), 68, 72–74,
　parameters for ideal system, 67
　special clinics (TB/chest/leprosy) card, 83, 84
Medical students, training of, 206, 207
Medical Superintendent, 3, 4, 9, 20, 21,
　committee role of, 21
　dealing with financial matter, 31, 32, 38, 40, 46
　pharmacy supervision, 174, 175
　purchasing role, 173
　responsibility for disciplinary procedures, 63
Midwives, 4
　training of, 204
Milk kitchen, 127–128
Money *see* Finance
Mortuary facilities, 129–131
Mothers' shelter, 168

National health administration, 231–237
National Insurance, 55
National Provident Fund, 55
Needles, (reuse after sterilisation), 110
Nepal, 182, 211, 240
Nigeria, 6, 13, 15, 178, 199, 237, 240
　Christian Health Association of (CHAN), 243
　community health projects, 225, 232, 233
　medical training, 207–210
NKST Hospital, Nigeria, 228
Nurse-aids, training of, 204
Nurses
　enrolled, training of, 205

registered, training of, 205
Nursing
　officer, 9, 10, *see also* Matron
　staff, 3, 4
Nursing training, 4, 222
Nyankunda, Zaire, HIV testing, 187

Occupational therapy, 195
Office staff *see* Hospital staff clerical
Ogbomosho, Nigeria, 227
Operating theatre services, 188
Ophthalmoscope *see* Auroscope/
　ophthalmoscope
Overdraft facilities, 31

Partnerships, 17
Payment vouchers (PV), 37, 38, 45, 46
Pension arrangements, 55
Personnel management *see*
　Management of personnel
Personnel qualifications/specification, 53
Petty cash vouchers, 26, 35, 37, 38
Pharmacist, 9, 10
　relationship with doctor, 175

Pharmacy services, 174–184
　annual tendering, 179
　drug issuing procedures, 182
　drug storage, 180, 181
　drug trolleys, 182
　emergency drug ordering, 180
　essential drugs for Primary Health
　　Care, 229
　in-house preparation of medicines, 183, 184
　national suppliers of drugs, 179
　ordering procedure, 178, 179
　stock control system, 181, 182
　ward drug cupboards, 182
Pharmacy staff, training of, 204
Philippines, District Health Service, 237
Physiotherapy, 194
Pikine, Senegal, 50
Plans and specifications, 163

　see also Floor plans
Post-mortem examinations, 130
Postal services, 121
Postgraduate training, 208
Power sources, 100–105
Power supply, dealing with rationing, 103
Prescriptions, 76, 175
Primary health care, 7
　outreach, 118, 213–230
　under-five's clinics, 81, 82
Primary Health Centre, 4
Principle Medical Officer (PMO), 9, 10, 13, 14
Private practice *see* Management, private practice
Problem summary card, 69, 76, 77
Professional associations, 241–243
Provisional diagnosis, 69
Public Service Hospital *see* Hospital, Public Service

Quorum, 19

Radiology, 190, 191
　equipment, 190, 191
　essential work, 192, 193
　film supplies, 191
Radiophone *see* Communications
Rain
　protection against, 148
　storm water drainage, 149–151
Receipts, 37, 45, 46
Refrigeration, 101
　for storage of blood, 187
Refuse collection *see* Waste disposal
Rehabilitation services, 194, 195
Remuneration *see* Salaries
Research, clinical, 241
Retention fee, 164
Retirement gratuity *see* Pension arrangements
Roof, 145–147
Rural Health Programme (RHP), 229

Salaries, 18, 30
'Samaritan Fund', 40
Save the Children, mobile team, 227
Sanitation, 99, 100, 131–141
    aqua-privy, 136–137
    bucket latrine, 132
    chemical closet, 132
    soakaway pit latrines, 133
    ventilated improved pit (VIP) Latrines, 133–136
    water closet (WC), 136–137
Savings group, 25
Screening of patients, 164, 185
Secondary health care, 6, 208, 234–236
Security, 32, 162, 180, 181
Self-accounting institutions, *see* Accounting practices
Septic tank, 136, 138, 140–141
    see also Sanitation
Servicing *see* Maintenance, routine
Sewage disposal, 138, 141
    see also Sanitation
Signposts within hospital compound, 121
Silicone parchment, use in instrument sterilisation, 189
'Sister Doctor', 5
Soakaway pit, 141
    see also Sanitation
Software *see* Computer equipment, software
Solar power, 33, 104, 105
    see also Power sources
Sphygmomanometer, maintenance of, 107–108
Spread sheets, 34, 3
    see also Computers and Computerisation
Staff *see* Hospital Staff
State Health Management Board (SHMB), 9, 10, 14
    autonomous powers, 14
Statement of account, provisional, 46, 47
Statements
    annual, 41–43, 45
    bank, 31, 36, 46
    interim, 45
Stethoscope, maintenance of, 107
Suction machines, maintenance of, 111
Sun, protection from, 144
Surgery, postgraduate training in, 208
Surgical instruments, maintenance of, 109

Tansen Hospital, Nepal, drug issuing procedures, 182
Termination of appointment, 63
Therapeutic community, 213
Toilet *see* Sanitation
Trade Unions, negotiation with, 64
Traditional birth attendants (TBA), 218, 234
Traditional healers, 218
Training, 197–212
    accountancy staff, 203
    clerical staff, 202
    doctors, 206, 207
    family medicine programmes (FMP), 211
    for primary health care, 216–218
    hospital, inspection of, 210, 211
    in use of computers, 203
    laboratory staff, 203, 204
    labourers, 201, 202
    legal bonding, 200
    medical records staff, 203
    medical students, 206, 207
    midwives, 204
    nurse-aids, 204
    personalised, 199
    pharmacy staff, 204
    policy, essential features, 201
    postgraduate, 208
    in general practice, 208, 211
    in obstetrics and gynaecology, 208
    in surgery, 208
Training cont.
    international acceptance, 211, 240
    ward attendants, 201

Transport *see* Hospital vehicles, Hospital drivers
Trial balance, 43
'Tropical general practice', 209, 211

Ultrasound scanning, 193, 194
Under five's clinics, 81, 82, 214,
Under-five's clinic cards *see* Medical records, infant and children's clinic cards
Uninterrupted power supply (UPS) Unit, 32
Unions *see* Trade Unions
Unpaid fees, 39

Vaccination
   record of 74,
   under-five's record of, 82
Vehicles *see* Hospital vehicles
Ventilation, 101, 143, 146
Village Health Workers (VHW)
   in 'blueprint' for rural health, 234, 236
   training of, 216–218
Voluntary agency hospitals, 3, 17
   drug purchasing, 179, 180
Voluntary Hospital Association of India, 20
Volunteers, 224

Ward pantries, 127
Waste disposal, 129–131
'Waste stabilisation pond' system, 138
Water, 93, 94
   distillation plant, 112
   for cleaning purposes, 113
   purification of, 100
   quality, 99, 100
   storage tanks, 93–97
   supply, 94–97
Water closet (WC) *see* Sanitation
Weighing scales (for infants and young children), 220–221
Wesley Guild Hospital, Ilesha, Nigeria, 7, 20, 37, 38
   air conditioning, 101
   community health, 214, 215, 226, 227
   drivers. 119
   energy sources, 101, 103
   financial procedures, 48–50
   floor plans, 167–171, 185
   kitchens, 125–127
   maintenance, 106–112
   medical records, 68–90
   mortuary facilities, 129
   pharmacy services, 175–181
   staff committee, 62
   staff housing, 56, 59
   staff training, 200, 202, 206
   telephone service, 112
Wind
   protection against, 148
   damage to roofs, 151, 152
Windows, 144–149
Wood *see* Power sources
Word processing *see* Computerisation, word processing
World Health Organisation (WHO)
   Director General, Dr H Mahler, 236
   Division for Strengthening Health Systems, 237
   model list of essential drugs, 177, 178
   recommendations on management structures, 15
   registration of notifiable disease, 223, 224

X-rays *see* Radiology

Zambia, 32, 211, 212, 237, 240
Zimbabwe, 134